Britain and the 1918–19 Influenza Pandemic

The period 1918–19 saw the end of the Great War and the eruption of the largest epidemic in history, a global epidemic, a pandemic of flu. Influenza struck half the world's population, killing 50–100 million people in less than a year. This work is the first examination of Britain's experience of the pandemic. But this work is not only concerned with the historical; as well as telling the story of the 'Spanish' influenza, the book looks forward and considers the possibilities of future pandemics, including the dangers of bird flu.

A 'total' history, this book ranges from the spread of the 1918–19 pandemic, covers the basic biology of influenza, and how epidemics and pandemics are possible, to consider the demographic, social, economic and political impacts of such a massive pandemic, including the cultural dimensions of naming, blame, metaphors, memory, the media, art and literature. In many countries the pandemic precipitated the creation and expansion of public healthcare as nothing else ever could. Despite this, in subsequent times, the role and impact of the pandemic has been overlooked, an oversight this work redresses.

The British story of the pandemic has never been told. *Britain and the 1918–19 Influenza Pandemic* tells that story but also places it in its fuller context with extensive material from around the world. The book provides the most recent tally of the pandemic's impact, including the vast mortality, as well as questioning the apparent origins of the pandemic. An inter-disciplinary study, it stretches from history and geography through to medicine in order to convey the full magnitude of the first global medical 'disaster' of the twentieth century.

Niall Johnson is a respected authority on the 1918–19 influenza pandemic. In addition to writing his PhD (Cambridge) on the British experience of the pandemic he has published and presented numerous research papers on this topic, including articles in leading medical, history and history of medicine journals, and has contributed pieces on influenza pandemics to various media outlets as well as being an expert consultant to Granada Media for a Channel 4 documentary on the pandemic.

Routledge studies in the social history of medicine

Edited by Joseph Melling
University of Exeter
and
Anne Borsay
University of Wales, Swansea

The Society for the Social History of Medicine was founded in 1969, and exists to promote research into all aspects of the field, without regard to limitations of either time or place. In addition to this book series, the Society also organises a regular programme of conferences, and publishes an internationally recognised journal, *Social History of Medicine*. The Society offers a range of benefits, including reduced-price admission to conferences and discounts on SSHM books, to its members. Individuals wishing to learn more about the Society are invited to contact the series editors through the publisher.

The Society took the decision to launch Studies in the Social History of Medicine, in association with Routledge, in 1989, in order to provide an outlet for some of the latest research in the field. Since that time, the series has expanded significantly under a number of series editors, and now includes both edited collections and monographs. Individuals wishing to submit proposals are invited to contact the series editors in the first instance.

1 **Nutrition in Britain**
Science, scientists and politics in the twentieth century
Edited by David F. Smith

2 **Migrants, Minorities and Health**
Historical and contemporary studies
Edited by Lara Marks and Michael Worboys

3 **From Idiocy to Mental Deficiency**
Historical perspectives on people with learning disabilities
Edited by David Wright and Anne Digby

4 **Midwives, Society and Childbirth**
Debates and controversies in the modern period
Edited by Hilary Marland and Anne Marie Rafferty

5 **Illness and Healing Alternatives in Western Europe**
Edited by Marijke Gijswit-Hofstra, Hilary Maarland and Has de Waardt

6 **Health Care and Poor Relief in Protestant Europe 1500–1700**
Edited by Ole Peter Grell and Andrew Cunningham

7 **The Locus of Care**
Families, communities, institutions, and the provision of welfare since antiquity
Edited by Peregrine Horden and Richard Smith

8 **Race, Science and Medicine, 1700–1960**
Edited by Waltraud Ernst and Bernard Harris

9 **Insanity, Institutions and Society, 1800–1914**
Edited by Bill Forsythe and Joseph Melling

10 **Food, Science, Policy and Regulation in the Twentieth Century**
International and comparative perspectives
Edited by David F. Smith and Jim Phillips

11 **Sex, Sin and Suffering**
Venereal disease and European society since 1870
Edited by Roger Davidson and Lesley A. Hall

12 **The Spanish Influenza Pandemic of 1918–19**
New perspectives
Edited by Howard Phillips and David Killingray

13 **Plural Medicine, Tradition and Modernity, 1800–2000**
Edited by Waltraud Ernst

14 **Innovations in Health and Medicine**
Diffusion and resistance in the twentieth century
Edited by Jenny Stanton

15 **Contagion**
Historical and cultural studies
Edited by Alison Bashford and Claire Hooker

16 **Medicine, Health and the Public Sphere in Britain, 1600–2000**
Edited by Steve Sturdy

17 **Medicine and Colonial Identity**
Edited by Mary P. Sutphen and Bridie Andrews

18 **New Directions in Nursing History**
Edited by Barbara E. Mortimer and Susan McGann

19 **Medicine, the Market and Mass Media**
Producing health in the twentieth century
Edited by Virginia Berridge and Kelly Loughlin

20 **The Politics of Madness**
The state, insanity and society in England, 1845–1914
Joseph Melling and Bill Forsythe

21 **The Risks of Medical Innovation**
Risk perception and assessment in historical context
Edited by Thomas Schlich and Ulrich Tröhler

22 **Mental Illness and Learning Disability Since 1850**
Finding a place for mental disorder in the United Kingdom
Edited by Pamela Dale and Joseph Melling

23 **Britain and the 1918-19 Influenza Pandemic**
A dark epilogue
Niall Johnson

Also available in Routledge studies in the social history of medicine series:

Reassessing Foucault
Power, medicine and the body
Edited by Colin Jones and Roy Porter

Britain and the 1918–19 Influenza Pandemic

A dark epilogue

Niall Johnson

Routledge
Taylor & Francis Group
LONDON AND NEW YORK

First published 2006
by Routledge
2 Park Square, Milton Park, Abingdon, Oxon OX14 4RN

Simultaneously published in the USA and Canada
by Routledge
270 Madison Ave, New York, NY 10016

Routledge is an imprint of the Taylor & Francis Group, an informa business

Typeset in Garamond by Wearset Ltd, Boldon, Tyne and Wear
Printed and bound in Great Britain by TJ International Ltd,
Padstow, Cornwall

British Library Cataloguing in Publication Data
A catalogue record for this book is available from the British Library

Library of Congress Cataloging in Publication Data
A catalog record for this book has been requested

ISBN10: 0–415–36560-0

ISBN13: 9–780–415–36560–4

Contents

Plates

Figures

Tables

Preface

This work draws on the approaches and literature of a number of disciplines, including medicine, history and geography, and takes a multi- and inter-disciplinary approach. As a history, this work is more a history of the larger population rather than an individualised history. But it is still a social history of sorts for, as Rosenberg stated, 'Every aspect of medicine's history is necessarily "social"' (Rosenberg 1992: 307).

The study of epidemics had often focused on their rarity, their abnormality and their drama. Social and economic histories have examined the impact of epidemics on society, particularly those oriented toward writing histories demonstrating the significance of medical factors (and the heroic medical figures battling them) throughout history. Another approach to medical history is that which regards disease as a function of social organisation, a more structural approach that moves the focus of disease from being external to society to being internal as a consequence of societal structures, particularly inequities and change. This change makes the disease a symptom of social pathology. Influenza has not been 'ordinarily studied' by social or economic historians, largely as it has been perceived not to exhibit these social dimensions, as it is 'too easily transmitted, too universal, and [generally] insufficiently lethal' (Rosenberg 1992: 110–1). Consequently, this work, along with those of the likes of Crosby, Phillips, and Rice (Crosby 1989; Phillips 1990a; Rice 1988) is attempting to address this neglect of a disease whose 'ordinariness' has rendered it almost invisible to historians.

This is not solely a social or economic history, rather it is an attempt to uncover more of the story of the pandemic, particularly in Britain, and may be considered an attempt at what Risse terms a 'total history' in examining how the 'environmental, geographical, political, cultural, biological, and medical aspects inextricably' bind together to constitute an epidemic (Risse 1991: 4–5). This work falls in the remit of both history and geography, but as it has progressed it is fair to say that it has leant slightly toward the historical rather than the strictly geographical. However, in many ways this is in keeping with the current trajectory of historical–cultural geography which has seen a broadening of what constitutes human geography. This is based on a broad, pluralistic view of geography, particularly at the junction of historical and medical geographies.

Attempting to bridge these multiple boundaries requires multiple sources, multiple approaches, and multiple 'gazes'. Foucault (1976) wrote that the 'analysis of an epidemic does not involve the recognition of the general form of the disease ... but the rediscovery ... of the particular process ... peculiar to this moment in time and this place in space' and that as 'an epidemic has a sort of historical individuality' there is a need to utilise 'a complex method of observation when dealing with it. Being a collective phenomenon, it requires a multiple gaze; a unique process, it must be described in terms of its special, accidental and unexpected qualities.' It is these multiple gazes that I have attempted to bring to this study in a 'search for an essential coherence, the subtle perception of a complex historical and geographical space' (Foucault 1976) of the 1918–19 influenza pandemic.

Acknowledgements

While many have played a part in this book's genesis, prominent among them has been Dr Gerry Kearns, Jesus College, Cambridge, who supervised the PhD this book stems from, and whose broad intellectual interests informed that work.

The staff and resources of the Wellcome Library for the History and Understanding of Medicine, the Public Record Office (now the National Archives), the British Library, the National Archives of Australia, the National Archives of South Africa and many other archives and libraries have been invaluable in the course of researching this book. A number of organisations, and their staff, provided access and resources that helped ensure the research progressed as well as it did, including the University of Cambridge, Macquarie University (particularly Dr Kevin McCracken) and the University of Toronto.

I would also like to thank all those who have contributed in so many different ways, including my fellow pandemic researchers who have freely exchanged information and opinions, and my friends and colleagues who offered their much-appreciated opinions and assistance, particularly Tristan Clayton, Emma Simone, Dr Mark Russell and C.A. Smith.

Picture credits

Plate 1: C.W. Broughton.
Figures 3.2 and 3.3: G.F. Pyle and Johns Hopkins University Press.
Plates 4 to 6: University of Cambridge University Library, by permission of the Syndics of Cambridge University Library.
Figure 5.1: National Archives of Australia.
Plate 7: Wellcome Trust, Wellcome Library for the History and Understanding of Medicine.
Plate 8: Nasjonal Museet, Norway/Viscopy. Photographer: K.Ø. Nredrum.

Abbreviations

ARRG	Annual Report of the Registrar-General
CAMC	Canadian Army Medical Corps
CB	County Borough
CBR	Crude Birth Rate
CDC	Centers for Disease Control and Prevention, USA
CDR	Crude Death Rate
CMAC	Wellcome Library for the History and Understanding of Medicine, Contemporary Medical Archive Collection
IMR	Infant Mortality Rate
LB or MB	London or Metropolitan Borough
LGB	Local Government Board
MJA	*Medical Journal of Australia*
MOH	Medical Officer of Health
MRC	Medical Research Committee
NAA	National Archives of Australia
NASA	National Archives of South Africa
PRO	Public Record Office, Kew (now the National Archives)
PROV	Public Record Office, Victoria
RAMC	Royal Army Medical Corps
RD	Rural District
RN	Royal Navy
RG	Registrar-General
SLNSW	State Library of New South Wales
SLV	State Library of Victoria
SRNSW	State Records of New South Wales
UD	Urban District
WHO	World Health Organisation

1 Introduction to an unregarded killer

Since the earliest descriptions of influenza-like disease by Hippocrates, influenza has infected billions and killed millions of people across the globe. A highly contagious disease, it is usually limited to just a few days' illness with a low fatality rate. However, in times of epidemic and pandemic it can become so prevalent, infecting the majority of the population, that these elevated rates give rise to massive surges in mortality as influenza strikes 'like a flash flood' (Stöhr 2005: 407). With pneumonia, influenza remains one of the ten leading causes of death in the United States of America (Crosby 1993: 807) and Australia (AIHW 2004: 45). These two respiratory infections are commonly tallied together and frequently interact – in 1918 it was the complications from pneumonia that killed so many, contributing to a death toll of tens of millions. In the UK the average annual influenza death toll is currently around 12,000, and in the first week of 1999 alone more than 3,000 Britons died of influenza (BBC 1999g) – an outbreak that forced one hospital to hire a refrigerated truck as a temporary mortuary (BBC 1999c) – and this was not officially regarded as an epidemic. The winter of 1989–90 saw an epidemic claim an estimated 29,000 British lives (Radford 1995). Even in non-epidemic years it can have a major impact; for example, in Britain an average of approximately three working days per patient are lost annually as a result of flu, and it may account for approximately 10 per cent of sickness absences (BBC 1999d). An average year in the USA sees approximately 36,000 flu deaths, with more than 200,000 hospitalised (CDC 2004) at a cost to the economy of US$71–167 billion (WHO 2003). The World Health Organisation (WHO) estimates that influenza causes 'between three to five million cases of severe illness and between 250,000 and 500,000 deaths every year around the world' (WHO 2003). But all this may pale against the possibility of a pandemic that many now regard as inevitable, if not imminent. Indeed, in early 2005 the British government apparently recognised that an influenza pandemic was a greater risk than terrorism, particularly in terms of the number of people directly affected and the potential to disrupt society (Hall and Sample 2005).

Rosenberg suggests that 'there is no human crisis more compelling than an epidemic', but specifies epidemics of diseases such as yellow fever, cholera and plague. Such epidemics are of such a scale and of such a terrifying nature that 'most physicians and historians have tended to view them as something alien, something outside of society and contending with it' (Rosenberg 1992: 110). Influenza is something with which we are well acquainted and rarely regard as a major threat to health, and even less as a mortal threat. This work examines the 1918–19 influenza pandemic and demonstrates how it was one of the most massive disease outbreaks in human history, and how influenza remains a threat. While the British experience is the focus, this was a true pandemic, a global epidemic, and as such necessarily detailed consideration is given to the global extent of the pandemic, often to highlight the universality of the pandemic, as well as drawing comparisons between the British experience and that experienced elsewhere. Given the very real possibility of future flu pandemics, the parallels and portents that can be drawn from the 1918 experience, and how they might be played out in a future pandemic, are also discussed. Thus the consideration of flu is not parochial but encompasses the scale of the pandemic, both in time and space.

The 1918–19 pandemic struck a Britain undergoing quite profound change, including a reappraisal of the nation's position in the world. From being the global superpower at the height of its imperial reach, there were already signs of the Empire breaking apart. For example, South Africa had been lost in the long, brutal South African War. This was a shock that had been compounded as Britain ground out what must have seemed a rather hollow and expensive victory in the Great War. The political and social order at home was also undergoing much change as Lloyd George's administration started to bring about many of the changes that were to give the state a greater role in the life of individual Britons. These changes from a laissez-faire state to a more interventionist state were by no means a smooth transition. Nor was the welfare state of the later twentieth century in place by any means. The Ministry of Health, while foreshadowed, did not exist and public health was largely the preserve of the local authorities and their MOHs. The Local Government Board (LGB), the national government's public health body, was little more than an advisory body rather than a service-delivery authority. Thus it was a very different place that influenza struck in 1918.

Influenza

Our acquaintance with influenza is centuries old and in our classifications of disease, influenza is one disease whose classification has remained essentially unchanged. This suggests a disease whose nature and symptoms we have long recognised, even if the actual causal organism, the flu virus, was not identified until 1933 (Smith *et al.*, 1993). Influenza is universal: all ages and both sexes are susceptible to the disease. During times of epidemic, between 15 and 40 per cent of the non-immunised are stricken and this figure can climb markedly under pandemic conditions. It is 'a disease of paradoxes' and is widely considered to be 'a disease of little consequence, one which is a nuisance but causes only minor illness. However, it is also a disease which kills' (Riordan 1986: III). Influenza is transmitted person-to-person, usually as droplets. These droplets of respiratory secretions are exhaled by an infected person and inhaled by others. Droplets can range in size, with the smallest remaining suspended in the air for as long as an hour. Factors such as the amount of virus shed, proximity, crowding and ambient conditions can all influence the efficacy of transmission. Furthermore, some sufferers can be 'supershedders', broadcasting masses of virus-containing droplets.

Symptoms and diagnosis

The symptoms of influenza are relatively easy to determine, but also make diagnosis difficult as many of them are shared with other conditions, including the common cold. But what exactly is influenza? We all have personal knowledge – every one of us has been struck by the disease at some stage. But what is the clinical description of the disease? In uncomplicated influenza, the first symptoms appear two to four days after infection. These first symptoms include headache, shivering and a dry cough accompanied by a sudden onset of fever. In adults malaise and an aching of the limb muscles and back can often occur. Nasal irritation or discharge can occur, as can a loss of sleep and dizziness. In some patients the symptoms subside rapidly after the first twenty-four hours. But the disease can have a prolonged course for some, with the temperature remaining high for up to five days, and with a residual weakness and/or a cough. Without complications, one usually recovers within ten days of the onset of illness. However, in some cases a persistent weakness or mental depression may require longer convalescence. Of the clinical features of influenza, the fever, a temperature of 38–40°C (100–104°F), is that which most typically distinguishes flu from the common cold (which is caused by a completely different type of virus) (Schild 1977: 350–1). Thus, influenza is an acute respiratory infection with an abrupt onset, and typified by high fever, sudden chills, muscular pain, dry cough and prostration that can also lead to diarrhoea, gastrointestinal pain, head cold, sore throat, nose bleeds and a fall in blood pressure.

Very young children, older people and those with weakened or damaged cardiovascular and/or respiratory systems are most prone to attack from influenza. Not only are young children the most likely to be attacked by the disease but they are also more likely to succumb. This pattern of mortality is reflected in the hospitalisation rates. While the highest incidence occurs in children and young adults, the rates of hospitalisation for 'severe or complicated influenza are lowest, around six per 10,000, in persons five to twenty-four years old' (Cate 1987: 16). The highest hospitalisation rates are in the extreme age groups – the youngest and the oldest – and 'age-related deaths due to pneumonia and influenza during epidemics tend to follow a pattern similar to . . . rates of hospitalization' (Cate 1987: 16). This age pattern, of illness and particularly mortality, is in marked contrast to that encountered in 1918–19.

Complications and sequelae

Influenza itself can pose a significant health problem. However, it is not always unaccompanied, and the complications and sequelae can be important in determining both morbidity and mortality. Significant proportions of the mortality associated with influenza may be caused by the sequelae and complications as even a 'low frequency of complications results in measurable increases in rates of hospitalisations, and often in mortality' (WHO 1999d: 34). Furthermore, the impact of the 1918 pandemic will be understated as long as the scale of these complications and sequelae is ignored. These complications usually involve the lower respiratory tract (tracheobronchitis, bronchiolitis and influenzal pneumonia or other secondary bacterial, mixed viral-bacterial, or viral infections), the cardiovascular system (often occurring through exacerbation of existing chronic conditions) and the nervous system. Our understanding of what conditions and diseases can be related to influenza has grown a great deal since the 1918–19 pandemic.

There are two major types of complication or sequelae for influenza. These are the cardio-pulmonary conditions, including other respiratory diseases, e.g. bronchitis, pneumonia and tuberculosis, and the neurological conditions, e.g. schizophrenia, encephalitis lethargica and Parkinsonism. The cardio-pulmonary conditions are often implicated in exacerbating the severity of influenza, whereas the neurological conditions tend to be sequelae to influenza. The dangers of both should not be overlooked, as the 'risk of serious and fatal disease is much higher . . . in patients with certain well-defined pre-existing underlying conditions. These conditions . . . predispose not to the risk of acquiring influenza virus infection but to the risk of suffering severe disease once infection is established' (Kilbourne 1987: 159).

Underlying cardiovascular disease can contribute to serious pulmonary manifestations of influenza. This can be particularly dire if the patient develops pneumonia, as studies have shown high mortality rates in such cases. The extra strain on an already damaged heart appears to lead to cardiac failure (Kilbourne 1987: 162–3). Changes in electro-cardiograph (ECG) reading seen in people with existing cardiac conditions during acute influenza have been ascribed to 'exacerbation of the underlying cardiac disease rather than direct involvement of the myocardium [heart] with influenza virus' (WHO 1999d: 35–6). Forms of carditis, such as myocarditis and pericarditis, are thought to occur as complications on occasion, and may also contribute to death. The Registrar-General noted in 1920 that in Britain an increase in certain types of 'heart disease' were linked to the pandemic and indeed that excess deaths in one form ('organic heart disease (No. 79)') were attributed to the pandemic (Registrar-General 1920: 3).

A range of pulmonary or respiratory conditions can cause complications and raise the risk of death. These can include infectious and non-infectious complications or conditions such as croup, pneumonia and any exacerbation of any of the chronic obstructive pulmonary diseases (e.g. asthma, chronic bronchitis and cystic fibrosis), with pneumonia being the greatest threat. Of the different forms of pneumonia, three types have been described in relation to influenza: bacterial pneumonia, combined viral and bacterial pneumonia, and pure viral pneumonia (WHO 1999d: 34–5). The prominent virologist Ed Kilbourne states that existing 'chronic bronchopulmonary disease is equal to pre-existing cardiac disease as a factor leading to severe or complicated influenza', and notes further conditions that can lead to pulmonary insufficiency or obstruction, including 'chronic bronchitis, bronchiectasis, pulmonary fibrosis, asthma, emphysema, or bronchopulmonary neoplastic disease.' For children, asthma is a particular concern, being recognised as a high-risk factor associated with increased hospitalisation (Kilbourne 1987: 164). All of these pulmonary or respiratory conditions can contribute to increased severity of an influenzal episode.

Pneumonic complications were widely described in the fatal cases of the 1918–19 pandemic. The dreaded diagnostic feature of the 'heliotrope cyanosis' indicated, almost invariably, terminal pneumonic complications (Abrahams *et al.* 1917, 1919; Cummins 1919; Frost 1919; Hammond *et al.* 1917; Levinthal *et al.* 1921; Lister and Taylor 1919; MacPherson *et al.* 1920; Ministry of Health 1920c; Opie *et al.* 1921; Royal Society of Medicine 1918, including 67–70). Pneumonic complications contributed a substantial proportion of the pandemic's total mortality. Burnet and Clark reported that 80 per cent of patients in the autumn wave of the pandemic still endured 'typical three- to five-day influenza without complication. . . . The only feature noted as unusual was the frequent occurrence of epistaxis [nose bleeds] as an initial symptom.' However, of the other 20 per cent of patients who 'developed pneumonic complications with a mortality of 40–50%', the pneumonic symptoms, other than the cyanosis, did not indicate the severity of illness, as the 'physical signs were irregular and usually slight in relation to the sickness of the patient' with the most obvious features of the severe cases being 'the rapidity of the respirations and the characteristic heliotrope cyanosis. There was little subjective distress and though some showed delirium and coma a majority were fully conscious to within an hour of death' (Burnet and Clark 1942: 88, citing Ministry of Health 1920c).

Whereas the cardiovascular and pulmonary conditions tend to be complications of influenza, making the disease episode more serious, the neurological conditions that have been associated with influenza tend to be sequelae, conditions that follow influenza infection with the assumption being that the influenza infection facilitates the later condition. It appears that many neurological conditions or maladies of the central nervous system (CNS) may be exacerbated, facilitated or otherwise associated with influenza, including asthenia, depression, mania, transverse myelitis, encephalitis lethargica,

Parkinsonism, senile dementia and schizophrenia (Kilbourne 1987: 171–7; Ravenholt 1993; WHO 1999d: 36). These associations have been noticed for some time, even if the mechanisms have not been fully understood. One observer, who on detecting such sequelae in 1918–19, 'recalled that influenza worsened existing neuroses and created "nerve invalids" who sometimes lost "their moral bearings" in theft and drunkenness. "Post-influenzal depression", "lassitude", "lethargy", "grippe catalepsy", "hysterical coma", "psychosis", "melancholy", "nona" (somnolence and absent-mindedness), "despondency", "neuritis", "neurasthenia", "shattered nerves", and "loss of grip" all became popular ascriptions of sequelae in the 1890s' (Smith 1995: 71). Similar observations were made elsewhere. For example, Phillips found these cases of

> Post-'flu debility and lassitude were by no means unusual. Recovery was often slow and uneven . . . 'impaired vitality', 'breathless', 'suffered palpitations', 'temporarily forgetful, deaf, blind or bald', 'anaemia', 'post-influenza melancholia' and 'several cases of suicide were attributed to this post-'flu melancholia' with others 'left with their health permanently impaired by, for example, deafness, weak lungs, heart trouble and a susceptibility to other diseases such as phthisis, tuberculosis, parkinsonism, nephritis, meningitis and encephalitis lethargica'.
>
> (Phillips 1990a: 189–91)

One set of neurological conditions that have been linked to influenza are those that fall under the term schizophrenia. Viral, behavioural, epidemiological and neuropathological evidence suggests that influenza, particularly in epidemics, can be 'neurovirulent' and can induce clinical schizophrenia in addition to 'manias', epidemic encephalitis, affective psychoses and Parkinson's disease (Maurizi 1984, 1985; Menninger 1994).

Charles Maurizi gave a first-hand account of influenza-related neurological disturbance. A serious influenza B infection induced a viral encephalopathy during which he 'could not complete abstract thought, had difficulty judging time, and had periods of intense anxiety'. Some two weeks following the initial onset of fever, his thinking and behaviour resumed a normal state and he began to feel better. Though much better (in fact he felt wonderful), this in itself was not good as he had 'a manic psychosis with elation, hyperactivity, poor judgement, grandiose delusions and decreased need for sleep'. Four months of treatment with lithium carbonate seemed to restore him to health. However, four weeks after stopping the treatment, the mania recurred before abating upon the resumption of the lithium (Maurizi 1984: 163). Maurizi drew parallels between his condition (and treatment) and that of an Australian soldier serving in Europe who was diagnosed in 1917 as suffering from 'cerebro-spinal fever'. Cerebro-spinal fever was certainly discussed in relation to the influenza at the time of the pandemic with little conclusive evidence (e.g. Hamer 1918: 2; Ministry of Health 1920c; Royal

Society of Medicine 1918: 6–7 and PRO MH 55 57). Apparently this soldier was the first patient to be treated with lithium following mild cerebro-spinal fever and after 'this encephalitis he was mentally disturbed'. Maurizi wonders if he had been infected by a 'neurotropic influenza virus' and considers it quite possible, if not probable. The soldier reportedly endured bouts of 'mania' for more than thirty years, including chronic mania for five years prior to the lithium treatment. It appears that the lithium treatment helped him, as it had Maurizi, at least to a point – he 'later died of lithium intoxication' (Maurizi 1984: 166).

Disruptions of the central nervous system caused by influenza do not have to be limited to those already born. There is some suggestion that influenza could have been the cause of some congenital deformities in the children of women who contracted influenza during their pregnancy. The influenza virus has been implicated as a cause of both maternal morbidity and congenital anomalies, particularly of the central nervous system (MacKenzie and Houghton 1974; Mattock *et al.* 1988). Graham attempted to determine if the pattern of schizophrenics tending to be born in late winter or early spring could be related to mothers being exposed to influenza, particularly during the second trimester of the pregnancy, and if this may lead to transmission of the virus or viral antibodies to the developing foetus 'leading to subtle brain damage which later manifests itself as schizophrenia' (Graham 1996: Abstract). The results of the study were somewhat contradictory.

Another CNS complication that, although rare, can be extremely serious, is Reye's syndrome. It tends to occur after viral infections, usually influenza B and almost exclusively in children, particularly where salicylates (aspirin, etc.) have been used. Occurring four to seven days after infection the symptoms include behavioural changes, nausea and repeated vomiting. Behavioural changes can progress from lethargy to disorientation, irritability and aggression to coma. It is a relatively rare condition (30–60 cases per 100,000 influenza B infections; 2.5–4.3 per 100,000 influenza A) (Kilbourne 1987: 176–8; Ravenholt 1993: 771).

One unusual neurological condition that was shown to have a possible connection with influenza is Guillain–Barré syndrome. This connection became apparent during the 1976 swine flu scare in the USA. It was feared that a swine flu that had been isolated from a dead soldier could lead to a large-scale epidemic. The American government mobilised for a national vaccination campaign. This campaign was halted after 'scores of millions of dollars were spent to devise a vaccine, to produce it in quantity (not without problems) and to deliver it into the arms of millions of Americans', with the result that, while no epidemic of influenza occurred, there was the appearance of a unusual number of cases of Guillain–Barré syndrome, 'a paralytic and occasionally fatal disorder' (Crosby 1993: 711). This incident severely dented the reputation of the CDC (Centers for Disease Control and Prevention) and contributed to its cautious initial response to HIV/AIDS.

The conditions and disease discussed thus far are by no means an exhaustive list of those that have been seen to have some (possible) association with influenza. Indeed, virtually all CNS conditions and many cardiovascular and pulmonary ones can be involved in an influenza infection. Some of these may be exacerbated or facilitated by influenza, while others can contribute to the severity of the influenza infection or combine to place a greater stress on the body. Yet other conditions have also been linked to influenza, for example, myopathy, nepropathy or nephritis (Collier 1974; Crosby 1989; Kilbourne 1987: 168–71; Mamelund 1998b; Phillips 1990a), while diabetes is 'often mentioned as a high-risk condition, but so it is in a variety of infectious diseases' (Kilbourne 1987: 164).

Some of the other diseases and conditions that show links or correlations with influenza were most prominently seen during or following the 1918–19 influenza pandemic, particularly encephalitis lethargica and bacterial pneumonia. During the pandemic, the most important related or complicating conditions were the pneumonic complications. It was these that contributed so greatly to the excessive mortality of the pandemic. It was the pneumonic complications that led to the widespread and usually tragic symptom of the heliotrope cyanosis that was such a feature of this pandemic – one of the great universalities of the pandemic.

To produce a more accurate figure for global mortality of the 1918–19 pandemic, it would be necessary to investigate the mortality that was attributed to these complications and secondary causes, particularly the excess deaths recorded for the pandemic period, and following it in the case of some conditions. Such work would need to include not only tracking the rise and fall in the mortality numbers, but may also need to pay heed to the age distribution of that mortality, as a rise in the young adult age groups may prove a useful indicator of mortality that could be associated with the pandemic. One example of these revisions of mortality suggests that if encephalitis lethargica deaths are counted, then another 'half a million deaths may be attributed to the pandemic' (Patterson and Pyle 1991: 20).

Treatment

Despite hundreds of years of experience with dealing with influenza, our pharmaceutical armouries are still bereft of any genuinely effective long-term weaponry. The WHO co-ordinates the Global Surveillance Programme for Influenza, which monitors what influenza strains are circulating at any given time, partly to watch for the first signs of a new strain that could potentially lead to epidemics or a pandemic (WHO 1999b, 1999e, 1999f, 2003). Another major role of this programme is to make recommendations on the composition of influenza vaccines for the influenza seasons in the northern and southern hemispheres (e.g. WHO 1999g). Each season's vaccine may be prepared to combat a number of strains of influenza.

The vast majority of the pharmaceuticals thrown at flu are for the topical treatment of symptoms, such as fever, coughing, nasal obstruction or discharge, myalgia and neuralgia. Antibiotics are designed to attack bacteria and have no effect on influenza, although they can be used to treat complications (such as the pneumonic complications that killed so many in the 1918 pandemic). However, there are some drugs that actually work on the virus itself, but these anti-virals are not widely distributed, nor are they a substitute for vaccines as preventive measures: vaccinations are considered more useful and cost-effective (Hayden 2001). Four anti-viral drugs are now available: amantadine, rimantadine, zanamivir and oseltamivir. These work by preventing influenza virus replication, and they vary in their pharmacokinetics, side-effects, target age groups, dosages, forms of administration and cost. If taken before infection or in the early stages these anti-virals can help prevent infection and may reduce the duration of symptoms by one or two days.

For some years the only anti-virals for influenza were amantadine and rimantadine. Whilst relatively inexpensive these are only effective against influenza A and can be associated with severe adverse effects, for example, amantadine can cause dizziness, headaches and insomnia (Dillner 1995) as well as 'significant neurological side effects, particularly in those with diminished kidney function, including generally healthy elderly persons' (WHO 1999d: 53). Research suggests that amantadine and rimantadine should have some effectiveness against any future pandemic strains of the virus (Oxford and Al-Jabri 1996). However, they do have be taken throughout the entire period of exposure, which is much less convenient than a single vaccination. Furthermore, the limited success that they have had can also be attributed to such factors as under-utilisation, the development of viral resistance and lack of efficacy on influenza B viruses (Calfee and Hayden 1998).

A newer class of anti-viral drugs, the neuraminidase inhibitors, have been developed (these work by preventing the release of the virus from cells). These drugs, zanamivir and oseltamivir (commercially known as Relenza and Tamiflu), have shown fewer adverse side effects (although zanamivir may exacerbate asthma or other chronic lung conditions) and have seen lower rates of resistance by the virus (BBC 1999a, 1999b, 1999c, 1999g; Elliott 2001; Roberts 2001; WHO 2003). Both these drugs have apparently demonstrated a reduction in the severity and duration of naturally occurring, uncomplicated influenza in adults (Calfee and Hayden 1998). However, these drugs are relatively expensive and currently are not available for use in many countries. The cost is also a consideration in determining whether stockpiles of these anti-virals can be held in case of a pandemic outbreak (Barnett 2001).

Research continues apace on influenza vaccines (Monto 2005; Stöhr 2005; Wood 2001). The rewards for the successful developer of an influenza vaccine, particularly one that remained effective against many virus strains, would be enormous. The successful production of a vaccine which conferred widespread immunity would be of enormous benefit in reducing the morbidity and mortality that influenza causes. Even a moderately successful vaccine could be beneficial for, as Riordan notes, an 'epidemic occurs only when a large proportion of the population has no . . . [immunity] or only a low level of it against an invading virus' and that, consequently, 'vaccinating a proportion of the population could produce a "herd immunity" effect' (Riordan 1986: 28), thus making it more difficult for the virus to find susceptible individuals through which to propagate.

Virus

So what is it that causes such suffering? What does the virus 'look like'? Concentrated study of the virus in the years since its discovery in 1933 (Smith *et al.* 1933) has revealed a 'spherical orthomyxovirus' that is approximately 75 to 100 nanometres in diameter (Plate 1).

Influenza is not a single disease. Rather, there are three main types of influenza viruses: A, B and C, 'alphabetically named in chronological order of their isolation and definition' (Kilbourne 1987: 26). Within these types there are dozens of known strains. We are primarily concerned with the various manifestations of the influenza A virus, for this is 'the most important and most interesting and so far as we know is the only one that causes serious pandemics and the only one that occurs naturally in animals' (Beveridge 1977: 9); it can infect pigs, horses, seals, whales and birds as well as humans. Type B is thought to be a human-only virus and tends to cause illness mainly in children of school age (Beveridge 1977; Stuart-Harris *et al.* 1985). Its impact is not as wide-reaching as Type A, but it can cause a significant public health problem; consequently the influenza vaccines are often prepared to combat the most common B strain as well as the most likely A strains. Type-C influenza belongs to a different genus and was considered to be a human-only virus, but has since been isolated from pigs in China (Stuart-Harris *et al.* 1985). However, Type C is relatively uncommon and does not lead to epidemics.

The influenza virus has a number of structural features that are of importance when it comes to epidemics and pandemics. These include the fact that the RNA (ribonucleic acid – the genetic material for the virus) occurs as eight separate segments. The other important structural features are the surface projections or 'spikes'. These spikes are antigenic glycoproteins with either haemagglutinin or neuraminidase activity.

The haemagglutinin spike, abbreviated to H or HA, is roughly triangular in cross-section and extends approximately 12 nm from the lipid membrane. This spike is responsible for binding the virus to red blood cells and host cells. In binding to the red blood cells it causes them to agglutinate, hence the name haemagglutinin. This attachment to the host cell facilitates the entry of the virus into the host cells (Nicholson *et al.* 2003). After infection, antibodies to the haemagglutinin spike are formed, preventing re-infection with the same strain of influenza virus. This is how the immune system 'learns' of the particular strain of the virus and is thus able to combat it should the individual ever be re-attacked by the same, or very similar, strain of the virus.

The second type of spike, the neuraminidase spike, usually abbreviated to N or NA, is shaped rather like a mushroom (Stuart-Harris *et al.* 1985: 9). This spike is an enzyme that 'cleaves terminal salic acid residues from glycoproteins and glycolipids' (Pyle 1986: 4), thus facilitating the spread of the virus from one cell to another in addition to the release of progeny virus from infected cells – it 'unlocks' cells to allow infection. It is the blocking of this exit from a cell that the recent anti-viral drugs are designed to achieve. After infection, antibodies against the neuraminidase enzyme are also formed.

Both the haemagglutinin and the neuraminidase spikes are highly variable and antibodies to these distinguish the different strains of influenza. When these 'spikes' change, our immune systems can fail to recognise a virus and thus not attack it immediately and successfully. When these changes are significant and the virus is able to evade the immune defences of the majority of people, epidemics and pandemics can occur. Changes in the 'spikes' occur when there are changes in the RNA of the virus. The segmentation of the RNA into eight single-strand pieces is unusual among animal viruses. This segmentation has major repercussions for the variability of the virus into a myriad of types, subtypes and variants, as this

> segmentation of the RNA means that genetic recombination, or reassortment, can occur readily during mixed infection with different influenza A strains. The recombination of RNA segments is probably of key importance in accounting for major antigenic variations of influenza viruses.
>
> (Kaplan and Webster 1977: 91)

It is the surface antigens (haemagluttinin and neuraminidase) that are used to identify and name the different subtypes of influenza. Fifteen forms of haemagglutinin and nine forms of neuraminidase have been identified to date, but only three haemagglutinin and two neuraminidase subtypes are commonly associated with human infection (Table 1.1). Within each subtype there can be a variety of strains. These are usually signified by a designation indicating influenza virus type, location where first isolated, isolate number, and the year of isolation, for example, A/Puerto Rico/8/34. Other examples come from the WHO recommendation of a specific Southern Hemisphere vaccine for 1999 that included components to combat three different strains of influenza, two influenza A and one influenza B, with the two influenza A strains being of different subtypes: A/Sydney/5/97 (H3N2 subtype), A/Beijing/262/95 (H1N1 subtype) and B/Beijing/184/93-like virus (WHO 1999g).

The next chapter examines our long-term association with this disease, its

Table 1.1 Haemagluttinin and neuraminidase subtypes

Haemagluttinin subtypes and hosts		*Neuraminidase subtypes and hosts*	
H1	humans, pigs, birds	N1	humans, pigs, birds
H2	humans, birds	N2	humans, pigs, birds
H3	humans, horses, pigs, birds	N3	birds
H4	birds	N4	birds
H5	birds	N5	birds
H6	birds	N6	birds
H7	horses, birds	N7	horses, birds
H8	birds	N8	horses, birds
H9	birds	N9	birds
H10	birds		
H11	birds		
H12	birds		
H13	birds		
H14	birds		
H15	birds		

Source: after Nicholson *et al.* (2003: 1734).

discovery, and how epidemics and pandemics can arise. That is then followed by examinations of the origins and extent of the pandemic (Chapter 3), its human cost, particularly the vast mortality caused (Chapter 4), and the impacts of the pandemic and the responses to it, including the imposition of quarantine and the responses of the public health authorities and the medical profession (Chapter 5). Chapter 6 describes a number of the cultural aspects to the pandemic before a consideration of the longer-term repercussions in Chapter 7. The concluding chapter looks ahead and considers the possibilities and dangers of future influenza pandemics.

2 The history of influenza

A long history of affliction

While influenza (and 'influenza-like' illnesses) occur throughout our medical history, they rarely appear in the written histories. For example, Cartwright's 1972 discussion of diseases and their role in human history contained no mention of influenza and William McNeill's 1977 study only just acknowledged the pandemic of 1918–19 and the potential for future epidemics. More recently, Peter Baldwin's examination of the divergent public health approaches of Sweden, Germany, France and England, as expressed in their responses to contagious disease in the period 1830–1930, managed to avoid any assessment of the single greatest outbreak of infectious disease in that timespan, focusing instead on diseases such as cholera, smallpox and syphilis (Baldwin 1999). Cartwright may have overlooked influenza in his earlier work, but this was corrected in later work (Cartwright 1983), where he ranked the influenza pandemic among the three worst pandemics in history, alongside the Justinian plagues (*c.*AD 540), and the Black Death (the fourteenth century).[1] Kenneth Kiple's lavishly illustrated history of disease summarises the salient points of each of these episodes (Kiple 1997). Kiple recognises distinct similarities between the plagues of the sixth and fourteenth centuries in terming the earlier event 'The Plague of Justinian: an early lesson in the Black Death' and noting that '[o]verall mortality was placed by contemporary observers at 100 million' (Kiple 1997: 29).

The fourteenth century saw recurring outbreaks of bubonic plague, reaching their zenith in 1348, and lasting for generations as the plague visited most Mediterranean towns and cities at least four times over the course of the second half of the fourteenth century and 'would occur in Europe every generation for the next three centuries' (Kiple 1997: 60). These visitations were frequently marked by very high mortality, with up to 60 per cent case fatality rates. Kiple argues that the Black Death killed as much as '20 per cent of a Eurasian population . . . and killed with unimaginable speed during the peak of the epidemic. Soaring death rates prevented any semblance of normal burial practice' (Kiple 1997: 61). This disruption of normal burial practices was seen in many parts of the world during the 1918–19 pandemic, another indication of how dramatically and rapidly these diseases could break over populations.

Kiple also claims that the fourteenth-century visitations of plague played a major role in changing conceptions of disease, changing them from being regarded as expressions of the will of God to conceptions based on the human body and its failings as, prior to the bubonic plague pandemic, a

> great plague was believed to reveal God's will. . . . Mechanisms to understand the timing, meaning or other particulars of a plague emphasized its spiritual and celestial origins. But the Black Death changed all that. From then onward . . . the focus increasingly turned toward the body, the terrestrial, the victims.
>
> (Kiple 1997: 60)

Kiple suggests that each of these three pandemics may have claimed as many as 100 million deaths. This is somewhat higher than the commonly cited estimates for mortality from the 1918–19 influenza pandemic. However, as will be seen, the estimate for mortality caused in 1918–19 due to influenza can be raised as high as 100 million: thus, these three events can legitimately be linked in terms of total mortality. In terms of the proportion of the population killed, influenza was a lesser threat to the population. However, the disease carved its path through humanity far more rapidly than the two other disease outbreaks; Kiple allows estimates of 100 million deaths for both earlier events, but over a span of decades, whereas the influenza pandemic claimed its victims in a period from 1918 to no later than 1920.

Despite the considerable conceptual difficulties in attaching modern labels to historical disease outbreaks, including problems of distinguishing influenza from outbreaks of the many diseases that can display similar symptoms, and also problems with the use of the term 'influenza' itself, more recent overviews of disease in history have started to recognise the scale of influenza mortality and to accord influenza its appropriate status in the pantheon of human disease. That status is attributable not only to the potential and past capability to cause suffering and death on a vast scale; it is also due to the persistence of the malady over thousands of years.

The 'new acquaintance'

While Mary Queen of Scots may have referred to influenza as her 'new acquaintance', influenza has certainly been recognised as a specific illness for a very long time. The earliest descriptions of influenza (or influenza-like illness) are commonly attributed to Hippocrates (or Livy) (Beveridge 1977: 25; Gallagher 1969; Kaplan and Webster 1977; WHO 1999d: 38). For example, the WHO noted that 'Influenza-like disease was well described by Hippocrates in 412 BC, and influenza-like outbreaks since AD 1173 were clearly tabulated by Hirsch (1883)' (WHO 1999d: 38). A summarised, and updated, version of August Hirsch's tabulation (Table 2.1) indicates how extensively influenza has spread during our recorded history.

Table 2.1 Major influenza epidemics and pandemics 1173–1977

Years	*Geographical extent*
1173	Italy, Germany, England.
1387	Italy, France, Germany.
1510	General diffusion in Europe.
1557	General diffusion in Europe.
1580	General diffusion over the East, in Africa and in Europe.
1593	General diffusion.
1693	General diffusion in Great Britain, the North of France, and the Netherlands.
1709	General diffusion in Italy, France, Belgium, Germany and Denmark.
1729–30	Europe, Global.
1732–3	Seemingly a general diffusion over the globe. True pandemic.
1742–3	Europe.
1757–8	General diffusion in North America, parts of Europe.
1761–2	General diffusion in North America and West Indies, Western Europe.
1767	Widely diffused over North America and Europe.
1775–6	Europe and Asia.
1781–2	Global. True pandemic.
1788–90	General diffusion over the Western Hemisphere.
1800–2	China, Europe, Brazil.
1815–16	General diffusion in North America.
1826	Widely spread over the Western Hemisphere.
1830–3	General diffusion over the Eastern and Western Hemispheres. True pandemic.
1836–7	Considerable diffusion in the Eastern Hemisphere, Europe, Africa. True pandemic.
1847–8	Generally diffused over the Eastern Hemisphere, Europe, Americas. True pandemic.
1850–1	Generally diffused over the Western and Eastern Hemispheres.
1857–8	Wide diffusion over the Western and Eastern Hemispheres.
1873–5	Widely spread over the Western and Eastern Hemispheres.
1889–92	Global. True pandemic. The 'Russian' flu.
1918–19	Global. Greatest pandemic. The 'Spanish' flu.
1946	Global pandemic.
1957	Global pandemic. 'Asian' flu. First indisputable pandemic of the virologic era.
1968–70	Global pandemic. 'Hong Kong' flu.
1977	Global pandemic.

Sources: Beveridge 1977; Garrett 1996; Hirsch 1883; Kilbourne 1977; Patterson 1986.

Hirsch, a German physician, medical historian and medical geographer, writing in the late nineteenth century, certainly recognised the importance of influenza, as it was the first disease he described in his three-volume opus *Handbuch der historisch-geographischen Pathologie* (1883: 6–54). The English physician and writer on medicine, psychology and society Francis Crookshank[2] recognised that Hirsch was largely responsible

> for our present notions concerning influenza. ... Hirsch regarded influenza as a specific disease, independent of 'weather' in its origins and dissemination, and no less independent in respect of climate, of telluric, and of cosmic conditions: a disease specific and infectious 'like cholera, typhoid, small-pox and others,' which has 'at all times and in all places borne a stamp of uniformity in its configuration and in its course such as almost no other infectious disease has.' Hirsch went further: he postulated a 'uniform and specific cause, of which the origin and nature are still completely shrouded in obscurity.'
>
> (Crookshank 1922: 52)

These origins were still very much shrouded when Crookshank wrote this in the 1920s and this perhaps explains why Crookshank rather derided Hirsch, who has subsequently been shown to be more accurate than Crookshank believed. In fact Hirsch went further than Crookshank suggests, as he recognised the following truisms about flu:

> Influenza['s] wide prevalence in space and in time; the history of the disease may be followed into the remotest periods from which we have any epidemiological record at all, and its geographical distribution ... extends over the whole habitable globe.
>
> (Hirsch 1883: 7)

> [I]nfluenza takes an exceptional place among the acute infective diseases; no other of them has ever shown so pronounced a pandemic character as influenza.
>
> (Hirsch 1883: 18)

> Conditions of race are entirely without significance for the distribution of influenza.
>
> (Hirsch 1883: 29)

While influenza has afflicted us for centuries, it has been claimed that it was in the nineteenth century that influenza 'became an endemic disease in the majority of the countries in the world, regularly producing large epidemic and pandemics', a claim that extends Crosby's contention that it is a disease of a humanity living in large communities (Zhdanov *et al.* 1958, read in translation United States of America 1960: 4; see Crosby 1997: 148).

Hirsch's tabulation was extended back through time with claims of influenza epidemics also occurring in 393 BC, 43 BC, AD 591–2, 837, 876, 889 and 932, as well as in 1307, 1529, 1551, 1647, 1718, 1727, 1793 and 1889–90 (Townsend 1933). In addition to these outbreaks, there were large-scale epidemics of what was termed the 'Russian flu' during the early to mid-1890s (Smith 1995). Hirsch's English translator, Charles Creighton,[3] also described the history of epidemics in Britain, adding further detail to and updating Hirsch's work, at least in the British context (Creighton 1965: 398, 402 and 407).

In Britain, the Registrar-General (hereafter RG) has been recording influenza mortality since 1838. Never before or since in the influenza record had there been such an upturn as was evident in 1918 (Figure 2.1). 1918 was, as the RG noted, 'the first time since the commencement of registration' that deaths exceeded births (*ARRG* 1918: xxvii), and influenza played a major role in this mortality. Figure 2.1 also shows how flu had largely disappeared as a cause of death before the 'Russian' flu of the 1890s and that, after the 1918–19 pandemic, it remained a threat for the following decades, albeit at a much lower level.

One advantage of working with a disease that has been recognised for centuries is that it appears as a single entity through all the changes to nosologies. The classification of 'diseases' came to prominence in the mid-eighteenth century and became an obsession of medical writers largely due to the impetus given to taxonomy by Linnaeus' *Systema Naturae* (1735). In 1768, Francois Boissier de Sauvages, botanist and physician, published a detailed *Nosologia methodica sistens morborum classes, genera, et species* based on Linneaus. He divided 'diseases' into ten classes, subdivided these into forty

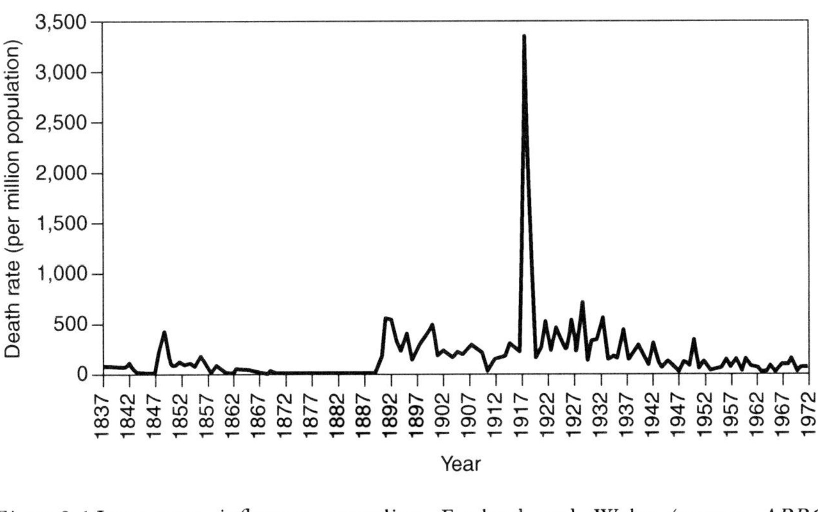

Figure 2.1 Long-term influenza mortality, England and Wales (source: *ARRG* 1837–1973).

orders, the orders into genera, and the genera into species – 2,400 in all; later workers extended this greatly (Caplan *et al.* 1981: 212). Michel Foucault wrote at some length on nosologies and how they reflect the conception of disease at a given time. In addition to reflecting the changing spatialisations of disease that Foucault discusses – changes that saw disease moved purely from the two-dimensional space of the nosology to the three-dimensional geography of the patient – the emphasis moved from the arrangement of disease in abstract form to a medicine driven by the gaze, by observation of disease in situ (Foucault 1976). Thus, as conceptions of disease and the focus of medicine changed – changes in the belief of disease causation and how disease is studied and attacked – the nosologies changed. Interestingly, influenza is one of those few conditions that appear consistently throughout this evolution of nosologies as it has long been recognised, even if its cause was unknown. For example, it has always been a single cause in the International Classification of Diseases. This makes tracking the long-term history of the disease much easier than is the case with other conditions, notwithstanding the problem of accurate diagnosis.

Nonetheless, disease diagnoses are a perennial problem. Riley, in discussing European health in the period 1600–1870, observed that the leading causes of death are in fact a 'comparatively short list' that included bubonic plague, cholera, dysentery, influenza, malaria, measles, pneumonia, smallpox, tuberculosis, typhoid fever and typhus (Riley 1989: 54). However, Riley also acknowledged that the list was 'open to objection' as the designation of a specific cause, when it was done, often 'occurred chiefly after the physician or, more often still, a lay person . . . had glanced or gazed' at the corpse or spoken with the family or friends (Riley 1989: 54). This is not what one could term a rigorous, reliable method. Furthermore, as cause of death is often multi-factorial, singling out a specific cause can be profoundly difficult even under the best of conditions. Obviously under conditions of extreme stress, as in an epidemic, diagnosis would often be done cursorily, and could possibly lead to an over-estimation of cases. It is also worth remembering that influenza is a disease that is frequently self-diagnosed, usually on the basis of severity of symptoms. This has consequences for measures of morbidity and also has meant that influenza continues to be overlooked. As the journalist and historian Brian Inglis dryly noted:

> The term 'flu' has consequently become 'probably the most abused and most meaningless term in the whole sphere of medicine' . . . little more than a synonym for a severe cold, because it is 'considered a more respectable excuse for a few days off work'.
>
> (Inglis 1981: 160)

Confirming the diagnosis of influenza is more difficult than just identifying a series of symptoms. This is partly because not all of the possible symptoms may be present in any given case, or they may be present to varying extents.

Additionally, there is the issue of sub-clinical infection – infection that does not display clinical symptoms – and therefore the individual is almost invariably unaware that they have been exposed to the influenza virus, but they have been exposed, and their immune system has 'learnt' about the virus and coped with it. The number of sub-clinical infections is often much the same as the actual clinical infections, but the ratio varies as much as 4:1 to 1:7; sub-clinical infections are thus important for both the spread of influenza and the level of immunity (Riordan 1986: 23). In epidemics and pandemics where the proportion of the population reporting infection can be higher than 50 per cent, it is plausible, with sub-clinical infection, that most, if not all, of the population has been exposed. This also helps to explain how influenza epidemics and pandemics can fade so rapidly as they run out of fresh susceptibles to infect.

Diagnosis of many conditions and diseases is often difficult, perhaps none more so than influenza. The WHO recognises that on 'clinical grounds alone it cannot be distinguished from other acute respiratory infection; laboratory tests are necessary' (WHO 1999a). In 1918 no one was sure what it was they were dealing with, as they had never seen the influenza virus itself. Accurate, certain diagnosis of influenza requires further medical technology, as exemplified in this extract from a WHO factsheet on influenza:

> Influenza infections can be diagnosed by serology using haemagglutinin-inhibition tests to detect antibodies during acute infections, more immediate diagnosis may be achieved by the direct detection of viral antigens in nasal secretions by inmmunoflourescence test. Diagnosis could also be done by polymerase chain reaction (PCR) or by antigen capture ELISA with monoclonal antibody to the nucleoprotein. Culture of the influenza viruses from nasopharyngeal secretions are preferred for further identification of strains.
>
> (WHO 1999a)

This level of medical technology is in fact rarely invoked for what is generally perceived individually as an insignificant disease.

As the medical profession has changed, the role and importance of symptoms in diagnosing and classifying disease have also varied. Medicine is a very visual science (or art) in which the eye is the critical tool, even if in modern times it has been augmented by technologies and techniques including x-rays, MRIs (magnetic resonance imaging), pathology, and so on. The gaze and its resolution have been enhanced in their dominance as these 'aids' have developed. Influenza has long been identified based upon the observed symptoms. Obviously as medicine has changed the credence given to clinical observation has varied over that time, as Foucault noted. The change in the emphasis given to symptoms relates to what is conveyed by them and how they relate to the body of medical knowledge (Foucault 1976: 92). For influenza, we have a long history, a long history of study and classification that has given significance to the various symptoms as signs (of the disease). Over time the symptoms observed converged and gave a more characteristic picture, but one that allowed for some variation. In the nosologies, in the description of the 'typical' form of the disease, 'variations cancel each other out, and the effect of the repetition of constant phenomena outlines spontaneously the fundamental conjunctions. By showing itself in a repetitive form, the truth indicates the way by which it may be acquired' (Foucault 1976: 110). Thus, from the wide array of symptoms eventually there emerged a 'core' or 'truth' that is influenza.

Foucault suggested that '[s]igns and symptoms are and say the same thing, the only difference being that the sign *says* the same thing that *is* precisely the symptom. In its material reality, the sign is identified with the symptom itself; the symptom is the indispensable morphological support of the sign. . . . But what makes the sign a sign belongs not to the symptom, but to an activity that originates elsewhere' (Foucault 1976: 93). Thus, there has to be a system or body of knowledge that attaches significance to a symptom, that makes it a sign. The system that existed in the early twentieth century could still not resolve what was the causative mechanism of influenza, but it was a question that had begun to be asked. The success (or otherwise) of the 'gaze' of early twentieth-century medicine in the 'discovery' of the influenza virus may be attributed to the existing body of knowledge. Opening the 13 November 1918 Royal Society of Medicine 'Discussion' on influenza, Sir Arthur Newsholme (then Chief Medical Officer of the Local Government Board[4]) argued that definition must precede diagnosis:

> The first difficulty is to define Influenza. Is it one disease or a group of diseases? And is the disease now prevailing the disease which prevailed in the spring? . . . These two questions cannot easily be separated. The symptoms were usually mild in the earlier than in the present outbreak . . . there is evidence that occasionally influenza kills rapidly by toxæmia, but more often by pulmonary complications. . . . There can be no doubt that all these bacteria, often acting in conspiracy, have contributed greatly to the recent mortality from influenza, but whether there is in addition a hitherto undiscovered virus to which influenza is primarily due is still a moot point.
>
> (Royal Society of Medicine 1918: 1–2)

Newsholme's questions reflected the lack of knowledge about the prevailing epidemic, the uncertainty about the nature of the disease, and its relation to prior influenza epidemics, including the first-wave outbreak in the spring of 1918.

Discovery

The discovery of the influenza virus was not made until 1933 by Wilson Smith, Christopher Andrewes and Patrick Laidlaw at the National Institute for Medical Research facilities at Mill Hill in north London (Smith *et al.* 1933), based on the American bacteriologist Richard Shope's earlier success in isolating and identifying swine flu (Shope 1931). Walter Morley Fletcher, the head of the laboratory where Smith, Andrewes and Laidlaw worked and Secretary (the analogous modern position is Chief Executive Officer) of the Medical Research Council from its inception in 1914 until 1933 (and later Sir Walter), had been very concerned about the influenza pandemic and he apparently instigated the research at Mill Hill. His wife, Maisie, wrote in his biography that, in 1918,

> [t]hat late summer and autumn saw the appalling ravages of the black influenza pandemic. Walter himself fortunately escaped, but he was terrible concerned about it, and from then on he initiated a real attack on the disease . . . and the starting of the Field Laboratories up at Mill Hill where the vast Laboratory of the Medical Research Council was to be built thirty years later.
>
> (Fletcher 1957: 143)

Why the virus was not isolated sooner can be attributed to a variety of factors, including technical reasons (for example, the difficulty in culturing the influenza virus, the small size of the virus being beyond the resolution of existing microscopes and being able to pass through filters that were impervious to known bacteria) and the more pervasive obstacle of prevailing theories of influenza causation and the bacteriological paradigm that ruled the research environment of the time,[5] established on the 'scientific and practical results of bacteriology', led by Louis Pasteur, Robert Koch and Joseph Lister (van Helvoort 1993: 6). At the time, the pandemic bacteriology, with its strict adherence to 'Koch's postulates', was in many respects hindered in looking for viruses. Basically, these four 'commandments' of bacteriology stated that:

1. The micro-organism must be found in every case of the disease and in such a way that explains the symptoms and the damage caused.
2. The micro-organism must be isolated and cultured in pure culture outside the host.
3. The pure culture must be able to produce the disease when transmitted to healthy animals/hosts, with identical symptoms as the naturally occurring disease.
4. The micro-organism should be recoverable from all experimentally induced cases.

In examining influenza cases in 1918 and 1919, 'whole zoos' (Crosby 1989: 265) of micro-organisms were found, including Pfeiffer's bacillus, staphylococci, streptococci and pneumococci.[6] Indeed, during the pandemic the real cause, the influenza virus, was never to be seen.[7]

In 1891–2, shortly after an influenza epidemic, the German physician and bacteriologist Richard Pfeiffer isolated the bacillus that was to carry his name for a long time. Pfeiffer was already a very important figure in the bacteriological world.[8] A colleague of Koch's, he was head of research at the Institute for Infectious Diseases in Berlin. His publications on a wide range of diseases were extremely well-regarded. Thus any pronouncement he made on influenza would carry much weight; if he got it wrong, his word would become 'an authoritative road sign pointing in the wrong direction' (Crosby 1989: 269). Crosby critiques Pfeiffer's approach, revealing the flaws in his research, but does recognise the 'keenness of hindsight' (Crosby 1989: 269). Pfeiffer first saw the bacillus in 1890, but did not begin his research on influenza until November 1891, by which time the Russian flu epidemic was waning. Crosby wonders if the organisms Pfeiffer examined actually came from that epidemic at all. Pfeiffer certainly found large quantities of the bacillus in the upper respiratory tracts of people who apparently had been ill with influenza, as required by the first of the Koch postulates. The second postulate was met in culturing the bacillus, but the third postulate was not to be clearly met as inducing influenza in susceptible animals proved very difficult. Pfeiffer was unable to induce influenza in mice, rats, guinea pigs, cats and dogs. The fact that influenza A does not infect many of the animals used in experiments conducted around the pandemic certainly did not help matters. He was able to induce a respiratory disease in monkeys, but this was not unambiguously influenza. The illness in rabbits was also not influenza and the growth of the bacillus in their lungs was isolated and inconsistent, thus failing the fourth of Koch's postulates. Pfeiffer, by the rules governing bacteriology, had not proved the role of the bacillus in causing influenza. However, while he stated his results and theories quite conservatively, such was his status that they were regarded as correct. The 1919 edition of Hans Zinsser's *Textbook of Bacteriology* stated 'the relationship between the clinical disease known as influenza or grippe and the Pfeiffer bacillus has been definitely established by numerous investigations' (Zinsser 1919: 540, cited in Crosby 1989: 270).

Consequently, when the first outbreaks were detected in 1918 Pfeiffer's bacillus was widely considered to be the culprit. Much of the literature before, during and shortly after the pandemic regarded Pfeiffer's bacillus as being the (or at least the most likely) agent (examples include Cummins 1919; Galli-Valerio 1918; King 1922; Léon 1921; Levinthal *et al.* 1921; Lister and Taylor 1919; McIntosh 1922; Ministry of Health 1920c; Opie *et al.* 1921).[9] One of the major publications that came down on the side of Pfeiffer's bacillus was Opie, Blake, Small and Rivers' *Epidemic Respiratory Disease* (Opie *et al.* 1921). They went on record saying their research confirmed Pfeiffer's assertion that the bacillus was invariably present in cases of influenza and that it was most likely that the bacillus caused pandemic influenza. Several decades later Thomas Rivers, reflecting on his long career, much of it with the Rockefeller Institute, freely conceded, 'Well, we were just one hundred per cent wrong, and it's a chapter I wish I had never written' (Benison 1967: 59).

Pfeiffer's theory (and 'his' bacillus) held sway. However, as the pandemic progressed, more and more doubts were voiced about this and support for the existence of a 'filter-passing agent' became more widespread and vocal, but proof for this view was not quickly forthcoming. It is readily apparent from the published material that many researchers were extremely uncertain and often seem to have avoided coming down on one side or the other, or wavered in their convictions, providing papers that supported both sides. One example of such vacillations was Sir Frederick Spencer Lister in South Africa. In 1919 he published two papers together (Lister and Taylor 1919). The first paper, 'The bacteriology of epidemic influenza on the Witwatersrand', offers Pfeiffer's bacillus as the crucial agent. However, the second paper, 'Experimental investigation of epidemic influenza at Durban', co-authored with E. Taylor, reveals far less certainty and could be read as suggesting the existence of a viral agent. Three years later, Lister shows a more decisive frame of mind; here he firmly nailed his colours to the 'filter-passing' mast with his article titled 'A filter-passing micro-organism associated with epidemic influenza' (Lister 1922). In this later work he briefly discusses the search for a 'filter-passing micro-organism', i.e. a virus, and how the medical community was divided as to whether influenza was caused by such a micro-organism or by Pfeiffer's bacillus.

This uncertainty of causality was evident elsewhere. During the Royal Society of Medicine's November 1918 'Discussion', there was much debate about the bacteriology, with support for both Pfeiffer's bacillus and a 'filter-passing agent' being expressed.[10] Contemporary reports in newspapers and the medical journals also reported the debate surrounding influenza aetiology.[11] Donaldson's chapter in Crookshank's 1922 collection of essays on influenza is yet another example of the confusion surrounding influenza aetiology. He suggested that the 'medical world was in a receptive mood, ready to accept as "causal" any organism which could claim the distinction of being new to bacteriology, even though its constant relationship to the disease could not be proved' (Donaldson 1922: 144). Donaldson concluded that Pfeiffer's bacillus could not be the cause of influenza. However, he also concluded that there is no evidence at all that influenza is caused by a 'so-called filter-passing virus'. It was to be more than a decade before this argument was settled (Smith *et al.* 1933). Pfeiffer was still defending his bacillus as the (likely) cause of influenza as late as 1931 (Pfeiffer 1931). The uncertainty about the causation of influenza and the mortality it had brought energised the medical research community greatly in the decade following the pandemic, as more than 4,000 books and articles on influenza were published between the pandemic and the discovery of the virus (Crosby 1989: 265).

F. MacFarlane Burnet[12] and Ellen Clark reported that Pfeiffer's bacillus was repeatedly not found in the first two days of illness, but quite regularly found, often in large quantities, in the later stages of the illness. Their explanation of this pattern was that this 'would be expected if it were an infection secondary to a primary virus infection' (Burnet and Clark 1942: 85). They concluded that there was nothing in all the published reports on bacteriological examinations that were made during the pandemic that would indicate that it was caused by anything other than an influenza virus and that 'Pfeiffer's bacillus was only one of the more important secondary invaders', along with pneumococci, staphylococci and streptococci. Some modern researchers suggest that much of the excess mortality caused in the 1918–19 pandemic may in fact have been caused by these secondary infections, especially pneumococci.[13]

Even when the existence of these filterable (or 'filter-passing') agents was starting to be canvassed, this did not lead to changes in how they were studied: as van Helvoort argues, these filterable viruses were 'considered to be small bacteria or "ultrabacteria" and this presupposition had a great influence on how research was carried out' (van Helvoort 1993: 5). This conceptual framework was not challenged until it failed. It was the influenza experience that weakened the bacteriological paradigm and helped bring about the viral era. In the meantime, however, it had hindered the search for the real cause of influenza. How much this was hindered is debatable as the technology to actually 'see' viruses was not available in 1918, but it is also possible that a search for a 'filter-passing agent' earlier may have spurred on such technological development and brought about those advances earlier.[14]

The ever-changing virus

There are three main types of influenza virus: A, B and C. Type A is the most important; it is this type that leads to epidemics and pandemics among humans. Within Type A there are many subtypes and they can be found in humans, pigs, horses and birds, especially chickens and ducks. The continuing battle we face with influenza is due to the virus' ability to change. There are two different mechanisms of change, antigenic drift and antigenic shift. Both of these are genetic changes, through recombination of the RNA leading to changes in the haemagglutinin and neuraminidase 'spikes' that can cause the (human) body's immune system to have difficulty recognising the invading virus. These changes produce a virus to which a significant proportion of the population has no immunological experience or knowledge and therefore they are susceptible to the 'new' virus.

Minor mutations of the genetic material, the RNA, can cause minor changes in the surface antigens. This is a continual process and this 'drift' eventually causes enough changes to the virus so that every few years each of us may be vulnerable to a virus that is now sufficiently different from ones we have experienced and the record left in our immune system. This antigenic drift is 'believed to be analogous to the phenomenon known as "genetic drift" in plants and animals' (Beveridge 1977: 71). That is, minor mutations of the genetic code for these antigens occur, resulting in slight alterations of their properties. Marguerite Pereira, one-time director of WHO's influenza section, described drift as a subtle change 'as if the virus manages "to change its coat in such a way that it is no longer recognised by the sentries"' (Inglis 1981: 162).

Far less subtle and more important for the emergence of pandemics is 'shift'. Influenza's genetic material consists of eight separate pieces of RNA. These eight segments can function as distinct genes, so a form of genetic re-assortment can occur if a host cell is infected with two (or more) strains of virus. Thus, if an individual is attacked by two influenza strains at once a new virus can be created with genetic information from both 'parents'. The new virus will have a new genetic arrangement, one that will be expressed in a novel arrangement of the surface antigens: these will show a distinct 'shift' (as opposed to a minor 'drift') in the virus' antigens, and thus the virus has a new 'face'. This is made all the more critical as it is possible for human, swine, equine and avian influenzas to re-combine into a new virus. This does not seem to happen often or to necessarily lead to a new virus to which humans are widely susceptible. However, when it does, it can give rise to new strains to which there is little immunity and thus the possibility of epidemics and pandemics increases. Thus, antigenic drift is caused by mutation in the genes coding for haemagglutinin and neuraminidase and antigenic shift is caused by genetic re-assortment resulting in completely different antigens. This propensity for change in the virus led the esteemed American virologist Ed Kilbourne to term it 'an unvarying disease caused by a varying virus' (Kilbourne 1980).

Epidemics and pandemics

While epidemic is a word we use quite frequently, pandemic is not so common. But what do they mean?

> Epidemic
> *adj.* 1 Of a disease: normally absent or infrequent in a population but liable to outbreaks of greatly increased frequency and severity.
> (*New Shorter Oxford English Dictionary* 1993 4th edn: I: 836)
>
> Pandemic
> *adj.* 1 (of a disease) prevalent throughout a country, a continent, or the world; of or pertaining to such a disease.
> (*New Shorter Oxford English Dictionary* 1993 4th edn: II: 2082)

Pandemic tends to denote a global involvement, whereas epidemic refers to large outbreaks at the national or smaller scale. It is worth noting that it is not a rise in lethality that denotes an epidemic or pandemic of influenza, rather it is

> the occurrence of many cases throughout the world within a short period that constitutes a pandemic. The case fatality rate of pandemic influenza may not differ from that of interpandemic influenza, but the sudden increase of total cases is reflected by an increase in total excess mortality.
>
> (Kilbourne 1977: 1225)

This may seem somewhat peculiar: if the disease is not more lethal, then why worry? Kilbourne's riposte is that 'A pandemic virus is dangerous and should be curtailed because it infects, sickens and acutely incapacitates millions and millions of people. Even if case fatality rates are low . . . total excess mortality will increase substantially beyond that occasioned by any other human condition' (Kilbourne 1977: 1227). In Britain the Association for Flu Monitoring and Surveillance uses the benchmark of 400 cases per 100,000 population to denote an epidemic (BBC 1999b).

It is the antigenic changes that have a major impact as they effectively change the immunological pattern. Such changes, both drift and shift, can result in a virus to which populations have less or even no immunity. This is particularly true of antigenic shifts where the virus is changed so markedly that we recognise it as being a new subtype. It is such a major change that is considered as being one of the necessary preconditions for the emergence of a pandemic. Kilbourne recognises three such preconditions:

> (1) major antigenic mutation of the virus, (2) . . . susceptible population on the basis of immunologic inexperience with the antigen, and (3) . . . disappearance of the immediately antecedent strain. . . . The remarkably constant clinical picture of disease from epidemic to epidemic is striking.
>
> (Kilbourne 1977: 1226)

It is widely held that all of these conditions were met in 1918. The belief is that a new virus emerged and it struck a population that had no immunologic experience of the new antigen(s) and that the prior strain of the virus was replaced. The changes to the 1918 virus are unclear as the influenza virus itself was not isolated until 1933 (Smith *et al.* 1933), but recent work has postulated whether the HA gene segment of the virus could have come from an avian source or whether some of the gene segments could have evolved in an intermediate host, perhaps swine, before becoming a human pathogen (Reid and Taubenberger 2003; Reid *et al.* 2001). Further, the clinical expression of the new viral subtype, whilst more severe, was manifestly consistent with other subtypes of influenza, both before and since (Beveridge 1977; Braithwaite 1953; Bryder 1982; Burnet and Clark 1942; Collier 1974; Crosby 1989; Fincher 1989; Kaplan and Webster 1977; Kilbourne 1977, 1987; Starr 1976; Stuart-Harris *et al.* 1985).

A new virus has an edge in survival; the lack of immunity in the host population gives it the competitive edge, and thus it supplants its predecessor. The antigenic changes keep influenza one step ahead, ensuring that the threat of epidemic and pandemic is ever-present. It is for exactly this reason that the WHO co-ordinates a global monitoring programme on influenza. This programme is built on a network of more than 100 National Influenza Centres in dozens of countries and the four WHO Collaborating Centres for Virus Reference and Research in Atlanta, London, Melbourne, and Tokyo. These four centres have the prime responsibility for characterising or identifying influenza strains. They also exchange strains, reagents and information to complete the understanding of influenza during each influenza 'season' (WHO 1999b). They provide expert advice on the composition of each flu season's vaccine based on their predictions of what strains are likely to be present. It is their role to react to and co-ordinate the response to any outbreak of influenza, particularly if a new strain should emerge. This surveillance scheme has been in operation for more than fifty years (WHO 1999e).

Reservoir pigs?

Some animals besides humans can also be infected by influenza A viruses. With the ability of the influenza virus to re-combine should more than one strain be present in a single host, animals may be a critical source or reservoir of new genetic material for the creation of new influenza A strains to which humans could have little or no immunity. Suggestions of connections between human influenza and similar diseases in some animals have long been made. For example, an 1890 pamphlet titled *The Coming Epidemic. Influenza: Its History, Symptoms, Treatment, &c.*, written under the pseudonym of 'Scrutator', which had a warning '1,000,000 cases in Paris' luridly prominent on the cover, raised a connection with horses ('Scrutator' 1890). Just a few years before, Hirsch had also raised the apparent coincidence in observations of a disease in horses occurring around the time of some influenza outbreaks (Hirsch 1883). In South Africa, the historian Howard Phillips noted that 'frightening tales . . . gained wide currency at the time' of the pandemic, 'tales that included accounts of baboons, pigs and birds dying all across the nation' (Phillips 1990a: 132). The baboon tales made *The Times* in London, who headlined their story 'Influenza among baboons' (5 November 1918: 6).

It had long been thought that the virus which caused the 1918–19 pandemic was related to a swine flu virus and suggestions that it was a recombinant virus that had components from a human flu virus and a swine flu virus had gained some currency (Beveridge 1977; Burnet and Clark 1942; Chan and Liu 1998; Crosby 1989; Dillner 1995; Dowdle and LaPatra 1983; Graves 1969; Kaplan and Webster 1977; Kilbourne 1977, 1987; Neustadt and Fineberg 1978; Pickrell 2001; Radford 1996; Stuart-Harris 1965; Stuart-Harris *et al.* 1985; Webster and Laver 1972; Webster *et al.* 1992;

Zhdanov *et al.* 1958). However, as Dixon observed, 'the presumption that swine flu was responsible for the 1918–19 pandemic has always been made on circumstantial grounds. A disease of comparable severity had hit millions of swine at the same time, and the connection seemed obvious' (Dixon 1994: 69). Studies have suggested that the swine influenza virus Shope isolated in 1930 and contemporary human viruses are not direct descendants of the 1918 human virus strain, but rather shared a common ancestor from which they may have diverged sometime around 1905. Other work suggests that common ancestor may have been the 1918 virus itself, which may have 'entered human or swine populations as a novel avian-like' virus (Taubenberger 1998: 3; see also Brownlee and Fodor 2001). Study of the matrix gene segment from the 1918 virus has revealed it to be 'mammalian adapted' and that the '1918 sequence is very similar to the common ancestor of all subsequent human and classical swine matrix segments' leading to the observation that a 'matrix segment may have been circulating in human strains for at least several years before 1918' (Reid *et al.* 2002: 10717).

Recent attempts to recover genetic material of the 1918 influenza virus from bodies or stored pathology samples are following the initial findings reported by Jeffrey Taubenberger's team in Washington, D.C. (Reid, Fanning *et al.* 1999; Reid, Taubenberger and Fanning 2001; Taubenberger 1998; Taubenberger *et al.* 1997, 2001). The success of that team, allied with the avian influenza scares, led to renewed (media) attention on influenza and saw two expeditions launched in attempts to recover further influenza 'fragments' from bodies of 1918 influenza victims that were buried under the permafrost of the northern latitudes. One of the main aims of this research is, through understanding the genetic sequence and the phylogeny of influenza viruses, to explain 'why this strain was so lethal, and the likely mechanism of its emergence in humans' (Taubenberger 1998: 3).

One of these expeditions was to Spitzbergen, where it was hoped that bodies buried in the hillside cemetery of the town of Longyearbyen would provide further specimens. The cemetery was known to contain the bodies of several victims of the pandemic. The expectation was that these bodies buried in the permafrost of this far northern location could still contain frozen remnants of the influenza virus. The large and well-equipped team attracted much media attention (including BBC 1999a, 1999e, 1999f; Gladwell 1997). However, the prospect of finding useful viral genetic material seems dim: the team found the bodies were not buried as deep as they had hoped. Consequently, it seems likely that they have been frozen and thawed too often for much viral material to have survived. It is thought that perhaps the bodies were simply not buried very deep (perhaps due to the frozen ground), had been moved up the soil column due to the action of freezing and thawing, or that perhaps there were actually two layers of bodies.[15]

The other expedition that went searching for fragments of the influenza virus was Johan Hultin's return to Alaska. He was part of a similar expedition in 1951, one that was unsuccessful in recovering any identifiable material. Upon hearing of the work of Taubenberger he offered to return to Alaska, obtaining permission from local Inuit people and attempting to find material that the new techniques and technology might be able to make better use of than he and his colleagues had some four decades earlier. His solo expedition to Alaska, organised and conducted in a matter of weeks, led to the exhumation of a well-preserved body of a thirty-year-old woman 'so obese that her fat had insulated her organs from the effects of decades of frost and thaw' (Larson 1998: 39). From this body the lungs were removed, sectioned and shipped to Taubenberger. Apparently fragments of the virus have been found in these samples. Hultin named the body 'Lucy' in recognition of the 'prehistoric Lucy who shed so much light on human origins' (Larson 1998: 39).

The preliminary results on the samples found in the US Army Pathology stores indicated that the 1918 strain had haemagglutinin (HA) of H1 mammalian type (not avian), neuraminidase (NA) of N1 type and nucleoprotein that generally fell into the human/swine grouping in the analyses. The conclusion was that 'the 1918 strain was an H1N1 virus, distinct from all subsequently characterized strains' and that it is closely related to early swine influenza strains, corroborating the archaeserological data from the 1930s. Phylogenetic analyses of influenza genes suggests a common avian ancestor for both human and swine H1N1 virus lineages. However, they argued that the common ancestor was not the 1918 strain and that the 'ancestral virus has entered the mammalian population at some point prior to 1918'. A suggestion has been made that the 1918 virus they have isolated and started characterising should be classified as Influenza A/South Carolina/1/8 (H1N1) (Taubenberger 1998: 9). Another avenue of research has examined the HA of the 1918 strain and suggests that it may ultimately have an avian origin (Brownlee and Fodor 2001; Reid and Taubenberger 2003) and that in experiments this HA enhanced the virulence of influenza strains and led to symptoms similar to those seen in 1918 (Kobasa *et al.* 2004).

Thus there is a possibility that in the not-too-distant future this work may lead to our knowing more about the genetic make-up and origin of the 1918–19 virus (Boseley 2000). One thing this may reveal is whether there was something special about the virus itself that made it so virulent and so lethal, especially for young adults. For now at least we have every reason to continue to fear influenza, and to hope that the WHO's global monitoring programme provides an effective early warning. If it was not something peculiar to the particular virus then it is quite possible that the excess mortality of the 1918 pandemic was largely due to the secondary infections, especially pneumonias. If this is the case, then our prospects for dealing with future pandemics are much brighter as pneumonias can be readily treated. What determines the virulence of influenza virus strains may be present in either the haemagglutinin or the neuraminidase, the nucleoprotein, non-structural protein or may be scattered throughout the genome; as such, further microbiological research may yet tell us if it was something intrinsic to that virus that made it so lethal.[16]

1976 swine flu

Due to the ostensible connection between swine flu and the 1918 pandemic there was grave concern in the USA during the summer of 1976. In February 1976 an outbreak of disease was reported at Fort Dix, New Jersey. The symptoms were apparently reminiscent of the 1918–19 pandemic and an influenza virus that resembled a swine flu virus was later isolated from some soldiers there, with another 273 personnel found to have antibodies, an indication that they too had been infected by the virus (Gregg 1983). The fear was that this was the possible start of a new pandemic. In fact, two types of influenza were detected amongst the troops. First, there was one of the influenza viruses commonly circulating the world at the time (Influenza A/Victoria/75). The other resembled a swine flu virus that had been found in swine in 1975 and 1976. No patients examined had antibodies to both types – they had only been infected by one or the other. One soldier died, David Lewis, and he was the last to have the swine flu as all the subsequent cases were of the human-only A/Victoria/75 strain (Gregg 1983: 38). Thus, at Fort Dix two viruses had been present, and only one survived, and that was the A/Victoria/75 strain. One of Ed Kilbourne's conditions for an epidemic was that any new virus had to replace the existing strain. In this case, the new strain failed to do this.

The fear of a pandemic on the scale of 1918–19 led the US government to embark upon a large-scale vaccination programme, and the prospect of a presidential election campaign apparently encouraged the implementation of this. Arguments that not to do so would leave President Ford open to criticism for failing to look after the nation's health might have helped sway the administration into paying for such a extensive plan in the face of an uncertain threat and with unknown benefit. The administration drew on the public profile of the Centers for Disease Control and Prevention and famous scientists, including Albert Sabin and Jonas Salk (both renowned for their work on polio vaccines), to launch the concept and lobby for Congress approval for funding (Dutton 1988; Gregg 1983; Neustadt and Fineberg 1978; Osborn 1977). For various reasons the feared epidemic never arose. The virus never spread as it was not as transmissible or virulent as had been feared (a situation paralleled with avian influenzas of more recent years). Production of the vaccines did not progress smoothly. There were delays as the manufacturers demanded indemnification from the government for the vaccines, and the vaccines that were then rather hurriedly produced were not always effective and led to some deleterious side-effects, with the best-known of these being Guillain–Barré Syndrome,[17] that caused cases of paralysis and even some deaths were recorded. The vaccinations started in October 1976 and an estimated forty million people were vaccinated.

Whether this was necessary or even well-executed has been debated subsequently (Dutton 1988; Neustadt and Fineberg 1978), but some of the major participants still believe that they adopted the correct course of action and a prudent approach anticipating a pandemic was justified. They believe they acted in an appropriate fashion and that they were better off having a vaccine and no infection to fight than having an epidemic with no vaccine available.[18] However, with the link of the vaccines to an increase in diagnosed cases of Guillain–Barré Syndrome, the programme is harder to defend. One critic considered the episode to be a farce whose limitations would have been exposed further in the event of an epidemic (Dutton 1988: 169–74).

Notwithstanding this, the various international and national bodies responsible for monitoring and reacting to influenza outbreaks have become more cautious about advocating large-scale activity before being absolutely certain of the nature of the problem than was the case in 1976. So, while there is a continual global monitoring campaign for current influenza virus strains and action is very quickly brought to bear when a new strain does appear (as seen with the avian flus), the advocacy of action is now more carefully considered. This could in fact lead to problems: should a new strain emerge and quickly develop into a full-blown pandemic, these agencies may not be in the best possible position, as the provision of resources, the provision of information and the manufacture of vaccines takes time, more time than may be available in pandemic conditions. A number of the relevant agencies are aware of these competing pressures and have recently re-examined their planning procedures in relation to influenza in light of past pandemics and epidemics. The WHO published their *Influenza Pandemic Plan. The Role of WHO and Guidelines for National and Regional Planning*, indicating what they believe their role is, and what should be done and by whom in the event of an influenza pandemic.[19]

Bird flu

Examination of the 1918–19 influenza pandemic has waxed and waned in the intervening years. The most recent stimuli to bring it back into pubic view have been the threats of SARS (Severe Acute Respiratory Syndrome) – which was initially thought to be a Type-B influenza – and the bird flus of the late 1990s and the early years of the new century (examples of media interest in the pandemic include Brown 2003; Channel 4/Granada Media 2003; Gladwell 1997; Higgins 1997; Larson 1998; Radford 1996, 1998). While most avian strains are of low pathogenicity and are 'widespread in migratory birds and water fowl' (Monto 2005) recent years have seen a number of outbreaks where people have contracted avian flu, with an unusually high level of mortality.

In May 1997, a new influenza virus strain was isolated from a child who died in Hong Kong with Reye's Syndrome. The strain was H5N1, a strain previously only found in birds, mostly ducks and chickens (Nicholson *et al.*

2003; WHO 1998a, 1998b; Yuen *et al.* 1998).[20] In 1997 there had been a serious outbreak that killed thousands of chickens in Hong Kong (Larson 1998: 34). This isolation of a previously exclusively non-human strain took a few days to be confirmed but it proved the efficacy of the WHO surveillance programme on influenza. Shortly after the confirmation of the new strain of influenza, actions were being taken. Detailed surveillance of southern China, examinations of all possible cases, extensive research and field work by Chinese, Hong Kong and WHO personnel were all brought to bear on this outbreak. The potential for an epidemic or even pandemic was widely appreciated. Intensive surveillance in Hong Kong and Guangdong Province, China, revealed a handful of further cases by the end of 1997, all in the Hong Kong Special Administrative Region of China (HK SAR) (WHO 1998a, 1998b). From the eighteen cases, there were six deaths (Nicholson *et al.* 2003: 1736; WHO 2004a). With the large number of deaths in poultry allied with the small number of human cases, and with the risk of more, it was determined that drastic measures had to be taken with regard to the poultry population. The disease was a grave threat to all poultry and a potential danger to people. Consequently, more than seventeen million birds died or were destroyed in the HK SAR (Gladwell 1997: 64). The WHO subsequently claimed that 'most influenza experts . . . agree that the prompt culling of Hong Kong's entire poultry population . . . probably averted a pandemic' (WHO 2004a).

It appears that the virus may have been a re-combination of human and avian flus occurring in southern China. China has previously been identified as a possible reservoir of influenzas due to the large numbers of birds and pigs, often in close contact with people. Alternatively, it may have been a 'drift' in an avian strain (H5N1) that led to an epidemic among chickens in southern China, including Hong Kong, and a small number of cases that were somehow transmitted to people in Hong Kong. It is also argued that there is evidence that China was the origin of the influenza viruses that 'caused the pandemics of H2N2 influenza in 1957, H3N2 influenza in 1968, and the re-emergence of H1N1 influenza in 1977' (Nicholson *et al.* 2003: 1735).

Late December 1997 saw the start of the massive cull of all poultry in the HK SAR and the cessation of imports from mainland China. These were later allowed to resume conditionally on 7 February 1998. The conditions included additional inspection and blood testing at chicken farms prior to export, with further testing for avian influenza on arrival in Hong Kong. Chickens were also to be segregated from live ducks and other water fowl in order to minimise any transmission risks to the chickens (Larson 1998; WHO 1998b). There are a number of parallels with the 1976 outbreak including the relatively small number of cases. The most important similarity was its failure to go beyond a handful of people. For whatever reason it did not appear to transmit from human-to-human effectively: as the WHO noted, '[a]lthough the exact means of transmission of H5N1 to humans have not yet been identified, there is no clear-cut evidence of any human-to-human transmission. Infection with the virus is believed to come through contact with infected birds' (WHO 1998a).

Since the 1997 outbreak there have been a number of further outbreaks, including a small number of cases in Hong Kong and Fujian Province, China, in 2003, where at least one person died (Monto 2005). Also in 2003, a bird flu of H7N7 strain proved highly pathogenic among chicken flocks in the Netherlands and one person was fatally infected (Monto 2005). Avian flus of H9N2 strain have caused a small number of mild human cases in Hong Kong in 1999 and 2003 (Nicholson *et al.* 2003: 1736; WHO 2004a). Of greater concern though has been the changes to the H5N1 strain, termed the Z-strain, which has spread to a number of countries in east and south-east Asia (Monto 2005). This strain has shown pathogenicity in a number of animal species and further cases of animal-to-human transmission and human fatalities have been recorded, with some fifty-seven deaths from 112 cases as of August 2005 (WHO 2005a). These are the conditions that make many consider that the potential for an influenza pandemic is higher than it has been for some time (Stöhr 2005). This strain has demonstrated a concentration in previously healthy children and adults and an usually high mortality rate: the WHO is concerned that the risk of more people being infected is high, particularly in rural areas in Asia with most households being in close proximity to poultry kept for food and income. That an avian strain is showing high pathogenicity and the potential for human-to-human transmission of this strain or a recombination of it with another (possibly one of the currently circulating human strains) have caused an elevated degree of concern among medical and flu professionals (Monto 2005; Stöhr 2005). Early 2005 saw the Chinese government announce the development of a vaccine for bird flu; however, questions remain over how this it to be administered to potentially millions of birds, what bird populations are to be targeted, how long such a programme remains in place, and so on.

The years of these bird flu outbreaks also saw the emergence of SARS. It is to be hoped that the experiences of SARS and the bird flus in east and south-east Asia have encouraged governments that surveillance and preparation for the possibility of large-scale outbreaks are necessary and that international co-operation is essential for a disease that is so easily transmitted, especially in our highly interconnected world where we saw SARS readily transferred from China and Singapore to a new outbreak in Toronto. SARS was eventually contained at great cost and great effort; but such costs and the human toll – at least 8,349 cases with 812 deaths (WHO 2003) – could fade into insignificance should a highly transmissible novel influenza strain emerge.

Evolutionary possibilities

Perhaps these latest evolutions of the virus have simply been a failure in evolutionary and survival terms. The influenza virus, as a 'species', has been a wonderful evolutionary success, managing to reproduce and spread in vast quantities over a very long period. Influenza's long-term success may stem from the lack of lethality, being an unregarded killer. As Joshua Lederberg[21] wrote when discussing 'Infectious disease as as evolutionary paradigm' – 'Long-term outcomes are most stable when they involve some degree of mutual accommodation, with both surviving longer' (Lederberg 1997: 421). Consequently, in many ways it can be argued influenza is a superior virus to some of those we are more afraid of, such as the ebola virus. In evolutionary terms ebola would not appear as successful, as it kills its host in a rapid and spectacular fashion and this makes it harder to effectively 'reproduce' and be transmitted, and therefore much easier to contain. Influenza, on the other hand, is very difficult, if not impossible, to contain. It is very easily transmitted from one infective host to another. Only a small percentage of hosts are killed, thereby ensuring a large population of potential hosts is always available for infection. In evolutionary terms influenza seems to be a very effective virus, one that contains within it the mechanism for creating 'mutants' that enable it to continue to survive in the face of threats such as increasing immunity or the creation of vaccines. The 'species', if not the individual virus, can overcome such hurdles in ways that are not available to many viruses. In 1918, influenza presented a face to humanity that had not been seen before – and thus was in no position to resist. The flu research and medical communities know full well that a flu pandemic remains a serious possibility. Indeed, early 2005 saw a WHO official write that 'conditions favouring the start of influenza pandemic' were emerging and that 'the probability that this potential for a pandemic will be realized has increased' (Stöhr 2005: 405). These remarks were published within days of reports that the British government were anticipating the possibility of an influenza pandemic that 'poses a far greater risk . . . than a terrorist threat' (Hall and Sample 2005).

It is the evolutionary advantages and possibilities that allow this constant affliction from the 'ever-changing virus' to continue to harry humanity. While medical science and treatments for many conditions have changed immensely since 1918, we still have relatively little success in beating influenza, especially a novel influenza. While we believe we can contain and stop the impact of secondary (bacterial) infections, the flu virus is still eluding us. A new influenza strain as virulent as that experienced in 1918 would still wreak havoc, claiming a terrible toll, especially if preparations have not been made (and maintained) for such a possibility. As Dixon rather dramatically wrote, 'As confirmed by our response to the emergence of AIDS, we are not in a strong position to deal with viruses that spring surprises' (Dixon 1994: 70–1). Henri Léon, nearly 80 years earlier, had noted that 'No other disease as yet known can rival it in these pandemic outbursts' (Léon 1921: 4). Nor can any other disease rival it for the way it continually stays ahead of humankind's efforts or our immunity.

Influenza (or any other virus) cannot be studied in a vacuum: they must be considered in their normal environment, particularly as it is the environment that provides the evolutionary pressure and stimulus that drives evolution, the stimulus that provides the need for change and the need for a survival advantage. Zhadanov *et al.* saw this stimulus, the factor that leads to variation in influenza, and specifically the changes in antigenic structure as being dependent on the 'specific immunity of the population' (Zhdanov *et al.* 1958, translated 1960: 344). Thus the level of immunity makes it harder for the widespread strain to persist, to spread, and to maintain a level of existence. This evolutionary pressure thus favours the rise of a new strain, to which the population has less immunity (and thus the new strain can replicate, spread, and find new hosts within the population). They also saw benefit in adopting the approach Burnet suggested in his 1944 lectures at Harvard (Burnet 1945), agreeing that 'infectious diseases should be studied primarily as an ecological problem of interaction between two species of organism' (Zhdanov *et al.* 1958, translated 1960: 344). This is much more an ecological/epidemiological/geographical view rather than a simple, reductionist, mechanistic, 'scientific' medical view that had tended to dominate biomedical research. This criticism was echoed by van Helvoort who, when discussing Burnet's monograph, also raised how some 'studied the organism in isolation' (what he termed the 'ontological way') while

> Burnet contrasted these methods with a study of organisms in their natural environment: the ecological approach. . . . According to Burnet the relation between virus and host could not be an antagonistic one. If a pathogenic agent – be it a bacterium, a virus or something else – were considered as a living organism, then its existence and the *continuous survival* of the host and agent could not depend on antagonism. Since this antagonism would imply destruction of either the host or parasite.
>
> (van Helvoort 1993: 20)

Thus, to paraphrase George Evelyn Hutchinson's famous title (Hutchinson 1965), the 'evolutionary play' must be seen in its context of the 'ecological theatre'; the evolutionary pressures on the virus have to be considered. But determining these pressures on viruses is not so straightforward. For example, in rising and more mobile global populations, what is more likely? More new viruses or fewer? One view is that more people means more hosts and more opportunities for new viruses (drift and shift opportunities). Alternatively, does more hosts mean less evolutionary pressure, i.e. widespread immunity is going to take longer to develop? Perhaps the latter is true if we accept that there are growing gaps between pandemics of influenza. But what is more important – opportunity or evolutionary pressure?

Could vaccines then act as an evolutionary trigger or driver for influenza? By boosting humanity's resistance and immunity do we hasten the evolution of new strains? This is not to advocate the non-use of what influenza vaccines are developed: we need the pharmaceutical defences we have and are attempting to develop. However, we cannot out-evolve or out-adapt a virus. An evolutionary 'race' with a virus is not one humanity is going to win, for as Lederberg drolly noted, 'We cannot compete with microorganisms whose populations are measured in exponents of 10^{12}, 10^{14}, 10^{16} over periods of days' (Lederberg 1997: 418–19). Thus the struggle between the human race and the influenza virus shall continue. The host–parasite relationship shall continue. The influenza virus shall then continue to 'drift' and 'shift' and to cause human suffering. Stephan Jay Gould, the late Harvard palaeontologist, evolutionary biologist and science historian, in giving a lecture on HIV/AIDS, said:

> We've had a couple of generations of great fortune: since the . . . flu epidemic of 1918, there has not been a [lethal] pandemic disease that struck the human population. If you look through human history, a pandemic is everyday biology. With our usual hubris we felt that we'd learned through technological advances to be free of it forever. But we're not.
>
> (Fincher 1989: 145)

This drives us to the rather depressing conclusion that humanity must be prepared for further assaults of influenza, with the possibility of massive morbidity and mortality. The following chapters depict how grave a threat influenza can pose by describing the huge toll that influenza wrought on humanity in the space of a handful of months early in the twentieth century as the Great War gave way to the 'Great Spanish Influenza' (Oxford 2001).

3 Pandemic geographies

The second decade of the twentieth century was not a good time to be a young adult – the Great War and the influenza pandemic came to end millions of lives and blight hundreds of millions more. In British (as well as French and German[1]) history and literature, the story of the war's 'lost generation' is well-known. But another story, not as well-known, is that of the 1918–19 influenza pandemic. This is a story of as many as one billion ill and 100 million dead.

The blame falls mainly on Spain

In a world at war, Spain was a land of peace, adopting a neutral stance in the Great War. One of the consequences of this was that the Spanish press were not living under the restraints that restricted their counterparts elsewhere. Thus, when the disease broke out there it was widely reported. These reports were then repeated elsewhere and so Spain became the first country to be widely reported as being afflicted by an epidemic of influenza, and overcoming those initial reports was to be a forlorn task. One of the first reports of the epidemic in *The Times* (25 June 1918: 9) carried the headline 'The Spanish Influenza – A Sufferer's Symptoms' and attempted to reason why Spain was the source: 'the dry, windy Spanish spring is an unpleasant and unhealthy season at all times. A spell of wet weather or of moist winds would probably check the progress of the epidemic.' Unfortunately these hopes are ill-founded – the English weather was not to save them. Other newspaper reports made much of the fact that the Spanish King, along with the Prime Minister and much of the Cabinet (Echeverri 2003: 173), was taken ill with influenza.[2] These reports spread rapidly; the term 'Spanish influenza' quickly gained universal currency.[3]

Certainly the British medical establishment saw Spain as the likely source of the scourge. One of the first items of correspondence received by the Medical Research Committee's Influenza Committee from the Local Government Board (LGB) was a request for information on any outbreaks of influenza, dysentery or diarrhoea in Spain (PRO FD 1 535). However, Spain was not alone in taking the blame. From the earliest days, the conditions that had been brought about by the war were seen as being possibly involved in causing and spreading the new illness. One Canadian newspaper wrote that:

> Not the best intentioned of nations can keep wholly out of this war. Even Spain, so established in neutrality, has contributed the Spanish grippe to the general misfortune which the war has brought to the countries of Christendom. From Spain this unpleasant malady has followed its persistant [*sic*] way to the armies on the firing lines, and is now scattered to the four winds.[4]

Not unexpectedly the Spanish authorities complained about the slanderous claims that the illness came from their shores. They vigorously argued that the disease had come to them from France, and apparently claimed that the development of the epidemic in Madrid 'coincided with the presence of a large number of visitors' (Graves 1969: 23). The possibility of the spread of the disease from the battlefields of France to the Iberian peninsula was recognised at the time and is plausible given that the armies in France were the victims of the first major outbreaks of the pandemic. Decades later some Spaniards still regard the colloquial name 'Spanish influenza' as offensive; for example, a chapter on the Spanish perspective of the pandemic started with the assertion that 'Indeed, Spanish Influenza had nothing "Spanish" about it. The names refers to the reputed origin of the pandemic of 1918–1919 and is *totally unjustified*' (Echeverri 2003: 173, my emphasis). Echeverri then contended that censorship elsewhere meant the epidemic was both censored and overshadowed by the war, a milder version of her earlier denunciation that the 'only possible explanation for this unfair imputation is that during that spring, other countries, involved in the war, didn't want it to be known that half it's army was in bed, with the flu' (Echeverri 1998: 1). However, at least one nation may have been justified in calling the malady 'Spanish': a Portuguese sanitary official claimed 'the only nation that could rightly call the pandemic "Spanish" was Portugal, as they received the infection from their neighbour' (Jorge 1919). Argentina could possibly make a similar claim as it was from there that *The Times* correspondent, in a telegraph sent from his sick bed, claimed that the 'country is paying for its carelessness in allowing the disembarcation [*sic*] from a Spanish steamer of passengers suffering from influenza' (*The Times* 1 November 1918: 7).

It is now generally agreed that Spain was not the origin of this virulent strain of influenza. While Spain was initially seen as the possible source of the disease, other locations were also suggested. These included Russia, Asia, particularly China, and the United States of America (Barry 2004; Beveridge 1977; McGinnis 1976; Marks and Beatty 1976; Pettigrew 1983; Schild 1977). This may have some support in that modern virologists regard Asia as a reservoir, with various influenza strains residing in the region's large poultry and swine populations. Their apparent close proximity to a great mass of humanity may allow for the meeting of two strains of influenza A in a single host, leading to the creation of a new strain. The attribution of an Asian origin ranges from possibly being the source of the milder first wave of the northern spring of 1918 (Beveridge 1977) and remarks that an 'influenza epidemic occurred also in Japan and China in the spring of 1918' (Marks and Beatty 1976: 271) to such sweeping statements as 'it seems probable that the infection spread from Asia to Europe' (Schild 1977: 366). There is some evidence that influenza epidemics may generally arise in Asia as 'three of the last pandemic strains of influenza have been isolated in Asia' and thus 'Southeast Asia could be regarded as a diffusion pole from which virus dispersion occurs to other areas' (Cliff *et al.* 1986: 27, 261). However, it has also been claimed that China was largely spared the 1918–19 pandemic, this claim being based on an apparent lack of evidence (Iijima 1998).[5]

It is well documented that influenza was rampant among the military forces in Europe by the middle of 1918 (Beveridge 1977; Burnet and Clark 1942; Butler 1943; Crosby 1989; Cummins 1919; McIntosh 1922; MacPherson *et al.* 1920; Ministry of Health 1920c). This has been regarded as indicating that the disease arose there among troops in France (Dowdle and LaPatra 1983; Marks and Beatty 1976). Russia, then in such turmoil, has also been named as a possible fount of the disease (Beveridge 1977: 40). However, this has been difficult to establish, due in no small part to the lack of adequate records, a problem obviously compounded by the political and social upheaval of the times.

Claims for Spanish, European or Asian origins have faded from view as support for the USA as the ultimate origin of this virus became the orthodox belief. This view suggests that the disease probably originated in the Midwest of the United States. Apparently, one of the first documented instances of influenza occurred at Fort Riley, Kansas, on 11 March 1918, with other almost simultaneous cases reported at military installations and locations in the United States (Barry 2004; Crosby 1989; Frost 1919; Stuart-Harris *et al.* 1985; Zhdanov *et al.* 1958). Burnet and Clark, in discussing the healthiness of the US military camps, noted that the autumn and winter of 1917–18 had seen 'severe outbreaks of measles with a high death rate from complicating streptococcal pneumonia' and that lobar pneumonia due to pneumococcal infection was common, but had shown no unusual features and a normal case fatality rate, although at Camp Funston (Kansas) a 'sharp epidemic of influenza commencing about March 5 was described' (Burnet and Clark 1942: 69). Thus there are documented reports of influenza among the US troops stationed in the Midwest USA early in 1918. This was followed by outbreaks of respiratory illness, particularly in eastern USA. This virus was apparently then transported by American troops to the battlefields of France from where it was to spread to the rest of the world (Barry 2004; Burnet and Clark 1942; Crosby 1989; Stuart-Harris *et al.* 1985).

Burnet and Clark postulated that an 'ancestral virus' caused the American spring epidemics and that 'in army camps and transports it found free opportunities for passage and for the development of any mutations either of virulence or antigenic character which might favour its survival' and that this process continued among the combatants in France (Burnet and Clark 1942: 70–1). This view is echoed in Paul Ewald's later suggestion that the 'environmental conditions associated with . . . trench warfare . . . could hardly have been more favorable', with crowding, the rapid addition of fresh susceptibles, the transporting of infecteds and susceptibles together, and the increased mortality in the trenches leading to the further influx of susceptibles (Ewald 1994: 110–13). Ewald argues that given conditions so favourable or so different from the norm, the virus became more virulent than normal conditions would allow. Under normal conditions, being too effective, too virulent may result in killing too many hosts too quickly and thus making the survival of the virus 'species' harder. Ewald believes that with the special conditions that existed in the trenches of France in 1918 these normal limitations were removed and as a direct consequence the virus evolved into a more virulent strain.

Certainly there is evidence that influenza was present in France as early as April 1918. A Colonel Soltau reported that 'About the middle of April the first outbreaks occurred. . . . The first outbreaks to come under my own notice occurred in the ill-famed Ypres salient, an area where disease of all sorts always seemed to flourish' (Royal Society of Medicine 1918: 27). Further localised outbreaks among British troops were recorded, and it was suggested that the troops returning to England from France in June introduced the disease to Britain (Burnet and Clark 1942: 70; Carnwath 1919). Other reports place cases among 'American troops at Brest and in a rest camp near Bordeaux. About the same time a mild epidemic occurred at Chaumont near the Swiss border involving American troops and the civilian population' (Burnet and Clark 1942: 70). General Thayer of the American Medical Corps noted that, late in April and into May, there

> appeared this sudden epidemic, possibly first at Bordeaux, then at another point on the Marne, another in the Vosges, followed rapidly by its appearance in various camps, and then by a more or less general epidemic in the region of Bordeaux. . . . The symptoms at first were very mild, so that the condition rapidly earned the name of three-days fever.
>
> (Royal Society of Medicine 1918: 28)

The Australian official history of the war recorded that 'the Chinese and Japanese delegates reported their first outbreaks in March and April of 1918' and among the British Expeditionary Force 'the pandemic appeared first in April 1918, and in May it was rampant in the British, French and German armies' (Butler 1943: III: 192).

Colonel Soltau later reported that while the disease spread during May, 'it was mild and subsided' by the end of the month. This quiescence was short-lived and from early in June 1918 the disease re-appeared, this time more widespread and virulent. The epidemic among the allied forces in France peaked in the third week of June with 'an increasing number of respiratory complications . . . [and] of the cases admitted to the special influenzal centres, some two per cent developed serious pulmonary lesions, of whom a very considerable proportion died' (Royal Society of Medicine 1918: 27). Thayer confirmed this experience among the American troops, as these later outbreaks lasted 'longer, and the complications [were] much more frequent' (Royal Society of Medicine 1918: 29). Thus the view has been that the virus was brought to France by the American troops (Barry 2004; Beveridge 1977; Burnet and Clark 1942; Carnwath 1919; Collier 1974; Crosby 1989; Ministry of Health 1920c; Royal Society of Medicine 1918; Zhdanov *et al.* 1958).[6] The argument suggests that the virus emerged in Midwest USA, possibly from a re-combination of swine flu and a human strain, before being transported to France. There it found a large supply of susceptibles who then acted as very effective vectors to re-distribute this novel virus. Alternatively, it could have been that the environment of war proved a stimulus for further evolution into a particularly virulent strain of the virus. Either way, it seems probable that the virus was re-distributed by the movement of troops, often to their home countries before further dispersal.

But is this true? How much is due to the availability of records, a consequence of the existence of American records and the absence or overlooking of records elsewhere? While the theory of an American origin is more plausible than 'Spanish flu', it may not be the full story. Evidence has now been (re)discovered that questions this assumption of a new strain which may have emerged from American swine early in 1918 (Oxford *et al.* 1999, 2001, 2002). Some of this evidence actually comes from those sources that have been used to support the theory of an American origin, and has been overlooked or disregarded. For example, in the 1943 *Official History of the Australian Army Medical Services, 1914–18* it was noted that a number of hypotheses had been advanced as to the 'genesis of the epidemic' and that these had included it being the 'result of a pandemic "constitution"', that it had come '(i) from east (China) to west, (ii) from west (Spain or America) to east', that it was an 'epidemic exacerbation of the endemic disease' or that it was 'a development from the local epidemics of "purulent bronchitis" in Europe and epidemic empyema in the camps of the U.S.A.' (Butler 1943: III: 194).

This was a pandemic in the strictest sense of the word – spanning the entire globe in a short space of time. A short period from late September 1918 to November 1918 saw the death of the US Army private, Private Vaughan, in South Carolina[7] and the deaths of another soldier at Camp Upton in the USA, of 'Lucy' at Brevig Mission, Alaska[8] and of six Norwegian coal miners in Longyearbyen, Spitzbergen.[9] This same period (as early as September 1918) also saw reports of influenza deaths in countries as widely spread as Norway, Sweden, Finland, Canada, Spain, Britain, France, Germany, Senegal, Tanzania, Nigeria, Ghana, Zimbabwe, South Africa, India and Indonesia (Åman, 1990; Brown 1987; Crosby 1989; Echenberg 1998, 1993; Echeverri Dávila 1993; Echeverri 2003; Ellison 2003; Johnson 1993, 1998; Linnanmäki 1998; Mamelund 1998a, 1998b; Mills 1986; Musambachime 1998; Ohadike 1981; Patterson 1983; Phillips 1990a; Registrar General 1920; Witte 1998). The geographical extent of these deaths suggests that the disease had spread around the globe prior to this time, suggesting that 'seeding' of the pandemic had occurred. The earlier wave, in the northern summer, had been as widely distributed, even if less pronounced.

The fact that what had been termed 'purulent bronchitis' had been prevalent among troops in Britain and France in 1917 became evident at the Royal Society of Medicine's 'Discussion' on influenza, held in London on 13 and 14 November, 1918. At this gathering a number of speakers recounted their experiences, including Professor John Eyre, Major Adolphe Abrahams, RAMC, and Major T.A. Malloch, Canadian Army Medical Corps, who said that the morbid anatomy and histology of the lungs of 1917 'purulent bronchitis' cases were very similar to the more recent influenza cases (Royal Society of Medicine 1918: 45–50, 93, 97–102). Dr R.G. Abercrombie noted that:

> Early in 1917 I had under my care in France a large number of soldiers suffering from a grave form of purulent bronchitis, proceeding in some cases to broncho-pneumonia. The cases exhibited dyspnoea, a heliotrope cyanosis, purulent nummular expectoration, pyrexia, and a high mortality; delirium was not a marked feature. Healthy young soldiers were usually attacked; in a few cases the condition occurred in association with acute nephritis. In about one-third of the cases broncho-pneumonic consolidation was recognizable either by clinical or post-mortem examination.
>
> (Royal Society of Medicine 1918: 91)[10]

These outbreaks displayed the same precise clinical and physiological descriptions as the influenza deaths of 1918–19.

These testimonies echoed a number of medical papers that had reported the 'purulent bronchitis' (Abrahams *et al.* 1917, 1919; Hammond *et al.* 1917). These early reports are now known to have come from the vast British military camp at Etaples, on the coast south of Boulogne in France (Oxford *et al.* 1999, 2002). This camp, with its hospitals, piggeries, poultry (Oxford 2001) and all the other logistical support war necessitates, held as many as 100,000 soldiers at any time with in excess of a million soldiers passing through between Britain and the Western Front in 1916–18. Hammond *et al.* (1917) described an outbreak of 'purulent bronchitis' in 1916 which was 'characterised clinically by heliotrope cyanosis' and a clinical microbiological review of the outbreak considers this to be classic influenza, and as 'being essentially similar to the extensive documentation of deaths in 1918–1919' (Oxford *et al.* 2002: 112). Abrahams *et al.* (1917, 1919) reported an essentially identical epidemic of purulent bronchitis with the same 'peculiar dusky heliotrope cyanosis' (Abrahams *et al.* 1917: 377) and high mortality occurring at Aldershot barracks in March 1917. The Ministry of Health's 1920 report into the pandemic noted that, in addition to the cases among the military in France, 'there appear to have been some small outbreaks of a similar illness in 1916 and 1917 among the civil population' (Ministry of Health 1920c: 225). Interestingly, Burnet and Clark noted these early cases, but subsequently these reports seem to have been neglected. This is curious as Burnet and Clark set out the connection quite clearly in writing:

> In France there was a good deal of serious respiratory infection amongst British troops in the winter 1916–17. This took the form of 'purulent bronchitis' and was chiefly interesting in that the severe cases showed the clinical picture of heliotrope cyanosis so characteristic of the pandemic cases in autumn 1918.
>
> (Burnet and Clark 1942: 70)

McIntosh also noted these earlier outbreaks in a 1922 MRC report, in which he raised doubts about the alleged Spanish origin of the pandemic as

> The exact place and date when the epidemic first appeared is very indefinite. The Spanish origin of the outbreak is doubtful, although a large epidemic did occur in that country in the early spring of 1918. But an examination of the literature shows that local epidemics of apparently typical influenza were occurring in the British Army at home and in France even earlier than this, i.e. during the winter of 1916–17.
>
> (McIntosh 1922: 6)

Thus, it appears that the form of the virus that caused so much illness and so many deaths in 1918 and 1919 was already present among the British forces in 1917. Work by Taubenberger and Reid and their group suggests that the pandemic strain may have arisen as early as 1915.[11]

Further evidence suggesting that this form of influenza was present prior to 1918 includes circumstantial evidence such as the biographies of military and civilian medical staff and official reports. A number of these simply provide further confirmation of the situation in France. One example comes from the memoirs of Harvey Cushing, then a US forces surgeon, who made these entries in his diary:[12]

> Thursday Oct. 18 [1917]
> 2 a.m. En route, Camiers. The man next me has awakened and sneezed. So have I. . . . All the world has a coryza – in Mendinghem, in Hesdin, in Paris.

> January 28th, 1918. Boulogne
> I saw Jack McCrae . . . last night – the last time. . . . A soldier from top to toe – how he would have hated to die in bed. A three days' illness.
>
> (Cushing 1936: 228, 280)

But deaths from this form of influenza before 1918 were not restricted to the military populations in Britain and France. The MOH for London County Council observed that influenza (and bronchitis) deaths increased in December 1917 in London. He went on to write in an appendix to his 1918 annual report:

> Suspicion that something new and special in the behaviour of influenza . . . had . . . been . . . aroused in December, 1917, on the occurrence of a sudden fatal illness in a reformatory school boy. The death was attributed to 'congestion of the lungs,' and it took place just prior to the time when the general death rate in London showed its first distinct rise. Four further deaths occurred at intervals of some weeks, among boys from this same school; one on the 28th January, registered as due to 'apical pneumonia,' one on the 23rd February, due to 'phthisis,' one on the 12th April, attributable to cerebrospinal meningitis, and one on the 11th July, which was registered as 'influenza'. . . . These deaths must be regarded with great suspicion.
>
> (Hamer 1918: 2)

There are further indications that influenza was being reported elsewhere earlier than has been generally recognised. Admittedly some of these reports give little indication of the symptoms of the disease, and could thus have been of 'normal' influenza. Finland, for example, saw few influenza deaths reported in 1917, but did record an elevated level of pneumonia deaths, and the Medical Officers in Viipuri and Rauma both reported high levels of influenza in their towns (Linnanmäki 1999). Other examples include India where there are reports of 'the existence of influenza cases in various jails in the [Bombay] Presidency during 1917' (Mills 1986: 4) and Germany where it has been claimed that influenza may have been present as early as 1916 (Witte 1998: 1, citing Levinthal *et al.* 1921). The British Ministry of Health was aware of activity prior to 1918 in Germany, for example, 'in a recent report of the Bochum Administration of Sick Insurance it is mentioned that in that area during 1915 there were 9,117 cases of influenza, and that in 1916 the number rose to 12,788' (Ministry of Health 1920c: 267). The United States was also known to have significant influenza activity prior to 1918, including a 'prevalence of a disease, clinically identical with epidemic influenza, which extended practically to all parts of the States' towards the end of 1915. This outbreak was regarded as 'noteworthy' as the 'spread of the disease was so rapid that much difficulty was found in carrying on business, owing to the simultaneous attack of so many persons' and that the 'account of the 1915–16 outbreak reads very much like that of the 1918 epidemic' (Ministry of Health 1920c: 281).

From these various strands of evidence it appears justifiable to claim that the pandemic virus actually emerged sometime before 1918. Just when and where it emerged it is not possible to say, and it may never be known. While many now agree that the pandemic virus of 1918 should not be called the 'Spanish flu' or the 'Spanish Lady' (Crosby 1989; Shortridge 1999), what should it be called? Shortridge suggests the 'Chinese Lady' due to the apparent proclivity of influenza for China. More recent work suggests other designations, asking the question, 'Who's that lady?' (Oxford *et al.* 1999). Based on what may be the earliest clinical and pathological descriptions of the pandemic strain, some contend that the virus could be designated, using modern influenza nomenclature, as A/Etaples/1/1916 or A/Aldershot/1/1917; thus transforming the 'Spanish Lady' into either the 'French Lady' or the 'English Lady' (Oxford *et al.* 1999: 1352).

Accepting an origin prior to 1918, possibly even some years earlier, means the spread of the disease does not have to be quite as rapid as previously supposed. Rather this scenario allows for the 'seeding' of the virus around the world in the intervening period. Thus the earlier reports of influenza cases could represent the 'herald wave' of the pandemic (Glezen *et al.* 1982), and it has been argued that 'all known . . . pandemics [have] been preceded by a number of smaller, localized flu outbreaks, a process known as "seeding" the virus in the population' (Dutton 1988: 130). The preceding discussion provides some evidence for such seeding of the 1918–19 pandemic. Further evidence comes from Norwegian data,[13] where the age distribution of mortality suggests that the upturn in influenza activity in 1915 and 1916 was associated with an unusual level of mortality among young adults – a feature that was to be so characteristic of the 1918–19 pandemic itself (Johnson 2001: 123). This upturn in influenza activity prior to 1918 is also frequently seen when influenza and/or pneumonia mortality are plotted, for example, for England and Wales, Scotland, Sweden, Denmark, Norway, Dublin, New York, Chicago, and the District of Columbia (Washington, D.C.) (Johnson 2001: 120–1).

Influenza is generally a seasonal disease, tending to be associated with the cooler months. However, in pandemics this seasonality may disappear. The 1918–19 pandemic is recognised as having generally taken place in three waves, starting in the northern spring and summer of 1918 (May–July). This relatively mild wave attracted minimal attention. The searing wave, the second wave, burnt its way around the globe in the northern autumn (October–December) and was followed by another less severe wave early in 1919. The three waves of pandemic influenza circumnavigated the globe in a little less than a year. It came upon the British in these three waves, bringing massive morbidity and mortality, disrupting normal life and carrying away many, especially young adults. This wave pattern is readily apparent when influenza mortality is plotted (Figure 3.1). It was the second wave that was most deadly, and in the UK 64 per cent of recorded influenza deaths

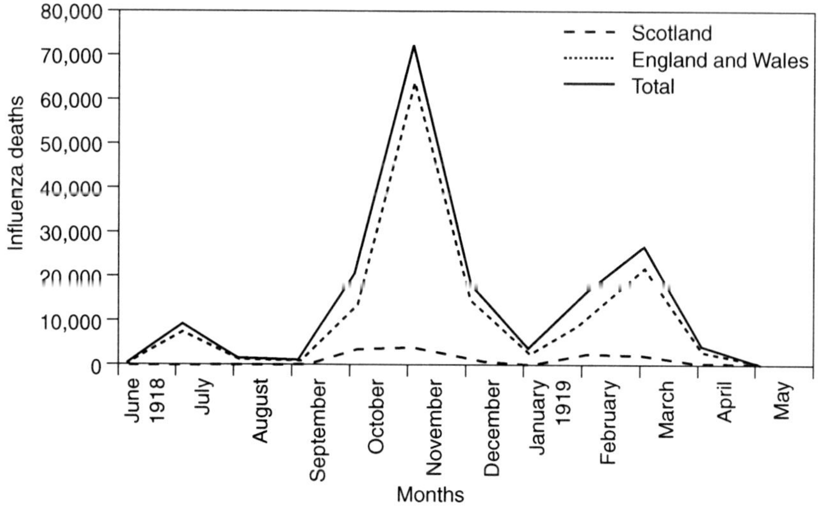

Figure 3.1 Monthly influenza deaths in Scotland, England and Wales, 1918–19 (sources: Registrar-General 1920; Registrar-General for Scotland 1919).

came in the second wave; 10 per cent in the first and 26 per cent in the last. This pattern of three waves with the bulk of mortality occurring in the second is all but universal. This timing and pattern hold true across almost every country in every continent, except Australia where maritime quarantine delayed widespread infection until early 1919. Neutral and belligerent nations, colonial powers and colonised lands, rich and poor nations, all shared a similar experience.

Each wave of the pandemic rarely lasted longer than a few weeks. The epidemic curves confirm this as an infectious disease with a short incubation period and of short duration, with the sharp rise in mortality maintained for a period of weeks before dropping away almost as rapidly as it rose. Different diseases produce different shapes in their epidemic curves. The curves are a function of factors such as incubation period, virulence and infectivity and there is a 'general tendency for propagative epidemics to be "right-skew", i.e. for the initial rise in incidence to be more rapid than the subsequent fall' (Fine 1982: 47), and this pattern is apparent in the mortality curves for this pandemic.[14] While this pattern of three waves is consistent, there were some locations that had a slightly different experience. For example, Australia, due to the partial success of maritime quarantine, experienced a single longer wave of influenza activity rather than the three sharp waves seen in most locations (McCracken and Curson 2003; McQueen 1976; New South Wales 1920; Rice 1989). While the Australian curve shows three peaks, it is notable that in between those peaks the level of mortality did not subside as it did in most locations. For most countries the waves were quite distinct and short-lived.

In some locations influenza seems to have persisted into or returned in 1920, most notably in Scandinavia. For example, this is apparent in the age structure of influenza mortality in Norway. Some regard this as a 'fourth wave', though this is not a consistent feature and it is debatable whether this should be considered a fourth wave of the pandemic or a new epidemic, possibly associated with a different strain of the virus (Åman 1990; Echeverri Dávila 1993: 64–5; Iijima 1998; Linnanmäki 1998; Mamelund 1998b; Ministry of Health 1920c; Pettit 1976). What is certain is that, by 1922, influenza mortality had reverted to a more common pattern of killing those at the extremes of age rather than young adults. England and Wales had a similar experience (for more details on age mortality, refer to Chapter 4) and, prior to 1918, influenza mortality was predominantly in the under fives and the older age groups. The change between 1917 and 1918 is remarkable, with mortality concentrated in the young adult age groups, continuing into 1919. However, 1920 shows a more mixed pattern at a much lower level of mortality. Burnet and Clark noted that 'age incidence of deaths returned fairly steadily toward the normal, but . . . it was not until 1929 that the pre-pandemic age incidence was regained' (Burnet and Clark 1942: 77).

'Cheerfully anticipated its arrival'

Infectious disease diffusion nearly always contains a component of contagious diffusion. Contagious diffusion requires close or direct contact for transmission and the spread of disease 'takes place in a centrifugal manner from the source location(s) outwards in a pattern which emphasizes the importance of proximity and interaction between actual adopters (acceptors, infectors, etc.) and potential adopters' (Goodall 1987: 126). Furthermore, contagious diffusion is an expansionary process and is strongly influenced by the 'frictional effect of distance' (Abler *et al.* 1971: 391). The 'neighbourhood effect' is very important in such diffusion, signifying the greater likelihood of spreading disease to someone or somewhere nearby than to a remote location. The pattern of diffusion is determined by the networks that encourage it and the barriers that modify that movement. For disease diffusion, factors including incubation period and infectivity are also of great importance. Diffusion of disease is considered a stochastic process and this has led to the development of models of diffusion that allow us to simulate the course of an epidemic. However, to produce such models it is necessary to have data that meet certain criteria. These include information such as disease origins, vectors, transmission rates, infectivity, population thresholds, the mechanism of spread and the probability of contact. Riordan claimed that the 'paucity of influenza research in geography' was a consequence of the disease's epidemiological characteristics, its unclear diagnosis and lack of predictable periodicity (Riordan 1986: 66). This position has changed slightly since, with the application of various forms of modelling. Forms of mathematical/geographical models that have been proposed or used for examining influenza at various scales include mass-action models, chain-binomial models, family models, large population models and the excess mortality models, but such modelling is beyond the scope of this work. However, the use of the pandemic as a worst case study could be an effective way of testing such models.[15]

Determining the spread of the pandemic is complicated if the origin is obscured. Until recently much of the literature has referred to an American origin preceding transportation of the virus to France where it apparently circulated among the warring armies and from there it was distributed throughout the world. Burnet and Clark, in supporting the idea of an American origin, wrote of a

> continuity of camp and civilian epidemics in United States in February and March, of very heavy troop movements from America to Europe at this time, of the appearance of the influenza amongst American troops at Brest and Bordeaux in April and later amongst the various armies in France. In Paris an epidemic of similar character to that of the first wave in England [May–June 1918] began at the end of April and almost simultaneously Italy experienced a similar epidemic. During May Spain, Portugal and Greece were involved, England and Switzerland toward the end of June, Germany, Denmark and Norway in July, Holland and Sweden in August.
>
> (Burnet and Clark 1942: 70)

Wherever the disease actually emerged, and whether or not it was seeded around the world in the years preceding this widespread outbreak, it is without doubt that by 1918 it was distributed throughout the globe. Following the first wave of the pandemic there was a period of quiescence. But the quiet was short-lived, as what Crosby has termed 'three explosions' of influenza in Boston, Brest and Freetown in August 1918 marked the beginning of the largest single wave of influenza morbidity and mortality in recorded history (Burnet and Clark 1942; Crosby 1989: 37). This wave flooded the world with an extremely virulent form of influenza. In the vast majority of countries the pandemic peaked in October and/or November 1918. It is the spread of the second wave that we can plot with greater certainty. Whereas the first wave is difficult to map due to the lack of awareness and a lack of reliable material, the second wave can be more accurately determined. Thus, mapping of the spread of influenza at this time can be accorded greater credence (Figures 3.2 and 3.3).

Human agency largely determined the spread of the pandemic. Once this new virus had launched itself, 'spread occurred to the rest of the world, and there can be little doubt that extension to the rest of Europe (excluding Russia), America, Australia and New Zealand was by human transport from the primary European–American centre' (Burnet and Clark 1942: 71). In Africa the disease spread out from Sierra Leone or by re-location, often by

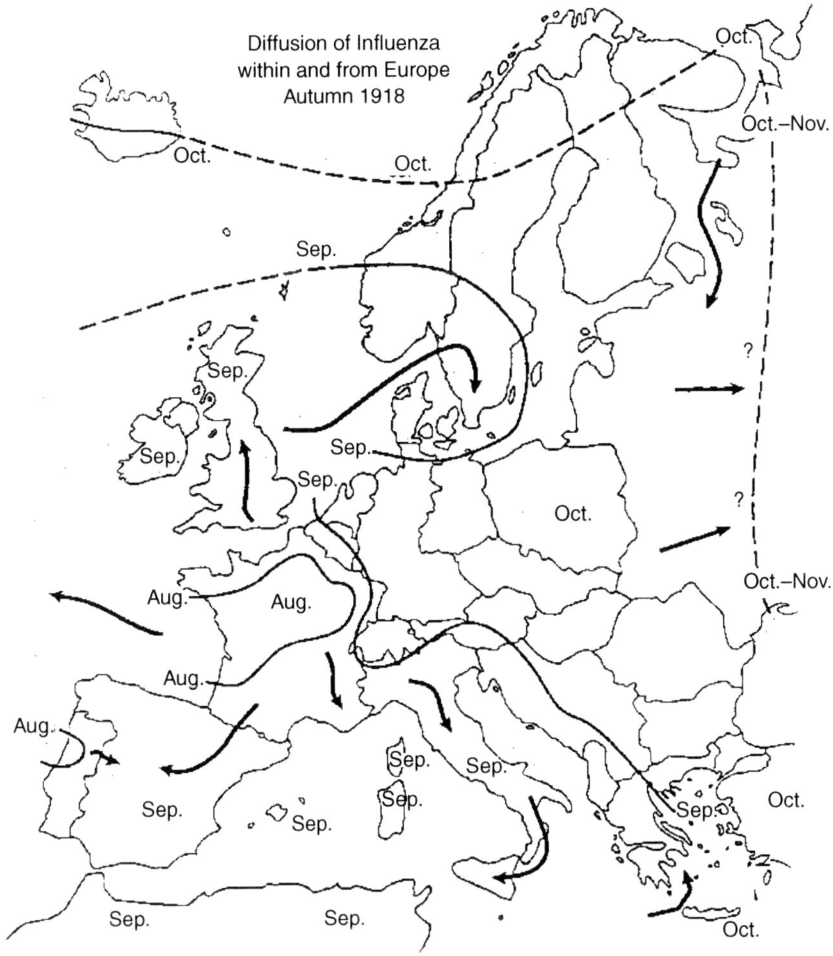

Figure 3.2 World-wide diffusion of influenza – second wave (source: Patterson and Pyle 1991: 12. Image reproduced courtesy of G.F. Pyle and Johns Hopkins University Press).

ship, into each country or region. War, and the use of native porters, was critical to the spread of flu in Africa (Cole 1994; Echenberg 1993, 1998; Ellison 2003; Killingray 1996; Mueller 1995; Musambachime 1998; Ohadike 1991; Page 1998; Phillips 1990a; Tomkins 1994). Spread of the disease through Asia and the Pacific was also greatly facilitated by human transport networks. For example, the introduction of the disease to New Zealand before being re-exported to large parts of the South Pacific has been demonstrated to the extent of being able to name the specific ships that introduced their lethal cargo.[16]

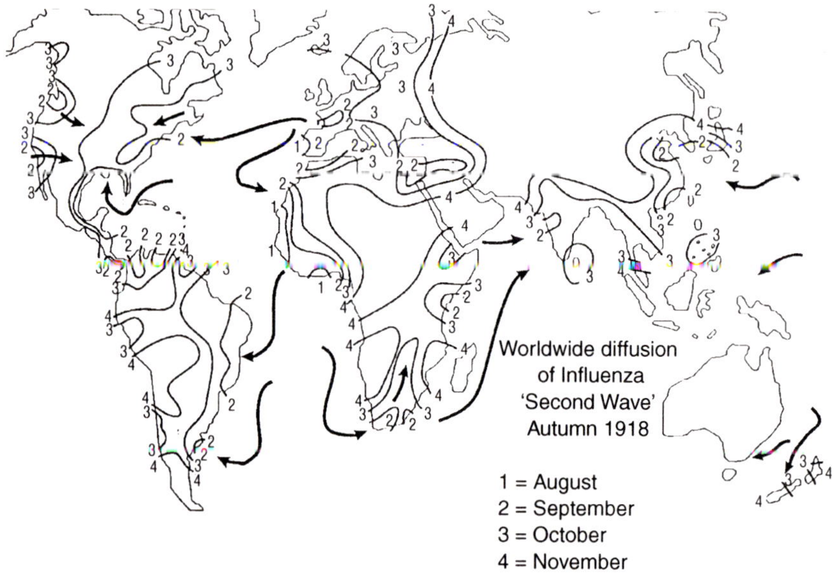

Figure 3.3 Diffusion of influenza into and from Europe – second wave (source: Patterson and Pyle 1991: 9. Image reproduced courtesy of G.F. Pyle and Johns Hopkins University Press).

The transport networks moving infective people are logically the most important and most visible of the linkages. Various forms of transport were of critical importance in the spread of the pandemic, the mechanisms by which lines of quarantine were crossed. Shipping was the most significant method for moving the disease between nations and, obviously, continents, with railways significant at the continental and national levels. While the causal organism of influenza was not to be found for some years, it was recognised that influenza was a disease that travelled with people. A letter to the Editor from a Clifford Allbutt of St Radegund's, Cambridge published in *The Times*, included a postscript that read 'During the influenza of 1891–1892 I studied with some care the records, so far as they existed, of the previous epidemics and came to the opinion that they ran on the lines of travellers' (31 October 1918: 7).

By far the most important form of transport in bringing the disease to further continents and countries was shipping. Ships, especially troopships, brought the disease into many countries. From the port cities the disease was moved throughout the continent or nation on the local transport networks, often the railways. The actions of the South African, Australian and New Zealand governments discussed elsewhere indicate how important they regarded shipping as the vector (using the term in a rather loose, non-technical sense) by which the disease was moved across much of the world. In work on

New Zealand, the *S.S. Talune* is seen as a 'death' ship delivering the pandemic to a series of south Pacific islands (Crosby 1989; Edwards 1986; Rice 1988). Elsewhere there are other cases where specific ships have been identified as the likely carrier of first infections. These include the cases of Iceland where three trawlers were linked to the initial introduction of the disease (Cliff *et al.* 1986: 147–9), Argentina where a Spanish steamer apparently disembarked stricken passengers into Buenos Aires (*The Times* 1 November 1918: 1), and Canada where the troopship *Araguayan* and the hospital ship *Med 1099*, along with the ships *Somali* and *Nagoya*, have been identified as being the first ships to bring influenza into Canada (Heagerty 1928: 215; Johnson 1998: 89–90). There are many other instances were shipping is considered the likely (even only) means by which the disease could have arrived, but where no individual ship has been or can be identified, including India, Mauritius, Indonesia, and much of west Africa (Brown 1987; Echenberg 1993, 1998; Fokeer 1921; Gill 1928: 252, 289; Mueller 1995: 2, 10).

Railways and, to a lesser extent, road networks played an extremely significant role in the dissemination of influenza at continental and national levels. Local transport systems spread the disease around individual cities and towns as well as providing increased opportunities for infection as people crowded onto the commuter routes; for example, reports of overcrowding appear in *The Times* during the period. In many localities where various forms of social and public activity had been suspended the public transport systems still worked and people still had to go to and from their daily activities. The importance of these transport networks at the national scale is widely recognised; for example, it was noted that once temporary workers from Portugal and Spain travelling between their homes and their work in France (where they were replacing enlisted workers) brought the disease across the border, the railways distributed it throughout the Iberian peninsula (Echeverri 2003). Similar accounts indicating the importance of railways and other transport networks in moving the virus down through the urban hierarchies exist for many countries, including Canada (Andrews 1977; Johnson 1993; McGinnis 1977; Pettigrew 1983), Norway (Mamelund 1998b), South Africa (Phillips 1990a) and Korea, where one observer attributed the transportation of the virus into Seoul to the Southern Manchurian Railway after the disease had arrived in the north from Europe, via Siberia.[17] In Britain, the crowded trains were recognised as being a problem and the Essex MOH, a Dr Thresh, attributed

> the spread of the disease along the lines of railway from London to Southend, Epping, Waltham, Colchester and Cambridge to overcrowding in railway carriages, and . . . while this continues it is useless to ask people not to attend churches, cinemas, and meetings where they do not get half so much crowded together as on the railway.
>
> (*The Times* 26 October 1918: 7)

The Ministry of Health later came to the similar conclusion 'that the overcrowding of trains and trams in 1918 helped the spread of the epidemic' (*The Times* 27 December 1919: 7). At the LGB Newsholme had also realised this as the

> crowded trains, trams, and omnibuses . . . doubtless, are prolific sources of infection, but the service cannot immediately be increased, and meanwhile the vast army of workers must not be impeded by regulations as to overcrowding of vehicles in their efforts to go to work and to return home.
> (Royal Society of Medicine 1918: 13)

The country had to 'carry on', the war effort had to be maintained at all costs. There was no consideration of possibly 'staggering' working hours to reduce congestion, an idea considered in Australia after hearing that it had been introduced in the American cities of New York, Chicago, Denver, Cleveland, Camden and Washington (NAA A2 1919/1328).[18]

The role of human transportation networks was not always seen as the critical element in the spread of influenza. Factors that were suggested included climate or weather, altitude, race and urbanisation. Gill's 1928 discussion of the epidemic, particularly in India, strenuously argues that climatic conditions were important in aiding or hindering the development of any epidemic, almost to the exclusion of other factors. Even when discussing the role of altitude, it was restricted to how altitude modified climate. His was a very environmentally deterministic view. Another noted environmental determinist, Ellsworth Huntington, also saw climate playing a major role in the spread of the disease in America (Huntington 1923), and such views were repeated in the press. For example, *The Times* employed various aspects of the weather to account for the flu: June 1918 saw it claiming that 'drought and high winds, which fill that air with microbe-laden dust' were spreading the disease in Spain (25 June 1918: 9); a December 1918 story was headlined 'New influenza "wave": effect of weather on disease', claiming that an apparent increase in flu deaths was linked to changes in the weather. While this resembles a re-stating of the older Italian concept of *influenza di freddo* (influence of the cold or cold wind), the paper's medical correspondent did rather hedge his bets:

> The increase, curiously enough, began just after the wind veered from east to west, and hot, damp weather succeeded to the cold, dry spell during which the disease had markedly declined. Too little is known about the relationship of weather to this disease to permit of any inference being drawn, but probably the effect, if effect there be, is on the individual rather than on the germ. In hot, damp weather, perhaps, the resisting power of the individual is lowered, he becomes depressed, and less well able to ward off the danger threatening him.
> (*The Times* 3 December 1918: 5)

Blaming the changes in the weather was again apparent at end of January, when the 'fresh wave of the influenza epidemic . . . corresponds . . . with a notable break in the weather' (31 January 1919: 5). But by February 1919 it was back to the cold weather, with the 'slush and snow always seeming to favour the spread of influenza' (19 February 1919: 8).

Whatever the weather, the impact of the pandemic was certainly felt all throughout Britain as the disease reached all parts (Plate 2); as the RG for Scotland commented, 'the most outstanding feature of the distribution of the mortality . . . is its universality' (Registrar-General for Scotland 1919: 5). Irrespective of the ultimate source of the virus strain, it is certainly true that major outbreaks occurred among the armies in France and among US troops in transit and at home early in 1918. Undoubtedly some of the first Britons to suffer from the 'new' influenza were those in the armed forces, both home and abroad. An MRC report later claimed that in May 1918 'there was a severe outbreak in the Grand Fleet . . . when about one-ninth of the total strength was affected.' This was shortly followed by the 'first large epidemic in the British Army [when] some 226,615 cases were reported' in May, June and July. Towards the end of this period the disease started to appear among the civilian population, 'although localized outbreaks were noted in May' (McIntosh 1922: 6–7). Thus, sometime in the first half of 1918, influenza was brought into Britain, probably by servicemen travelling through the ports, and probably through many ports more-or-less simultaneously.[19] Glasgow, Portsmouth, Southampton and Liverpool were all suggested as likely ports of entry as they apparently reported influenza cases (and deaths) earlier than many other centres. It is interesting that London, itself an important port, does not figure prominently early in the epidemic. *The Times* reported that the Navy's Grand Fleet had experienced cases at Scapa and Rosyth in April (raising doubts over McIntosh's later claim), and suggest that Glasgow was 'the seat of the first outbreak among the civil population – and that occurred in May, 1918' (15 January 1920: 9).[20] The RG recognised the 'association of the early stages of the second wave with ports . . . [was] . . . as well marked in the North as in the South', suggesting that the ports served as early foci in at least the first and second waves of the pandemic (Registrar-General 1920: 19).

It is difficult to confirm the early pattern of introduction and spread in Britain as the number of cases was presumably quite small and attracted little attention. Deaths occurring at this time may well not have been recorded as influenza deaths and it would have only been when the number of deaths started increasing that attention was drawn to the disease. Certainly *The Times* portrays a country hardly cowering before this threat, as

> Everybody thinks of it as the "Spanish" influenza to-day. The man in the street, having been taught by that *plagosus orbilius*, war, to take a keener interest in foreign affairs, discussed the news of the epidemic which

spread with such surprising rapidity through Spain a few weeks ago, and cheerfully anticipated its arrival here.

(25 June 1918)

The RG retrospectively dated the start of the pandemic in England and Wales to the week ending 29 June 1918, with its marked increase in influenza deaths, most of which came in the younger age groups, but certainly cases were being reported prior to this date. However, the start of the pandemic in England and Wales could possibly be dated from about 19 May 1918. That week saw 511 deaths attributed to influenza, whereas the previous week had recorded seventy-nine influenza deaths. Furthermore, prior to that date, influenza deaths at ages over fifty-five exceeded those under fifty-five. From 19 May to 15 June, deaths above and below age fifty-five were about equal; from the week ending 22 June, the younger ages showed more deaths.

Hierarchies and contagion

Research into influenza diffusion suggests that there may be two components to the spread of influenza: a hierarchical component and a contagious component (Cliff *et al.* 1981, 1986; Patterson and Pyle 1983; Pyle 1986; Selby 1982). For example, the Canadian experience of the 1918 pandemic saw the disease first percolate down the urban hierarchy before contagious diffusion assumed greater importance at the city or neighbourhood level (Johnson 1993). The first, hierarchical, relocation is responsible for the dispersal of the disease across the country, while the second, contagious diffusion, sees the illness spread throughout neighbourhoods, towns and cities.

Hierarchical diffusion is generally based on the premise that everywhere is equally vulnerable but those urban centres at the top of the hierarchy are the first to come into contact with the disease for various reasons. It has been argued that it is the relative location in the social and political hierarchy, and not just geographic location, that may be more important (Sattenspiel and Herring 2000). In this case the initial points of contact were the ports through which infected people were returning to or entering the country. From the ports the transport networks relocated the disease to the top of the urban hierarchy, then the transport networks distributed it progressively down the urban hierarchy. The UK being a more compact nation than many others, this process was likely to take less time than that experienced in a number of countries where the role of the transport networks in spreading the disease has been noted.[21] Being a more compact nation with a greater homogeneity of contact with, and access to, the upper tiers of the urban hierarchy may also help to explain why variations in the mortality across Britain were smaller – the mortality pattern was more homogeneous than in some other nations (Plate 2).

Britain's urban hierarchy was well-established by the time of the pandemic, Law argued that the 'rapid and large scale urbanization [was] ... nearly complete by the First World War', by 1911 the population of England and Wales was 78.9 per cent urbanised (Law 1967). Furthermore, the vital statistics registration system reflected this urban pattern with their new boundaries. The *ARRG* and the Census of 1911 both noted the change in reporting areas; the RG changing from registration districts to the new administrative areas. Bernard Mallett, the RG at the time, argued that the new areal classification of RDs, UDs, CBs and the London boroughs not only separated urban and rural more accurately, but also distinguished three different forms of the urban (*ARRG* 1911: Preface).[22]

In Britain the disease entered via certain ports before relocating to the upper levels of the urban hierarchy, then percolating down that hierarchy via the transport networks to the cities, towns and villages where contagious diffusion, the person-to-person transmission, spread the disease at the local level. This is reflected in the contemporary reports. A December 1918 report in *The Times*, for example, stated that:

> the ports were first involved. ... Next the disease reached London, to which no doubt it was brought by travellers in the through trains. From London it radiated again, visiting Birmingham, Nottingham, and other centres. It is still raging at full fury in the smaller country districts which have now become involved.
>
> (18 December 1918: 5)

This pattern of some ports first, London next and then descending down the urban hierarchy can be seen in Figure 3.4, showing the epidemic curves for a number of cities. It is clear that certain ports, here represented by Portsmouth and Liverpool, saw mortality peak earlier than London with smaller and/or more distant centres showing the later peaks (examples included here are Birmingham, Bradford, Manchester and Nottingham). Notably this pattern was not apparent in the third wave.

Examining the spread of the disease by mapping the mortality recorded in each week (Johnson 2001), it is apparent how little influenza activity there actually was in most weeks of the pandemic period. The peaks of mortality were all relatively short-lived. This pattern of 'one or two weeks of rapid spread followed by two or three weeks of high morbidity and mortality, whereafter the epidemic rapidly subsided' was by no means unique to Britain (Galishoff 1969: 249). These patterns confirm what the RG concluded from the mortality data, in that the first and third waves were slightly stronger in the north, as was the pandemic overall, while the south, particularly London, saw greater mortality in the second wave (Table 3.1).

The disease spread across the country rapidly, with some northern centres reporting high mortality quite early, as the RG noted: 'The North ... suffered most at the commencement, as it did also throughout the whole course of the first wave' (Registrar-General 1920: 12). However, the activity of the

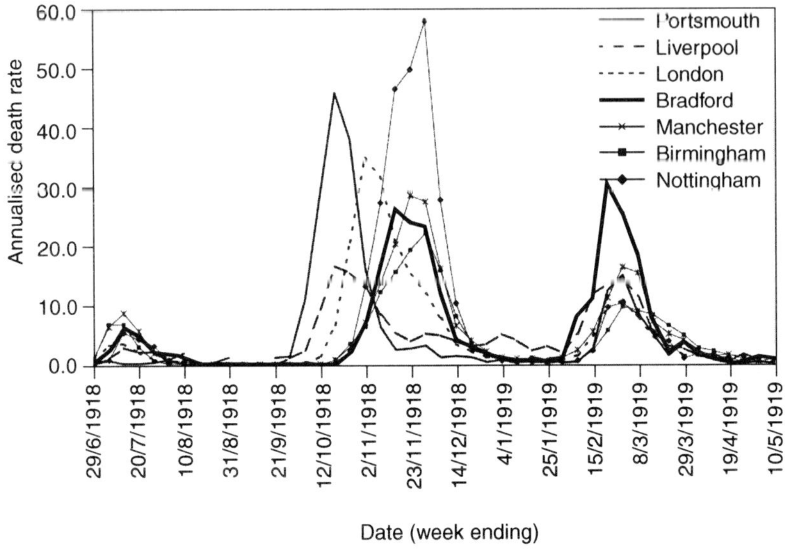

Figure 3.4 Influenza mortality in selected cities, 1918–19 (source: Registrar-General 1920).

Table 3.1 Regional mortality variation

Location	*Influenza death rate (annualised)*			
	Pandemic	*1st wave*	*2nd wave*	*3rd wave*
London	4.9	1.1	8.6	3.3
North				
CBs	5.3	2.0	7.6	5.1
All areas	5.4	2.0	7.8	5.0
Midlands				
CBs	5.1	1.5	8.6	3.6
All areas	4.9	1.1	8.6	3.3
South				
CBs	4.3	0.7	7.3	3.4
All areas (including London)	4.4	0.8	7.6	3.1
Wales				
CBs	4.1	1.3	6.1	3.7
All areas	4.3	1.5	6.6	3.5
England & Wales (all)	4.9	1.4	7.9	3.8

Data source: Registrar-General 1920: 24, Table IX. Influenza: Annual Mortality per 1,000 living in various parts of the country during each wave of the epidemic.

first wave never reached particularly high mortality levels. The week ending 19 October 1918 saw the heightened influenza activity in London, the north-west and some Midlands centres that marked the upswing at the start of the second wave of mortality. By the following week, ending 26 October, the north-west, London, Midlands, south coast and north Wales were all involved. By the end of the following week, great swathes of the country exhibited high levels of mortality, including those areas adjacent to the areas active the previous week as the disease continued to diffuse out from the major centres. The following week, ending 9 November, the disease had brought elevated mortality to all parts, but with higher levels in a belt running north-west from London and the south-east through the Midlands to the north-west (Plate 3). This was the week of peak mortality for England and Wales as a whole, and the widespread nature of the elevated mortality underlines this.

The RG claimed the 'tripartite division of England . . . proves . . . to be inappropriate . . . and a simple partition into North and South would have corresponded better with events', and that the Midlands tended to split into either a north or south pattern (Registrar-General 1920: 20). However, the mortality seen in the week ending 9 November 1918 and the total pandemic mortality (Plate 2) suggest not so much a north–south pattern as one that may follow the busier lines of communication and links along the urban hierarchies as the south-east and London connect with the Midlands and the north-west, while the less well-connected areas, such as the south-west and East Anglia, experienced the pandemic later and at lower overall levels. This is a finding that concords with the argument that connectivity and place in the social/national hierarchy are important determinants of influenza activity (Mamelund 1998b).

The second wave of the pandemic subsided in the week ending 16 November with only parts of the Midlands, Wales, Yorkshire and the north-east showing higher mortality. Again, these could be seen as being further along the lines of communication and further down the urban hierarchy, so experiencing the peaks of mortality slightly later. This argument is then supported by the more peripheral areas, such as the north-east, Scottish border areas and Wales reporting influenza mortality as the second wave petered out in the weeks ending 23 and 30 November and 7 December.

The third wave exhibited even lower levels of activity than the first, only bringing elevated levels of mortality in some northern areas in the week ending 22 February 1919. The following two weeks (ending 1 and 8 March) saw an increase in activity in the north-west and parts of the Midlands which then becomes restricted to the Midlands.

London

The passage of influenza mortality in London also supports the hypothesis of two stages in the spread of influenza: following the introduction or relocation of the disease into a location, contagious diffusion then assumes a greater role. The first London boroughs to display increases in mortality were those that host the capital's docks and/or major railway termini. For example, in the week ending 19 October 1918, there was a rise in mortality apparent in Woolwich (a borough east of the city bounded by the Thames with a significant proportion of the workforce employed in and around dockyards, as indicated by the 1911 Census) and in the City of London, St Pancras (including many of the major railway stations) and Battersea. From these boroughs, the flu radiated out in the following week, intensifying in Woolwich and St Pancras and spreading from the four boroughs into the neighbouring areas, including Islington, Stoke Newington, Hackney, Bethnal Green, Poplar and Greenwich.

The week ending 2 November 1918 saw further intensification and spread, moving into South London (Camberwell and Lewisham). By the week ending 9 November, it was subsiding in most of those boroughs first affected, but peaking in some of the later boroughs (Holborn, Finsbury, Bethnal Green and Poplar) and in some of the south London boroughs (Bermondsey, Southwark, Camberwell) and to the west (Battersea, Fulham, Chelsea). The following fortnight saw a drop in most boroughs with only Bermondsey still showing significant activity in the week ending 16 November. However, it is not until the week ending 23 November that the pandemic penetrated Westminster. These peaks of influenza had ensured that in '1918, for the first time in records going back nearly a century, the deaths in London exceeded the births' (Hamer 1918: 1).

The third wave displayed a distinct north–south pattern in London. It emerged in the week ending 22 February 1919 and was apparent from St Pancras through Marylebone, Holborn, Westminster to Chelsea and Battersea. Once again, these boroughs contain many of the major railway stations linking the capital with the rest of the nation (King's Cross, St Pancras, Euston, Victoria, Paddington, Marylebone, Charing Cross). By the following week it spread to the (mostly) neighbouring boroughs, including Islington, Stoke Newington, Paddington, Kensington and Lambeth. But this wave was fairly short-lived and by the following week it had subsided with only Chelsea and Shoreditch (neighbouring boroughs to some affected the previous week) showing significant mortality rates.

Regions

Pandemic influenza reached into every corner of the world with little exception. It was not to spare any part of the British Isles, even reaching the Western Isles eventually. Eigg, for example, was hard-hit when the disease reached there in March 1919 (*The Times* 31 March 1919: 9). But while it did reach everywhere, there was some variation in terms of the impacts it had, as evidenced by the mortality (Plates 2 and 3). It is apparent that the north and the Midlands experienced a higher level of mortality. The RG concluded that while 'more populous centres suffered very slightly more . . . the incidence upon town and country was very nearly equal. The northern parts of the country . . . suffered decidedly more, on the whole, than the southern' (Registrar-General 1920: 24). Indeed, Plate 2 shows that the Midlands suffered as much as the north, and of the south it was the south-west and East Anglia that seems to have escaped the worst of the pandemic. This pattern supports recent work that suggests that urban areas, coastal areas and areas well-served by mass communication and transport links suffered higher mortality than rural, inland and isolated areas (Mamelund 1998b).

Further evidence of the difference in the experience of the north from the south comes from the epidemic curves, for example Figure 3.4. The epidemic curves for many northern centres show higher rates of mortality in all three waves of the epidemic. This is usually most pronounced in the second wave, where the curves show an extended second wave, often showing a biphasic pattern (two peaks) with the second peak of the wave often equalling or exceeding the first. This pattern holds throughout the north. The RG found such patterns when plotting the mortality by regions for total population, county boroughs, 'Other towns over 20,000' population and for the 'Remainder of Counties' (Registrar-General 1920: 45–7, diagrams XI–XIV). This pattern was also found in the Welsh figures, most markedly in 'Other towns over 20,000' (Registrar-General 1920: 44, diagram X).

It was one of these Welsh UDs that recorded the highest actual peak of mortality for any given week. Ogmore and Garw in Glamorganshire recorded an annualised influenza crude death rate of 106.4 per 1,000 population in the week ending 30 November (actually after the peak for England and Wales as a whole, again suggesting a hierarchical and distance effect). However, Ogmore and Garw's annualised rate for the entire pandemic was 6.3 per 1,000, while the lowest rate was recorded in Sutton UD, Surrey at 1.9 per 1,000, and the maximum at Hebburn UD, Durham, where the annualised rate for the entire pandemic was given as 11.9 per 1,000. The epidemic curves also show that in some northern areas the third wave quite often reached the same heights of mortality as the second. This also occurred in Scotland, where many of the largest burghs experienced their peak mortality in the third wave, early in 1919.

Scotland

The epidemic curve for Scotland (Figure 3.5) appears to suggest that Scotland actually preceded the rest of Britain in reaching the peaks of mortality. Mortality rose in October, before peaking in November, with an apparently more sustained peak than in England and Wales. It also appears that Scotland suffered the third wave earlier, reaching a peak in February 1919, whereas England and Wales reach their maximum in March 1919. However, this is largely an artefact of the Scottish RG summarising the data by

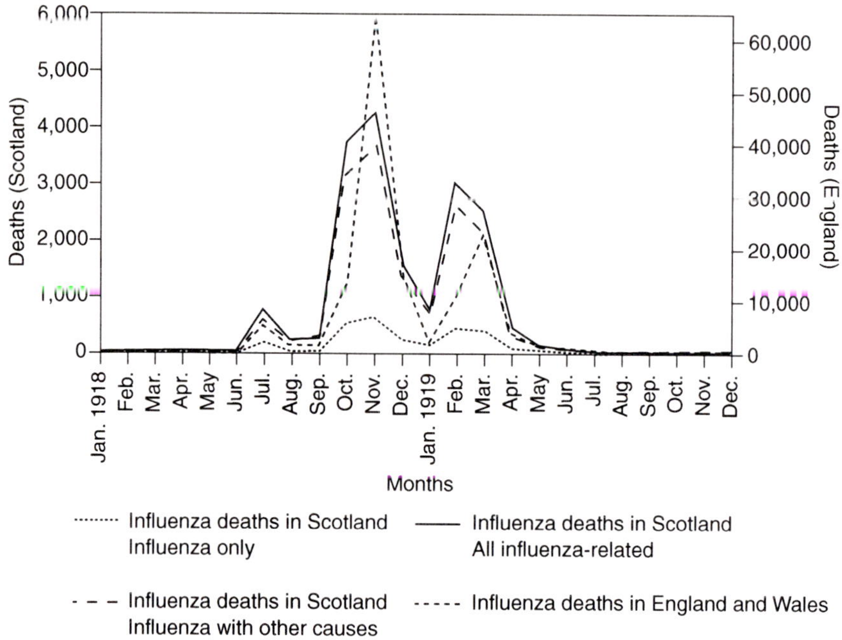

Figure 3.5 Influenza deaths in Scotland, England and Wales, 1918–19 (sources: Registrar-General for Scotland 1919; Registrar-General 1920).

month. Using weekly data, readily available for England and Wales, the lags and leads are less pronounced. For example, the English maxima for the third wave is reached in the week ending 1 March 1919, thus actually peaking in February, as in Scotland (Johnson 2004a).

A more significant point does not relate to the timing of the three waves, but the relative importance of the three waves. In England and Wales, the bulk of the mortality associated with the pandemic occurred during the second wave. Figure 3.5 clearly shows that the third wave, while not of greater magnitude (greater mortality) than the second, was of relatively greater importance in Scotland than in England and Wales. This variation in the relative importance of the waves of influenza is also apparent when examining the pandemic in Scotland's sixteen 'Principal Towns'. Some of these attain their highest death rates in the second wave, and others in the third wave (Table 3.2). Yet there appears to be no underlying (or overriding) geographic rationale as to why there is this variation. There is a slight tendency for the higher rates to be associated with those towns which had their mortality peak during the third wave. The Ministry of Health recognised this in noting that, '[r]elatively, the mortality of the third wave exceeded that attributed to the same phase in England and Wales'. However, the

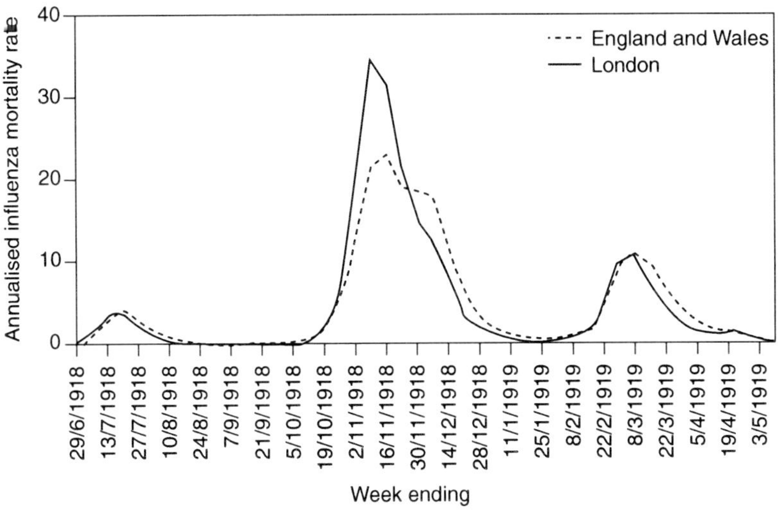

Figure 3.6 Influenza mortality, London and England and Wales, 1918–19 (source: Registrar-General 1920).

Table 3.2 Mortality peaks in Scotland's 'principal towns'

Principal towns	*Maximum reached in week ending*	*Wave*	*Death rate (official)*
Hamilton	12 October, 1918	2nd	2.8
Clydebank	19 October, 1918	2nd	3.7
Coatbridge	26 October, 1918	2nd	5.3
Motherwell	26 October, 1918	2nd	3.1
Aberdeen	2 November, 1918	2nd	3.2
Kilmarnock	2 November, 1918	2nd	3.1
Kirkcaldy	2 November, 1918	2nd	4.2
Dundee	9 November, 1918	2nd	4.1
Perth	9 November, 1918	2nd	4.0
Leith	15 February, 1919	3rd	4.9
Edinburgh	22 February, 1919	3rd	5.3
Paisley	22 February, 1919	3rd	3.4
Falkirk	1 March, 1919	3rd	5.0
Glasgow	1 March, 1919	3rd	4.1
Greenock	15 March, 1919	3rd	3.0
Ayr	22 March, 1919	3rd	2.7

Data source: Registrar-General for Scotland 1919: 7, Table C.

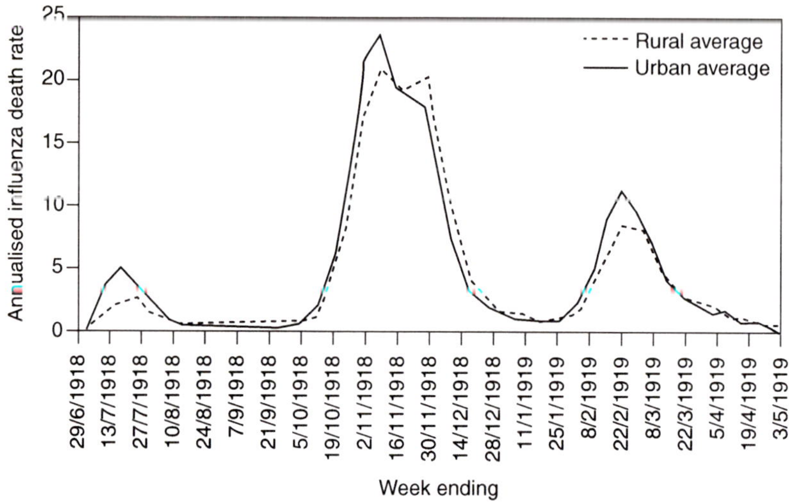

Figure 3.7 Urban and rural influenza mortality, England and Wales, 1918–19 (source: Registrar-General 1920).

Ministry dismissed this as of being of 'no epidemiological significance' (Ministry of Health 1920c: 50–1).

Urban–rural

The RG noted, as quoted earlier, a slight disadvantage to those living in the larger urban centres, a disadvantage that has been suspected elsewhere (Åman 1990; Ohadike 1991; Phillips 1988; Rice 1988). For example, London experienced considerably higher levels of mortality than the national average (Figure 3.6). London was also attacked and reached the peaks of mortality earlier than the national average, further supporting the role of the urban hierarchy in the spread of the pandemic.

While London has long been at the top of the British urban hierarchy, the rest of the hierarchy was shaped as the British population grew more urbanised in the latter half of the nineteenth century. At the start of the century only one-third of the population in England and Wales was urbanised; this reached 54 per cent by 1851, nearly three-quarters by 1871 and 78.9 per cent by 1911 (Law 1967). Law considered that this change to large-scale urbanisation was essentially complete by the start of the First World War. This is borne out by the fact that in the forty years from 1911 to 1951, the proportion of the population living in urban centres only grew from 78.9 to 81.2 per cent (Lawton and Pooley 1992: 91). Thus the pattern of urbanisation was established before the pandemic, and suggests the boundary changes made to the administrative areas, particularly in the larger centres such as Birmingham, Glasgow, Liverpool and Manchester in the period 1894–1911, may well have captured the real extent of that urbanisation. Superficially there are similarities between the pattern of influenza mortality (Plate 2) and the distribution of the principal urban centres (Lawton and Pooley 1992: 197, Figure 11.1). However, pandemic influenza mortality returned low correlations with either population or density measures (persons per acre) from the 1921 Census (0.031 and 0.086 respectively) when examined across the administrative areas of England and Wales (Johnson 2001).

The influenza mortality data published in the RG's report included detailed figures for some 290 urban areas (LBs, CBs and some UDs, generally with populations greater than 20,000, whereas Law's classification of urbanisation used a minimum population 2,500), along with a 'remainder of' county figures (or, in the cases of some smaller counties, total county figures). From these it is possible to calculate a rough average mortality for the broad categories 'urban' (those 290 specified areas) and 'rural' ('remainder of county' values) and plot epidemic curves (Figure 3.7). Obviously, these being average figures they hide a great deal of variation, for example different urban centres (at different hierarchical and geographical distances from London) can also exhibit great variation in the local timing of the pandemic waves. Notwithstanding these caveats, this figure suggests that rural localities experienced a marginally lower mortality and a slight lag in the timing of each wave (in keeping with the hierarchical and distance hypotheses), with the rural average also exhibiting the biphasic second wave seen in the north. These observations are complemented by the descriptive statistics (Table 3.3) that show the rural averages (mean and median) are slightly lower and the rural values are less variable (smaller range, standard deviation and skewness). As the RG concluded, 'It is not that the towns suffered excessively, for the rates for all classes of area throughout the whole epidemic were much the same, but the towns suffered first' (Registrar-General 1920: 12). Urban penalty may still be alive and (un)well in early-twentieth-century Britain,[23] however, it is not a penalty of large proportions.

Table 3.3 Urban–rural influenza mortality – descriptive statistics

	Urban	*Rural*
Mean	4.9	4.6
Median	4.8	4.3
Standard deviation	1.278	0.803
Skewness	0.962	0.328
Range	10.0	3.1
Minimum	1.9	3.2
Maximum	11.9	6.3

4 The human cost

Early in the twentieth century a new influenza washed over the world in three waves, alien to the immune systems of everyone. Such an unrecognisable virus, it went unchallenged by the sentries of the human immune system and claimed one of the greatest death tolls in recorded history. The first decades of HIV/AIDS have yet to slay the vast masses that influenza slaughtered in a year.

Manifestation: 'mix some heliotrope, or lavender, or mauvey-blue with red'

In many ways, the 1918–19 pandemic was similar to many influenza outbreaks, but on a vast scale – orders of magnitude greater than other epidemics and pandemics. The case fatality rate was similar to that found in other influenza epidemics, generally in the range of 1 to 3 per cent. The morbidity, based on what little information is available, seems to have been high; the published figures range from 25 to 90 per cent. This again is not dissimilar to that found in subsequent influenza epidemics, as is how it manifested itself in the majority of the afflicted population. The vast majority of the hundreds of millions of people who contracted influenza suffered in the same way we do now and have done for centuries. Most people displayed the symptoms of 'normal' influenza – fever, aches and a running or blocked nose. These symptoms ran their normal course and passed after three to five days. In many cases the onset seemed more abrupt and the symptoms seemed more severe, more sudden or were joined by other symptoms, such as violent nosebleeds and greater quantities of sputum but, as Stuart-Harris noted, 'Epidemics come and epidemics go, but the clinical picture of influenza remains remarkably unchanged' (Stuart-Harris 1960, cited in Spink 1979: 214). It has been recognised that the 'irregular' epidemics of influenza since 1890 and the pandemic form were little different from 'ordinary influenza' (Burnet and Clark 1942: 69). The first wave in 1918 was characterised by very typical flu symptoms – contributing to the lack of attention paid to the disease at the time. The later pandemic waves showed a greater proportion of fatal cases, but a number of the contemporary reports recognised that the vast bulk of cases seen took 'an ordinary simple uncomplicated course with fairly speedy recovery and without sequelæ' (Royal Society of Medicine 1918: 97). The American General and pioneering medico from Johns Hopkins University, W.S. Thayer,[1] gave a detailed clinical description that mirrors what we still recognise as 'normal' flu when addressing the Royal Society of Medicine's 'Discussion':

> suddenness of . . . onset . . . accompanied by severe headache, sometime chilly sensations, pain in the neck, general pain in the limbs, an aching pain throughout the body, and rapid rise of fever, usually to 103°F or more. The respiration and pulse as a rule are not much accelerated. The pulse is often rather slow as compared with the fever, and the appearance of the patient is noteworthy, the general flushing of the face, the injection of the conjunctiva, and the rather heavy and dull expression, so that patients with influenza can be picked out from the end of the ward by their flushed expression and their rather dull and heavy eyes. [Plate 4] There was very little cough; nose-bleeding at the outset was very common, but the respiratory symptoms were often unimportant, though sometimes later on there would be a dry pharyngitis, and sometimes a little coryza. After two to four days the temperature usually fell from crisis to normal, and in these early cases there was no mortality and there were few or no complications.
>
> (Royal Society of Medicine 1918: 61–2)

While by far the greatest proportion of those ill had 'typical' influenza, a significant number developed much more severe cases. In a period of vastly increased numbers of cases, the absolute number of serious cases and cases developing complications will also be much greater. A Medical Research Council (MRC) report on influenza among the British forces in France recorded that they had observed

> two major and serious forms of complications and sequelae: toxaemic and pulmonary. Toxaemic symptoms included: early cyanosis, early delirium, sudden rise in pulse rate, late onset or persistence of vomiting, epistaxis and constipation. Such patients had high mortality. Pulmonary symptoms included oedema, broncho-pneumonia, pulmonary haemorrhage, pleural effusion and bronchiectasis or abscess of lung.
>
> (Cummins 1919: 52)

Pulmonary symptoms, bronchitis and cardiac failure were among those symptoms noted quite frequently (Abrahams *et al.* 1919; Frost 1919; Hamer 1918, 1919b; MacPherson *et al.* 1920; PRO FD 1 533). General Thayer had also described the clinical features of the severe complications to the Royal Society of Medicine's 'Discussion'. He told the meeting that the

> fever did not fall. . . . Perhaps there were chilly sensations; the expectorations become blood-stained, sometimes extremely so, and then rusty. . . . The respiration was somewhat accelerated, the pulse not much accelerated. As a rule cyanosis developed early. The patient became dull and apathetic. . . . Very often suddenly, a few hours or a day before death, the evidences of pneumonic consolidation rapidly spread.
>
> (Royal Society of Medicine 1918: 63)

The South African historian, Howard Phillips, provides an even more vivid description of some of the symptoms encountered in the severe cases when he wrote of the

> laboured breathing, crackling sounds from the lung, bloody expectoration [or sputum], a furry coating of the tongue, heliotrope tingeing of the skin, bleeding from nose or mouth, delirium, sleeplessness and a host of gastric symptoms including diarrhoea and vomiting. Distinctive too, was an odour like very musty straw . . . 'so pungent . . . it just came into your nostrils with a bang'.
>
> (Phillips 1990a: 129–30)

While the (dis)coloration of many of the fatal cases was widely noted, this malodour is only rarely mentioned. The RAMC's Adolphe Abrahams had also mentioned it when speaking at the Royal Society of Medicine meeting as being another 'distinctive feature . . . a characteristic stench which appears to exude from the body as a whole' (Royal Society of Medicine 1918: 99).

Associated with many of the pneumonic complications was a most vivid cyanosis, a purple-blue tinge to the face (Plates 5 and 6). It could be confined to the lips and ears or generally diffused to the entire face. This 'heliotrope cyanosis' was one of the most commonly remarked features of this pandemic. One definition of the cyanosis was given in a 1921 booklet on influenza:

> Cyanosis – (Greek, Kyonos = blue) – The 'Blue disease' an affection in which the whole surface of the body exhibits a blue or purple colour, generally resulting from a communication between the aortic and pulmonary cavities of the heart or from some obstacle to the circulation in the former.
>
> (Léon 1921: 27, fn K)

The *Medical Journal of Australia*, Saturday 25 January 1919 edition, was an 'Influenza Number' and, in reporting the experiences on-board the *Medic*, Captain A.P. Derham, Army Medical Corps, AIF, described a very marked cyanosis of the face and hands, '[t]he lips were blue or purple, face blue and almost livid in appearance' (25 January 25 1919: 66). To see someone turn blue or even a dark purple and die is not an image easily lost, even in a world where death may have been much more part of life than is the case now. But even in a world where death was something all were closer to and more aware of, through the carnage of war, the domestic dealing with livestock, or simply because those parts of the human lifecycle dealing with disease and death were more likely to be played out in the home, this vivid mark of death was a shock. This discoloration of the dying and dead led many to wonder if this was not a form of black death.[2] Indeed this cyanosis was the most striking and memorable feature of the pandemic as it impressed itself upon many of those treating the ill (for example, Abrahams *et al.* 1919; Barry 2004; Collier 1974; Crosby 1989; Henrikson 1956; Hyam 1963; King 1922; Levinthal *et al.* 1921; Luckingham 1984a; Millard 1936; Ministry of Health 1920c; Phillips 1990a; Rice 1988). One of the earliest recorded observations of this striking development was that of the American nurse, Shirley Millard. On 1 April 1918, she wrote in her diary:

> we are swamped with influenza cases. I thought influenza was a bad cold, something like the grippe, but this is much worse than that. These men run a high temperature, so high that we can't believe it's true, and often take it again to be sure. . . . When they die, as about half of them do, they turn a ghastly dark grey and are taken out at once and cremated.
>
> (Millard 1936: 30)

In Sydney, Australia, the MO at City Road Emergency Hospital reported she had seen people turn purple, lilac and red, the latter 'more often seen in big, fat women'. Apparently the

> purple cyanotic colour' was 'very marked in some cases and often accompanied by jaundice . . . the face might be jaundiced, with intense blueness of the lips and round the mouth and chin. The hands and arms might be jaundiced and the fingers blue . . . so marked in some cases as to make even the dying patient remark on the strangeness of it. Very few of these patients recovered.

Distinct from this was a lilac tint 'often accompanied by a particularly ashed or leaden tint of the arms and chest'. The lilac tinge could extend half-way down the chest and the patient was 'constantly wet and clammy'. This colour was a dire sign, as Lucy Gullet felt 'the prognosis in the "lilac" cyanosis was worse than in the purple'. The red cases, 'a sort of magenta-coloured erythematous flush' that extended 'down the face and neck over the front and back of the chest', fared far better (*MJA*, 30 August 1919: 170–1). Gullet was also struck by how suddenly many patients succumbed as, in some of the worst cases,

> the patient had no pain and no distress. . . . Very many of those who died . . . would brighten up as the end approached and evince a very

> strong desire to live. It was this consciousness . . . that made the disease so very terrible. There is nothing very distressing in a death where a patient gradually sinks and becomes comatose and death comes while he is unconscious. But it is horrible to see patients either suffocating or dying of collapse who are acutely aware that they are dying.
>
> (*MJA*, 30 August 1919: 171)

Another to encounter such distressing scenes was the RAMC's Major Adolphe Abrahams. Older brother of the Olympic sprinter, Harold Abrahams (famously portrayed in the film *Chariots of Fire*), pioneer of sports medicine (he was honorary medical officer to the British Olympic athletic team for many years and founder of the British Association of Sport and Medicine) and later knighted, Abrahams had been one of the first to see the symptoms as he treated men at Aldershot barracks in the earlier outbreaks (Abrahams *et al.* 1917). His view had been that once the colour appeared 'the patient's condition may be regarded as desperate' and that all 'blue' cases were doomed. Later he and his colleagues found that some would recover, but that

> [t]he 'blue' cases which recovered were quite indistinguishable in any features from those which died. Cases regarded as beyond redemption recovered, encouraging the determination never to abandon hope while there was life, and we have even had the curious experience of thrice regarding as hopeless one man who recovered, relapsed, recovered, relapsed, and then finally recovered. An even more painful indication of one's prognostic deficiency was afforded by cases which, not only upon admission but even for several days of treatment in hospital, appeared to run a comparatively trivial course, and to give rise to no legitimate anxiety; the patients then suddenly took a turn for the worse, rapidly developed cyanosis, and died within a few hours of being only trivially ill
>
> (Royal Society of Medicine 1918: 101)

Abrahams continued to declare that the colour of the patient was critical and as long as the face, especially the lips and ears, remained red (Plate 4) there was 'ample room for hope of recovery, no matter what the lung signs, the temperature, the pulse rate, or the respiration rate', as Gullet had also suggested. However, as soon as one 'would need to mix some heliotrope, or lavender, or mauvey-blue with red' to create an accurate tint (Plates 5 and 6), then the 'prospect is grave indeed' – and even if the patient appears comfortable, 'has no signs of consolidation in either lung, is sleeping fairly well and taking nourishment, has no more than an ordinary degree of pyrexia [elevated temperature], a good pulse rate, not unduly fast, and a respiration rate that may not strike one as being unusual in the circumstances', this was a sign of the most unwelcome sort, as these cases were 'likely to be dead in a day or two' (Abrahams *et al.* 1919: 4).

The causality of such a cyanosis naturally provoked discussion. Was it a pulmonary phenomena or a change in the blood? One report claimed 'that the so-called cyanosis is in reality an erythema' and that in 'well-marked cases it is an intense dusky, reddish-plum coloured erythema' (*MJA* 5 April 1919: 280–1). Speaking to the Linnean Society of New South Wales, H.S. Halcro Wardlaw said '[t]his colouration was as first described as a cyanosis, and was attributed to the most likely cause of such a condition: a deficient oxygenation of the blood in the lungs.' However, he disputed whether it was a true cyanosis as many cases did not show signs of 'respiratory distress' (Wardlaw 1919: 514). A November 1919 report in the *MJA* on the 'The physiology of cyanosis' reported on studies into the cause of the cyanosis, concluding that '[t]he violet and heliotrope tints were seen to indicate a definite diminution in the amount of oxygen that the arterial blood carried' (*MJA* 1 November 1919: 370). By the start of the following year, 1920, a 'Retrospect' on the pandemic noted that *Bacillus influenzæ* or Pfeiffer's bacillus was no longer regarded as the causative agent as 'it is [now] generally recognised that the virus of the disease is still unknown', though some were claiming 'the discovery of a filter-passing virus in connexion with influenza', while also stating that the primary cause of cyanosis was 'an increase in the oxygen unsaturation of the blood in the peripheral capillaries' (*MJA* 17 January 1920: 59–60).

Mortality

In 1920 the RG declared that during the forty-six weeks of the pandemic in England and Wales, some 151,446 people had died of influenza, of whom 141,989 were civilians. From this toll the annualised civilian death rate for influenza in England and Wales was 4.774 per thousand (Registrar-General 1920: 3). In Edinburgh, the RG for Scotland stated 17,575 Scots had died at a rate of 4.3 per thousand (Registrar-General for Scotland 1919: 2). However, these are deaths allocated to influenza only. It is apparent that this was an outbreak of disease attended by a vast surge of mortality. The RG's report on the pandemic states that 'No such mortality as this has ever before been recorded for any epidemic in this country since registration commenced . . . the cholera epidemic of 1849 . . . [killed not more than] 3,033 per million population' (Registrar-General 1920: 3). While comparisons of the lethality of disease outbreaks may be odious, it is illuminating to recall that in Britain, plague killed 'a gross figure of 650,000 . . . between 1570 and 1670' and this is 'at least four times the known number of deaths caused by cholera in the whole of England and Wales in the nineteenth century' (Slack 1985: 174). Influenza makes these earlier outbreaks almost pale into insignificance as, in less than a year, at least 220,000 influenza-related deaths occurred in Scotland, England and Wales. Of course, the population at risk had risen by 1918, but the scale of the influenza was orders of magnitude greater than cholera or plague. However, this pandemic may not be without precedent in the British context. John Moore, when re-assessing Jack Fisher's work, argued that flu had contributed significantly to 'a marked population decline' in the sixteenth century, 'of the order of 20 per cent, as a result of two "catastrophic harvests of 1555 and 1556 . . . followed by one of the major influenza epidemics in English history"' (Moore 1993: 280).

This was a vast pandemic of influenza, but one in which other infections contributed to the morbidity and mortality. Pneumoccocus, streptococcus and staphococcus infections are considered to have been quite commonplace. Some argue that the pandemic was made so severe by the combination of the influenza virus and additional pathogen(s) (Kilbourne 1977, 1987; Pyle 1986; Stuart-Harris *et al.* 1985), especially pneumococcus, as influenza 'epidemics are notoriously associated with an increased incidence of bacterial pneumonia . . . bacteria were major contributors to influenza complications and mortality' (Kilbourne 1987: 174). Certainly, much of the mortality associated with this pandemic was not directly attributed to influenza. Indeed, in some locations much of the mortality was attributed to other causes, such as pneumonia, bronchitis, other respiratory diseases and various cardiovascular conditions. A chapter in *A Short History of Some Common Diseases* (1934) regarded the pandemic in terms of being a pneumonia pandemic, as 'the severe pneumonia of 1918 . . . was a form of influenza. Many patients had a brownish or cyanosed appearance' (Brockbank 1934: 57). These pneumonia deaths are now regarded as being very much part of the influenza pandemic experience, as the pneumonic complications of influenza became so prevalent and so pronounced.

The English RG's report explicitly recognised that there was likely to have been an understating of influenza mortality:

> It is well known that during influenza epidemics the mortality attributed to the disease does not represent the whole of that caused by it. The entries under other headings, especially those of respiratory disease, are always found to increase during an epidemic . . . it is still necessary to make allowance for these increases in mortality, allocated to other causes but really attributable to influenza, in endeavouring to measure the loss of life
>
> (Registrar-General 1920: 3)

Consequently, the RG devised three 'excess' deaths methods for estimating the total mortality attributable to the pandemic (Registrar-General 1920: 3–7). These methods were first applied to the female population, due to the 'profound modification of the male civilian population' (Registrar-General 1920: 3).

The first method involved comparing the deaths for each quarter of the pandemic against deaths in the previous five years (1913–1917) for specific causes of death. Several causes of deaths were examined for 'excess' deaths based on annualised death rates and these deaths then re-allocated as influenza-caused deaths. The causes included were pneumonia (all forms), bronchitis, 'organic heart disease' and pulmonary tuberculosis (phthisis). As the RG's report noted, 'Doubtless others might be added to this list, but the four above, and particularly pneumonia, are of such outstanding importance that the result could not be substantially affected by further refinements' (Registrar-General 1920: 3). The excess mortality derived was then added to the recorded influenza deaths to reach an estimate of total pandemic mortality. The result of this calculation was still regarded as too low by the RG when the estimate was done for the third quarter of 1918. This is seen as being a consequence of that third quarter, like the first two quarters of the year, being part of quite a healthy year (apart from influenza) as the death rates for all other causes were markedly lower in 1918 than in the previous five years, and the list of selected causes not being exhaustive as deaths actually caused by influenza 'may have been attributed to almost any cause' (Registrar-General 1920: 3).

The second method employed was to assess the comparative healthiness of 1918 to the average for the previous five years for the 'other causes' (excluding influenza and those causes listed above) and then to assume that in the absence of influenza the total mortality would have been in the same ratio as between these other causes in 1918 and in the previous five years. The 'excess' mortality could thus be regarded as influenza-related. From this method, 1918 was found to have 86.89 per cent of the mortality of the average for the previous five years for those 'other causes' (94.2 per cent in Scotland), making it a relatively healthy year. Taking this figure, the 'expected' mortality could be calculated and deducted from the recorded mortality with the remainder again considered to be the excess influenza mortality. This figure could then be added to the recorded influenza figure to obtain another estimate of total pandemic mortality.

The third estimation method was based on the assumption that total mortality would have been similar to that found in the first and second quarters of 1918. In England and Wales total mortality for the first quarter of 1918 was 86.5 per cent of that for the 1913–17 average, while in the second quarter of 1918 it was 89.6 per cent, an average of 88.0 per cent. In Scotland the figures are 81.3 per cent and 87.4 per cent respectively, an average of 84.4 per cent. From there it was possible to calculate expected mortality and compare it with actual mortality. Again the excess can be claimed to be influenza-related.

Using these three methods the RG's report calculated that female influenza mortality in the fourth quarter of 1918 (not the entire pandemic period) to be in the order of 60,000 to 65,000 (Registrar-General 1920: 4). The number of female deaths actually attributed to influenza for the quarter was 50,840.

The RG first calculated these excess mortality estimates for the female population due to the wartime changes in the male population. The available male population data was for civilians only. Furthermore, this civilian population had undergone major structural change during 1913–17. For these reasons, the RG made estimates for male deaths for the civilian population only and just used 1917 data for comparisons, rather than the five-year period used for the female calculations. The argument made for using the 1917 figures was that the 'alteration in the male civilian population between 1917 and 1918 must have been much less than earlier in the war, for the reduction in the numbers of civilians of military age was almost trifling compared with what had occurred before' (Registrar-General 1920: 4).[3] However, given the importance of the young adult population to the pandemic and their involvement in the war, and consequent likelihood that they were the most disturbed segment of the population, this 'disturbance' should be borne in mind. Further, the use of a single year as a comparison seems somewhat insecure, and comparisons with the female estimates are less robust as the sets of estimates are derived from different bases. Bearing in mind these limitations, the RG's report re-calculated civilian male influenza mortality in the fourth quarter of 1918 at about 51,000. The number of civilian male deaths actually allocated to influenza for the quarter was 39,205 (Registrar-General 1920: 5).

These re-calculation methods were then applied to the total mortality of the pandemic period in England and Wales where 151,446 deaths were recorded as being due to influenza, with 141,989 of these being civilian deaths. The recalculated mortality estimates were approximately 100,000 female deaths, 84,000 civilian males and 14,000 non-civilian men, some 198,000 deaths. This figure was rounded as 'in view of the uncertainties of the estimation the round figure of 200,000 deaths attributable to the epidemic . . . may be accepted' (Registrar-General 1920: 7). The originally allocated figure of 141,989 deaths gave an annualised civilian death rate due to influenza of 4.774 per thousand. An adjusted tally of 185,000 civilian deaths raises this to 6.264 per thousand for England and Wales (131 per cent of the original figure).

The RG for Scotland stated that the official (registered) mortality for the pandemic was 17,575, giving an annual death rate of 4.3 per thousand population. These figures included 'not only those deaths of which influenza was the sole named cause, but also those deaths of which influenza was one of two or more named causes, the latter being far more numerous' (Registrar-General for Scotland 1919: 2). Thus the official figures are based only on those deaths recorded with influenza as a cause of death. The RG for Scotland adopted a simplistic approach to determining what could be considered the maximum possible mortality attributable to the pandemic, by comparing the total registered mortality for Scotland during the influenza 'period' (July 1918 to April 1919) with the previous July to April period. Total deaths in the epidemic were 79,131 while in the comparable period there were 52,932. From this, the RG suggests that

> the difference, no doubt largely attributable to influenza, amounting to 26,199, which number is fully 8,624 or 49.1 per cent. more than that

> obtained by a count of the deaths of which influenza was a named cause. Taking 26,199 as a maximum number, and [the reported] 17,575 as a minimum, and assessing the true mortality from influenza at the mean of these numbers, a statement that the probable number of deaths caused by the epidemic amounted to nearly 22,000 appears justifiable.
>
> (Registrar-General for Scotland 1919: 5)

This approach does not take into account that the first half of 1918 was a period of markedly reduced mortality in all of Britain, including Scotland. When the English RG's excess methods calculations are applied to the Scottish data, the result is an upward revision of the mortality figures to between 27,650 and 33,771 (Johnson 2004a). These figures indicate that the recorded influenza mortality in Scotland of 17,575 is a marked understatement of the total mortality associated with the pandemic and the higher re-calculations of total mortality are near to doubling that figure. These new estimates of mortality give annualised death rates of 6.8 to 8.3 per 1,000 (158 to 193 per cent of the original figure). Consequently, the total mortality for the 1918–19 influenza pandemic in Britain would appear to be of the order of 230,000 rather than the recorded 169,021.

The RG selected five specific causes to include in their re-calculation of influenza mortality. One way to investigate whether these selections were justified is by examining the relative importance of each of these causes to total mortality and by examining the age–sex structure of the mortality caused by these specific causes. The relative importance of each specific cause of death can be revealed by obtaining the number of deaths from these causes and total deaths for males and females in England and Wales for each year in the period 1911–19, and by determining the proportion of total mortality caused by the specific causes.[4]

The relative importance of the five specific causes for female mortality in England and Wales is shown in Figure 4.1. These trends indicate how important each disease was through this period while reducing the problems of changing populations and population structure. The female population figures are considered more reliable than those for males that were much disrupted by the war. The trends for males (Figure 4.2) exhibit the same patterns as shown for females. It is apparent that influenza mortality rose steeply, particularly in young adults. Bronchitis displayed similar patterns of mortality in both periods, as did phthisis, with only some increases in female mortality at certain ages, notably young adults. Pneumonia claimed more lives in all age groups among both men and women, whereas 'organic heart disease' actually showed a decrease during the pandemic period. From these two examinations of the causes it seems that deaths attributed to bronchitis and organic heart disease may not have been particularly influenced by the pandemic. A link between phthisis deaths and the influenza seems more problematic, while pneumonia deaths appear to have risen in concert with the pandemic, as expected.

Examining the age–sex mortality for each cause would reveal any changes in

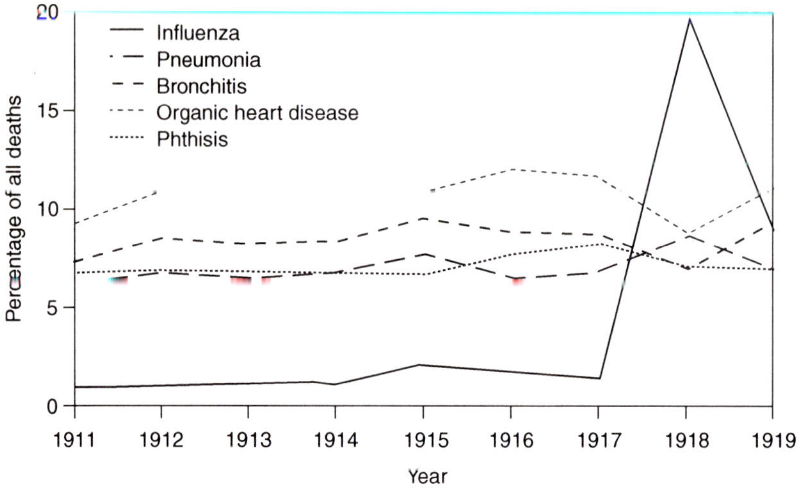

Figure 4.1 Proportion of female mortality by specific causes 1911–19, England and Wales (sources: *ARRG* 1911–19).

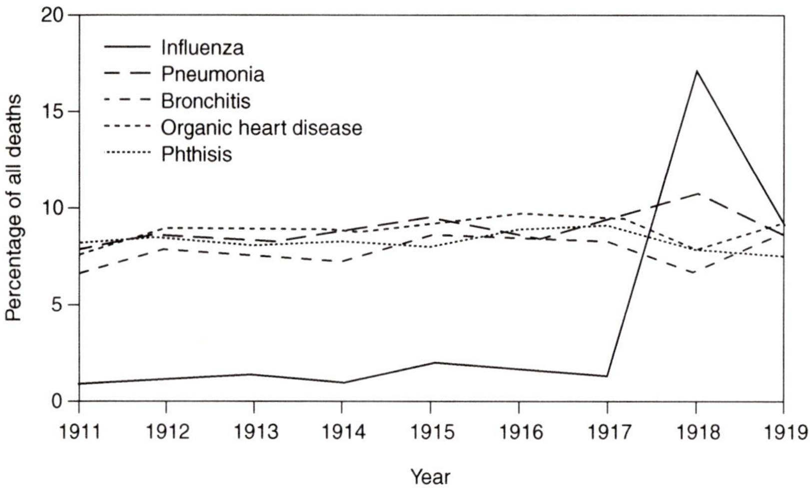

Figure 4.2 Proportion of male mortality by specific causes 1911–19, England and Wales (sources: *ARRG* 1911–19).

the age–sex distribution of these causes of death.[5] For all causes it was apparent that deaths were up in all age groups. Influenza deaths rose incredibly, especially in the young adult age groups, as we already know. Bronchitis, somewhat surprisingly, displayed similar patterns of mortality in the two periods. This contrasts somewhat with pneumonia, which saw increased mortality in

1918–19 for almost all age groups (not just young adults). Phthisis displayed increases in female mortality in certain age groups, particularly among young adult women. The cause termed 'organic heart disease' saw deaths actually dropping during the pandemic period. Were those likely to have died of these cardiac causes being claimed by influenza instead? From these two examinations of the causes there may be a case for removing bronchitis and organic heart disease from the further re-calculations and analyses, while pneumonia mortality was undoubtedly affected by the mortality of the pandemic. The case for removing or retaining phthisis is less obvious.

Encephalitis lethargica

It may be that pandemic mortality can be adequately calculated using influenza, pneumonia and possibly phthisis, and without bronchitis and 'organic heart disease'. But is there a case for adding any other causes? The RG, working on the 1918 and 1919 mortality data, concluded not. However, one condition has been identified as being related to influenza and also as having a distinct time lag between onset and death. Shortly before the end of 1918, the Local Government Board (LGB) issued regulations about and conducted an enquiry into an 'obscure disease'. The obscure disease in question was encephalitis lethargica.[6] Whereas it was previously a very unusual disease with few cases reported, it was noted that reports increased markedly following the pandemic and continued for a number of years. These early reports were followed by consideration of the disease and its possible relationship to influenza at meetings of the Committee of the Office International d'Hygiène Publique, Paris and of the Health Committee of the League of Nations.[7] Towards the end of the 1920s the Ministry of Health produced another enquiry report into encephalitis lethargica (Ministry of Health 1928). While this report has little discussion of influenza, the graphs for encephalitis lethargica notifications and mortality indicated an almost perfect six-year lag from the influenza pandemic. Encephalitis lethargica displayed a rapid rise in mortality during the 1920s before an almost equally rapid descent which resulted in its removal as a separate cause of death in the *ARRG*s.

The connection between the two conditions was much disputed and then gradually forgotten. A paper in *The Lancet* in 1982 renewed interest in the connection between influenza, encephalitis lethargica and Parkinsonism (Ravenholt and Foege 1982).[8] This article, on influenza and encephalitis lethargica in Seattle, and comparing the experiences in the two Samoas, was seen as conclusive. The Seattle work provided compelling evidence that encephalitis cases once considered independent of influenza were in fact sequelae, while the Samoan case studies demonstrated that

> whereas Western Samoa suffered heavily from both influenza-pneumonia and encephalitis lethargica during the years 1918–22,

> America Samoa was remarkably free of both these diseases during these years. The evidence, then, is compelling that the pandemic of influenza . . . and the pandemic of encephalitis lethargica . . . had a common aetiology. Both pandemics were globally distributed and were closely related in time.
>
> (Ravenholt 1993: 711)

Ravenholt and Foege looked beyond 1918–19 for evidence to support the hypothesis that encephalitis lethargica was related to influenza and demonstrated a clear lag in mortality of several years. This was seen for previous influenza epidemics, particularly with the 'Russian' flu of 1889–92. However, the sheer scale of the 1918–19 pandemic helped bring out the relationship because of the consequent massive rise in encephalitis lethargica. As Ravenholt later noted, 'the global pandemic of encephalitis accompanying and following the 1918 influenza pandemic was in a class by itself with respect to its virulence and sequelae' (Ravenholt 1993: 709).

The relatively long interval between the two conditions 'generated confusion and skepticism' as to the role of influenza in encephalitis lethargica as, apparently, '[l]ong latent intervals and slow viruses were not well-recognized in 1918; hence encephalitis epidemics occurring a year or more after attacks of influenza were perceived as evidence against rather than supportive of influenza as the cause.' Furthermore, the lack of infectivity of encephalitis, as opposed to the highly contagious nature of influenza, was taken as indicating that the two were unrelated and not 'different manifestations of the same viral agent'. However, as noted above, the sheer scale of the 1918–19 influenza pandemic led to epidemics of encephalitis lethargica in many countries, including Britain, Germany and the USA. Ravenholt asserts that the 'main causative agent of epidemic encephalitis lethargica during the pandemic years 1917–26 was the respiratorily spread influenza virus' and that as many as half-a-million people died as a direct consequence of encephalitis lethargica following the influenza pandemic, and others died of 'parkinsonism and other complications following the acute illness stage', with as much as '80 per cent of the survivors developing parkinsonism during ensuing decades' (Ravenholt 1993: 712, 710, 708).[9]

In England and Wales encephalitis lethargica only appeared as a separate cause of death in the period 1920–1930.[10] In Scotland, reporting was slightly more restricted, appearing from 1921 to 1930. It was only after the influenza pandemic that encephalitis lethargica became apparent in significant numbers, peaking in the mid-1920s (Figure 4.3). Total recorded encephalitis lethargica deaths for the period 1920 to 1930 in England and Wales were 10,673, with the annual crude death rate ranging from 0 per million (1918) to 36 per million people (1924) before steadily falling during the rest of this period. The Scottish records give another 1,203 deaths for the period, with death rates ranging from 1 to 4 per 100,000 population. Thus, if one were to accept that most of these deaths

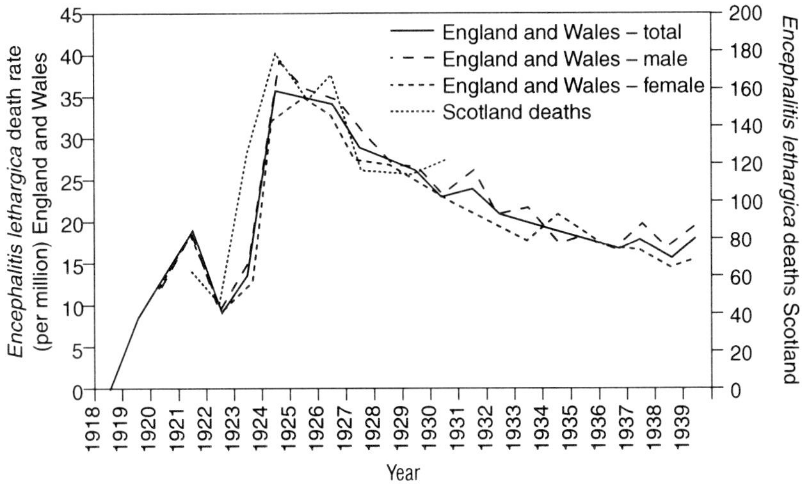

Figure 4.3 Encephalitis lethargica mortality in Britain (sources: *ARRG* 1918–40).

were related to the pandemic, they raise the British pandemic mortality to approximately 242,000.

Global mortality

The marked revision of mortality related to the 1918 influenza is by no means restricted to Britain. Global mortality was computed, by Jordan in the 1920s, to be in the vicinity of 21.5 million (Jordan 1927).[11] Successive upward revisions of the estimated mortality have been a feature of recent literature on this pandemic. Jordan's estimate stood for decades, and is still reported as fact, but does seem almost ludicrously low, especially when Mills has estimated Indian mortality alone at 18 million (Mills 1986). A more recent tally revised the mortality to being in the range 24.7–39.3 million, while suggesting that 'a conservative total of roughly 30 million victims' was their preferred figure (Patterson and Pyle 1991: 15). Given the time – and scholarship[12] – since that survey was published, it is timely that the tally should be re-visited and an updated account of the mortality occasioned by the pandemic provided (Table 4.1). This table is by no means a definitive record of the mortality brought about by the pandemic, and it must be accepted that much of the mortality may not have been recorded and the figures that do exist vary greatly in coverage and reliability.[13]

From Table 4.1 global mortality from the influenza pandemic is of the order of 50 million. However, even this monstrous figure may be substantially lower than the true toll. There are vast areas of the world for which we have little or no information, and often what information we do have is of dubious quality and contradictory. Sometimes this data only covers certain

Table 4.1 Global influenza mortality

Location	Population	Published death toll	Published death rate (per 1,000)	Re-calculated death rate
Africa				
Belgian Congo		~300,000	~50	
Botswana		7,000	40–50	
Cameroon	561,000 (1921)	250,000		445
Chad			21.4	
Egypt	12,936,000	138,600		10.7
Gambia	211,000 (1921)	>7,800	~50	37
Ghana (Gold Coast)	2,298,000 (1921)	88,500–100,000	~40	43.5
Kenya	2,596,000	150,000	40	57.8
Madagascar	3,388,000		35	
Mauritius	377,000	>12,000		31.8
Nigeria	18,631,000 (1921)	~455,000	30	24.4
Senegal		37,500	30	
Sierra Leone	1,541,000 (1921)		30	
Somalia			25.6	
South Africa	6,769,000	~300,000	43.97	44.3
Southern Rhodesia	873,000		27.3	
North Africa		200,000–248,000	7.5–10	
All sub-Saharan Africa		~2,175,000	~23.1	
Total Africa		**~2,375,000**	**~18.2**	

Americas				
Argentina	8,517,000	10,200	1.20	1.2
Brazil	26,277,000	180,000	6.00	6.8
British Caribbean		~30,000		
Canada	8,148,000	~50,000	6.25	6.1
Caribbean		~100,000		
Chile		35,000	11.00	
Guatemala	1,241,000	48,600		39.2
Mexico	14,556,000	300,000	23.00	20.6
Uruguay	1,439,000	2,050	1.40	1.4
USA	103,208,000	675,000		6.5
Other South America		~100,000		
Total Latin America		766,000–966,000	8.4–10.6	
Total North America		725,000		
Total Americas		**~1,540,000**		
Asia				
Afghanistan		~320,000		
Ceylon (Sri Lanka)	5,109,000	91,600		17.9
China	472,000,000 (1920)	4–9.5 million		8.4–20.1
India	305,693,000 (1921)	18.5 million		6.1
Indonesia	49,350,000	1.5 million		30.4
Japan	55,033,000	388,000	~6.7	7.0
Philippines	10,151,000	93,686	8.00	1.7
Taiwan	3,670,000	25,394		6.9
Southwest Asia		215,000–430,000	5-10	
Other East and Southeast Asia		220,000–1.3 million	5–30.6	
Total Asia		**26–36 million**		

continued

Table 4.1 continued

Location	*Population*	*Published death toll*	*Published death rate (per 1,000)*	*Re-calculated death rate*
Europe				
Austria	6,131,445			
	(post-war)	20,458	3.00	3.3
Croatia		109,000		
Denmark	3,010,000	12,374	3.50	4.1
Eire	4,280,000	18,367	4.04	4.3
England & Wales	34,020,000	~200,000	~4.9	5.8
Finland	3,120,000	18,000	5.8	5.8
France	32,830,000	240,000	3.9	7.3
Germany	58,450,345			
	(post-war)	225,330	3.70	3.8
Prussia		236,662	4.5	
Hungary	7,880,000	~100,000		12.7
Iceland		484	5.4	
Italy	36,280,000	390,000	11.0	10.7
Malta		588		
Netherlands	6,750,000	48,042		7.1
Norway	2,580,000	14,676	5.7	5.7
Portugal	6,010,000	59,000	9.7	9.8
Russia/USSR	184,000,000 (1917)	~450,000	5.00	2.4
Scotland	4,850,000	27,650–33,771	6.8–8.3	5.7–6.9
Spain	20,880,000	257,082	12	12.3
Sweden	5,810,000	34,374	5.41	5.9
Switzerland	3,880,000	23,277	6.00	6.1
Total Europe		**~2,300,646**	**~4.8**	

Oceania				
Australia	5,304,000 (1919)	14,528	2.8	2.7
Fiji	164,000	9,000	52	54.9
Guam		858		
Nauru			160	
New Zealand	1,158,000		<20	
Pakeha		6,413	5.8	
Maori		2,160	42.4	
Pacific Islands			>50	
Tonga	23,000 (1921)		42–84	
Western Samoa	36,000 (1921)	8,500	220	236.1
Total Oceania		**~85,000**		
Global		***>48,798,038***		
		~50–100 million	~2.5–5	

Sources: Åman 1990; Brown 1987; Cavina 1959; Chan and Liu 1998; Cliff *et al.* 1986; Cole 1994; Collier 1974; Collins 1932; Collins and Lehmann 1953; Crosby 1989; Echenberg 1993; Echeverri 2003; Eichel 1923; Garner 1921; Hartwig and Patterson 1978; Herda 1998; Iijima 1998; Jordan 1927; Killingray 1994; Linnanmäki 1998, 1999; McCreery, 1992; McGinnis 1977; Mamelund 1998a; Martin 1921; Mills 1986; Ministry of Health 1920c; Mueller 1995; Müller 1996; Ohadike 1981; Palmer and Rice 1992; Patterson 1983; Patterson and Pyle 1991; Phillips 1988; Phimister 1973; Rice 1988, 1989; Tomkins 1992b. With additional communications and calculations by Juergen Mueller, University of Hanover and the author (particularly figures for Scotland, England and Wales). In producing this updated tally of influenza mortality several dozen researchers into the 1918–19 pandemic were canvassed for their opinions on the figures, particularly for their areas of expertise, much as how AIDS mortality was/is derived – the so-called 'Delphi method' (Mann and Tarantola 1996: 487). Population figures from Mitchell (1992, 1995 and 1998) and *Census of England and Wales* (1921: 17).

cities or populations: often indigenous mortality has never been considered. In some cases, the figures given are only those that were recorded as influenza deaths, while others recorded both influenza and pneumonia deaths. Consequently, total pandemic mortality may fall in the range 50 to 100 million, but it would seem unlikely that a truly accurate figure can ever be deduced. Notwithstanding this, the scale of mortality undoubtedly makes it one of the largest outbreaks of disease in recorded history. Furthermore, these deaths occurred in a very short time, from early 1918 to, in some cases, 1920. The bulk of them actually occurred in less than a year, from mid-1918 to early 1919. However, it is a disease which has little resonance in the collective memory. As Camus asked:

> But what are a hundred million deaths?. . . since a dead man has no substance unless one has actually seen him dead, a hundred million corpses broadcast through history are no more than a puff of smoke in the imagination.
>
> (Camus 1947: 38)

The pandemic killed an estimated 50 to 100 million people and is thought to have infected half the world's population, some one billion people. Just prior to this, the First World War ended with an estimated death toll of less than ten million (Steiner 2005: 4). Nature had demonstrated most forcefully that while humankind had mechanised killing and had recently slaughtered millions in the prosecution of this war, humanity was still far from being as 'efficient' as nature could be. Nature had perfected mass killing in a way that we could not emulate. This was, as an editorial in the South African newspaper *The Friend* put it, 'Nature in her most maleficent mood' (*The Friend* 22 October 1918, editorial, quoted in Phillips 1990a: 203). Indeed, this pandemic may well have claimed more lives than both World Wars combined.[14]

In many instances the case fatality rates in epidemic and pandemic influenza are no greater than in 'normal' years, ranging between 1 and 3 per cent. However, in 1918 morbidity was so much greater that the resulting mortality was tremendous. But some countries and some peoples suffered dreadfully. Throughout the Pacific, for example, more than 5 per cent of the population of almost every island died. Western Samoa suffered one of the greatest losses as a nation, losing 22 per cent of its population: 30 per cent of the adult males, 22 per cent of the adult female population and 10 per cent of its children (Tomkins 1992b). The *Medical Journal of Australia* carried a report on the Samoan experience claiming that 'incidence amongst the natives . . . was 80% and . . . the total deaths number almost exactly one fifth of the entire population (to be exact, 7,264 out of 34,405)' (*MJA* 3 May 1919: 360). The report noted that local behaviours compounded the problem as, when someone was ill, the entire family would come into the hut, lower the blinds and lie down by the ill person. Further, the storing of food was apparently not common practice, so when many people were ill there was little food available. In some isolated cases, such as among the Canadian Inuit, even higher fatality rates were found, with entire communities felled (Crosby 1989). However, it is recognised that much of the mortality in such events was not a direct result of infection with influenza. Some of the mortality has been attributed to the possibility of 'innate susceptibility' (or 'virgin soil' epidemics) and a lack of care when all members of a community are incapacitated at the same time leading to deaths from thirst, starvation and hypothermia (Burnet and Clark 1942: 76; Crosby 1989: 227–64).

Age and death

The two most notable features of this pandemic were the heliotrope cyanosis that tainted so many victims and the age distribution of the dead. Influenza is a killer, usually of the young and the old and those with impaired health. While influenza may have high attack rates in adults, their mortality tends to be very low. Plotting influenza mortality by age characteristically produces a 'U' shape emphasising how mortality is largely confined to the extremities of age. The pandemic of 1918–19 exhibited a very different age mortality distribution. While young and old were still hard-hit, there was one extremely significant difference and it was this that contributed much to the huge excess mortality. This time young adults bore the brunt of mortality. Here the age distribution produces what has been termed a 'W' curve – with a massive spike of mortality in the young adult age groups (Figure 4.4 and Figure 4.5). An MRC report on influenza among British forces noted that, while they were discussing a male population aged 19 to 50, they

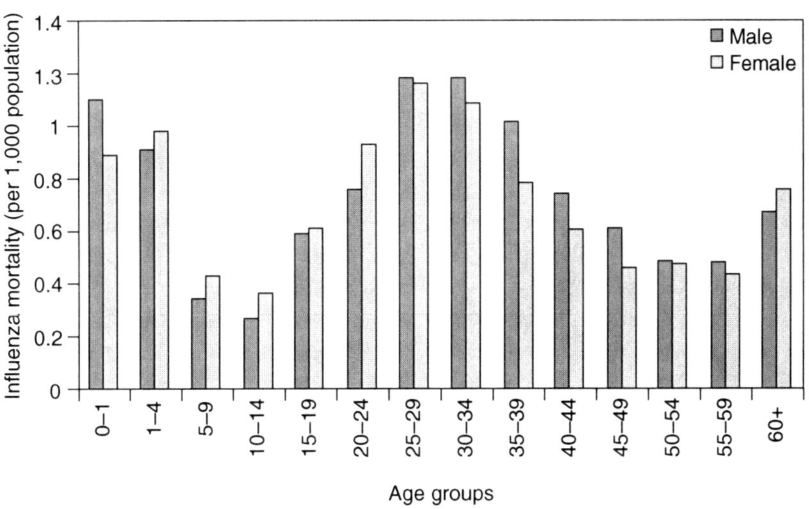

Figure 4.4 Age–sex distribution of influenza mortality, Spain 1918 (source: Echeverri 2003: 185).

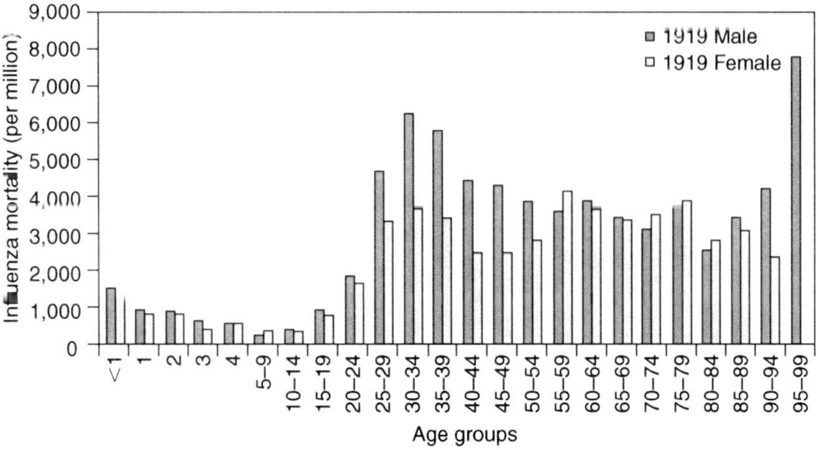

Figure 4.5 Age distribution of pandemic mortality, Australia 1919 (source: *Official Yearbook of Australia* 1920: 1131).

could still state that it was more prevalent among younger men and that the 'severe type of the disease was much more prevalent among the younger than among the older men' (Cummins 1919: 47).

Britain's 'lost generation' came from both the war and the influenza,[15] whereas in some countries they came more (if not exclusively) from the influenza, for example, Norway, whose neutrality meant its young did not die in war. In South Africa, 56 per cent of the recorded mortality fell in the age range twenty to forty-four (Phillips 1990a: 168). Such a proportion of the mortality falling upon the young adult sector is a universal characteristic of the epidemic. This is true even where the introduction of the virus was much delayed and the pandemic played out differently, for example in Australia (Figure 4.5). Britain, despite having an epidemic that peaked later than much of western Europe, the United States and even New Zealand and South Africa, again saw the young adult population bear the brunt of the pandemic's mortality. Once more there is the characteristic 'W' age–mortality curve, the peaks coming in the young and the old with a massive spike in the middle covering the young adult age brackets (Figures 4.6 and 4.7). This pattern is found consistently whether examining numbers of deaths by age, proportions of total mortality by age, or death rates (Figure 4.8).

The basic statistics led the Ministry of Health to conclude that 'the mortality in England and Wales, as a whole, attributable directly or indirectly, to influenza, is without any precedent in magnitude . . . the toll taken at the young adult ages of life is without any know [*sic*] West European or North American precedent' (Ministry of Health 1920c: 40). Similarly, in Scotland, the RG there wrote that the 'most conspicuous feature of this distribution is the great frequency of death at the younger adult ages, 20 to 40' (Registrar-

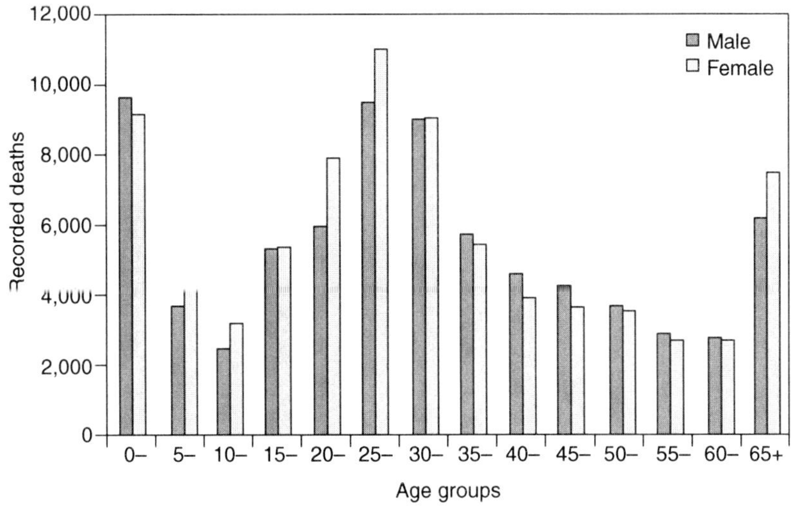

Figure 4.6 Age distribution of pandemic mortality, England and Wales 1918–19 (sources: Registrar-General 1920, *ARRG* 1918 and 1919).

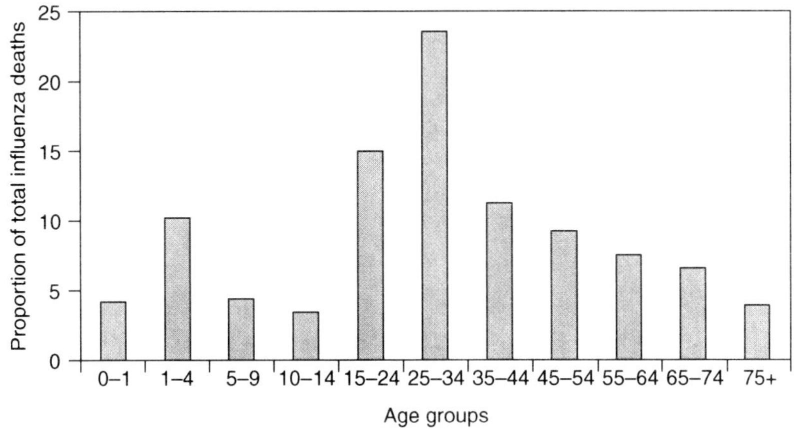

Figure 4.7 Age distribution of pandemic mortality, Scotland 1918 (source: Registrar-General for Scotland 1920).

General for Scotland 1919: 8). Indeed, that report goes on to note that 'fully 50 per cent. [of the mortality occurred] between ages 15 and 44' (1919: 12). During the last quarter of 1918, mortality among women aged twenty-five to thirty in England and Wales was almost 600 times higher than the average for that quarter over the previous four years (Reid 2005: 32). It can be readily appreciated how dramatic the change in this distribution of

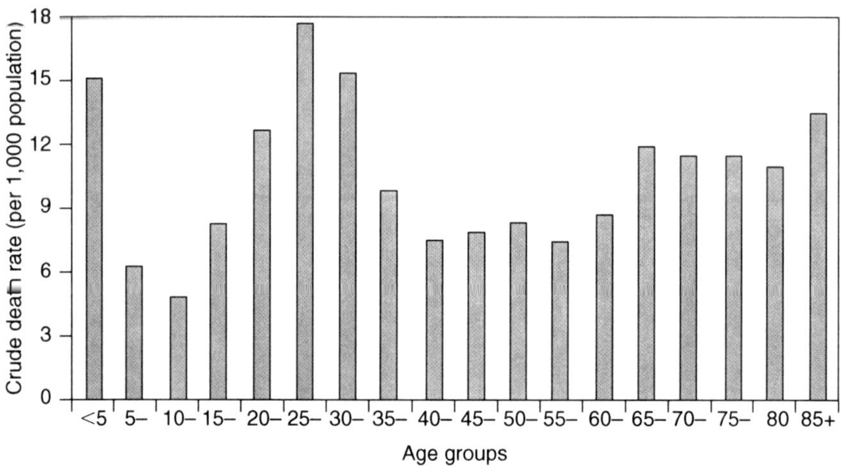

Figure 4.8 Female influenza mortality, England and Wales (source: Registrar-General, 1920: 8).

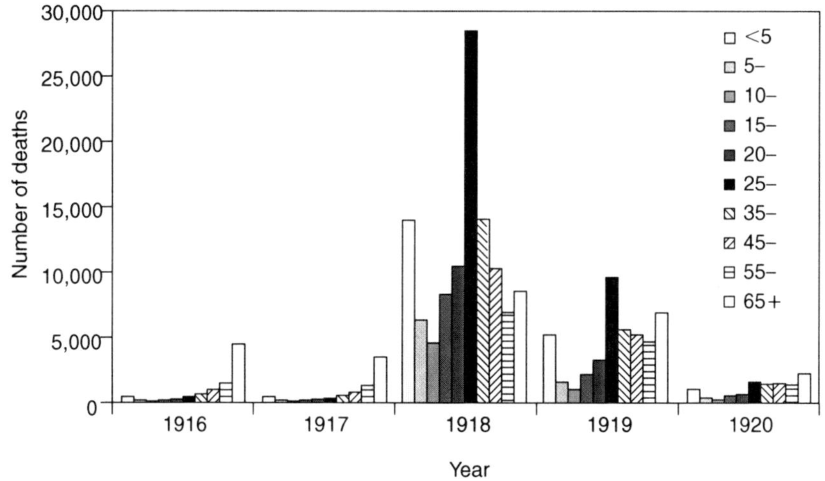

Figure 4.9 Age structure of influenza mortality, England and Wales 1916–20 (source: *ARRG* 1916–20).

mortality is when it is displayed graphically and Figure 4.9 shows the age distribution of influenza mortality for 1916 to 1920. These figures are dominated by 1918, and to a lesser extent 1919, both in terms of the scale of mortality and in the change in the age distribution.

Influenza mortality in England and Wales from 1890 to 1917 exhibited a very consistent age distribution, with mortality restricted to the age extremes, even during the 'Russian' flu epidemic of the early 1890s. The years 1918 and 1919 produced a strikingly different experience. Prior to 1918 there was a distinct predominance of mortality in the under-five and the older age groups. The change between 1917 and 1918 is remarkable, with mortality now concentrated in the young adult age groups (Figure 4.9) and this continued into 1919. However, 1920 showed a more mixed pattern at a much lower level of mortality incidence. Here the young adult mortality was still very important, but mortality among the elderly and young children resumed a more 'normal' share of the total mortality. The changed age distribution of mortality first appeared in the first wave of the pandemic and was disappearing by 1920. It is this pattern of influenza mortality by age that can be used to determine the duration of the pandemic and to confirm that there were three waves of the pandemic in Britain, and that there was not the fourth wave as detected in some countries.

The novelty and scale of the young adult mortality has rather obscured the pandemic's impact on other age groups. Young children and infants are inherently a vulnerable group, and it has been shown that their 'relative mortality . . . increased dramatically' (Reid 2005: 53). Further, the 'supreme dependence' of young children on their parents, particularly their mothers, means that an illness that has a particular impact on young adults may have a very severe follow-on effect for children. Effects can range from influenza in the first or second trimester of pregnancy provoking delivery, leading to greater risk of stillbirth or early death, to the reduction in ability to care for and nourish children (including breast feeding) (Reid 2005). Such factors may have led to many child deaths being attributed to other causes, including 'prematurity', 'wasting' or other causes, and thus the full impact of the pandemic in terms of childhood mortality may be greatly understated (Langford 2002; Reid 2005).

Correlating pandemic influenza mortality and population cohorts in England and Wales reveals the strongest positive correlations with the youngest age groups (male and female 0–4 and 5–9) and the strongest negative associations with the older age groups (all groups above age fifty) (Johnson 2001: 254–7). This may be indicative of the association of young children with dying parents as well as the possible role of children in transmitting the disease, reinforcing suggestions that children are a major risk factor in influenza.[16] It would also support Burnet and Clark's assertion that the highest morbidity rates were among children and adolescents when they claimed that 'curve of age incidence is quite unlike that of mortality. The highest incidence is in children and adolescents' (1942: 81). The fact that the strongest negative correlations are for the age groups above fifty emphasise how this was a pandemic of young adult death. Studies of the excess mortality of the pandemic claimed that there was in fact 'negative excess mortality' among the elderly and attributed this to previous exposure to an 'influenza strain similar to the so-called Spanish influenza' that conferred some degree of immunity (Luk *et al.* 2001: 1375; see also Schoenbaum 2003; Langford 2002). There is some evidence to suggest that this pattern of elevated young adult mortality was seen in the epidemics of 1781–82 and 1890 (Kilbourne 1987: 8; Pyle 1986: 27; Smith 1995). However, it is certainly unusual and has never been recorded to the extent it was to dominate the mortality of this pandemic. Indeed, it has been argued that it is 'in fact, the only satisfactory criterion by which pandemic influenza can be recognized as distinct from the pre-existing influenza of the 1890 epoch' (Burnet and Clark 1942: 69).

Many theories have been put forward as to why the young adults were taken at such a rate, including immunity for the older age groups due to exposure to earlier influenza strains, bacterial infections working symbiotically with the virus, or a particularly virulent strain of the virus that effectively turned the victim's immune system against the host by triggering such high levels of inflammation that the respiratory system was overwhelmed by the body's own defences. There was even a behavioural explanation: that young adults are more prone to trying to keep on working through illness and thereby maximising their risk. Unfortunately none of these theories explain why this pattern was true across all nations and all variables, and how rarely this pattern has been seen before or since. As Crosby was also forced to conclude, 'no completely satisfactory answer to that question has yet been offered – or may ever be offered' (1989: 221). The virus seems to have been unusually pneumotropic and a very significant proportion of the deaths involved secondary bacterial pneumonia or pneumonic complications. But why was it so prevalent on this occasion? And why so fatal for the young adult population of the world? Was it something inherent to the virus? Was it the bacterial complications? Was it something to do with the population? It is unlikely to have been something related to the war as it is a pattern that holds true across belligerent and neutral nations. These questions vex many of those working on the 1918 pandemic and drive their work. For example, the virologists (and others) working on the 'resurrection' of the virus from cadavers and preserved specimens state that one of their goals is determining if there was something in the composition of the virus that made it so virulent (Basler *et al.* 2001; Brownlee and Fodor 2001; Kobasa *et al.* 2004; Duncan 2003; Fanning *et al.* 2002; Gibbs *et al.* 2001; Oxford *et al.* 1999, 2002; Reid *et al.* 2000; Reid and Taubenberger 2003; Taubenberger 1998, 2002; Taubenberger *et al.* 2001; Tumpey *et al.* 2002; Worobey *et al.* 2002).

Variations in mortality

One of the outstanding features of this pandemic was its universality. The commonality of the pandemic across all sorts of boundaries – national, social, racial, climatic – is arresting. The vast majority of diseases, even in times of epidemic and pandemic, are differentiated along such dimensions. The striking feature of all the accounts of this pandemic is how common and universal the experiences are; the experience of illness, the experience of mortality, the actions debated and taken. However, there are some conflicting claims about the mortality. Many suggest that this was a uniform and egalitarian killer, whereas others see variation. For example, the Canadian historian Margaret Andrews argued that while 'Certain groups – gasworks employees and Cornish tin miners – were only lightly touched by the epidemic; others – coal miners and pregnant women – suffered high mortality rates' (Andrews 1977: 24–5). Al Crosby attempted to account for these variations, the apparent correlation between influenza mortality and both pregnancy and coal mining, by noting that 'A pregnant women has one set of lungs to handle the affairs of two bodies, and a coal miner often has something less than a fully efficient set of lungs to handle the affairs of one often overworked body' (Crosby 1989: 227). There do emerge some interesting variations in mortality, but often they are as contentious as they are illuminating. Rather than giving us any great insight into the pandemic and the virus that wrought it, they tend to further cloud the picture. This is due to the fact that they tend to be inconsistent, rarely holding from one location to another.

Nations and peoples

It has been noted that certain nations suffered greatly, including native peoples in Western Samoa,[17] Alaska and Labrador.[18] There is evidence of elevated levels of morbidity and mortality among small, isolated, and often indigenous groups. While high levels of morbidity are not uncommon in influenza epidemics and pandemics, the high mortality levels are unusual. It is worth bearing in mind that, in these relatively small, isolated communities, the disease itself was probably not the sole killer, as Crosby postulated:

> Almost total isolation from humanity and its common respiratory illnesses . . . would have been enough to assure that flu would attack an immunologically defenceless population, that the majority of those infected would fall sick at the same time and the individual illnesses would be quite severe, and that for at least several days few in the infected villages would be healthy enough to provide even the barest necessities of life for the helpless. High morbidity and mortality rates are then to be expected.
>
> (Crosby 1989: 231–2; similarly, see Burnet and Clark 1942: 76)

Thus high levels of morbidity could have rendered so many ill that adequate care could not be maintained and a significant proportion of the fatalities can be attributed to starvation, dehydration and, in some cases, hypothermia. Studies of an earlier epidemic, smallpox in the eighteenth-century Americas, also attributed much of the indigenous mortality to a lack of care, lack of food, customs and behaviours (including sweat bathing and plunging into ice-cold water) as well as the possibilities of a lack of innate, inherited or acquired immunity, or a lack of diversity in that immunity (Fenn 2002: 23–7). These are similar conclusions to those of a study of the 1918 influenza among ethnic minorities in Norway where it was suggested that the 'lack of inherited and acquired immunity' in the Sami people, largely as a consequence of their isolation, saw them endure greater levels of mortality than either the majority Norwegian population or another minority, the Kven people (Mamelund 2003: 83). A lack of immunological awareness of influenza may have played a role in some locations. However, the long history of influenza, the prior existence of pandemics (since at least the eighteenth century), and the centuries of colonial expansion meant few places were genuinely isolated, thereby rendering the possibility of virgin soil outbreaks limited. This has not stopped the question of virgin soil epidemics and also whether the influenza pandemic can be regarded as an 'imperial disease' being debated (Herda 1998; Herring 1994; Herring and Sattenspiel 2003; Kelm 1998; Killingray 1996; Mueller 1998; Musambachime 1998; Page 1998).

These instances of large numbers of indigenous peoples dying in remote locations are not the only reports of ethnic or racial variations in mortality. In South Africa, the black, Indian and 'Coloured' populations all recorded higher influenza mortality rates than the white population, and reasons proposed for this include socio-economic factors or factors related to the social practices, particularly around illness and death, among these various groups (Phillips 1990a: 158–60). These suggestions are similar to those postulated to explain high levels of mortality among the Maori population in New Zealand and across western Polynesia (Pool 1973; Herda 1998). In the USA, certain immigrant communities also exhibited differential mortality, particularly those born in Canada, Austria–Hungary, Poland and Russia, along with Italian–Americans. One interpretation was to conclude that it is probably no more than that

> some groups could afford more spacious quarters than others, and that the most recently arrived groups had a higher proportion of people of the ages most liable to pneumonic complications than groups which had arrived early. Perhaps differences in the customs of the different groups were the cause of the different death rates.
>
> (Crosby 1989: 227–8)

Crosby is left gesturing vaguely in the direction of an undefined set of behavioural and socio-economic factors to explain variations in mortality.

However, the mortality of the Afro-American population in America disputes such a socio-economic dimension to the pandemic's mortality. In examining disease, particularly epidemics, among the urban black population in the USA, David McBride made only brief mention of the 1918–19 influenza, perhaps because it exhibited a differential mortality pattern contrary to almost every other disease (McBride 1991). That is, whereas for many diseases Afro-Americans suffer more than other groups, this was apparently not the case during the influenza pandemic as 'influenza deaths among blacks ran askew of the national patterns for whites' (McBride 1991: 38). This lower influenza mortality occurred even though at the time 'Black Americans, locked in a caste of poverty, invariably have had a much higher death rate from respiratory disease than whites' (Crosby 1989: 229). McBride argues that incidence rates, even after adjustment for sex and age distribution, were consistently lower than those recorded in the white population. Indeed, there are claims that for black males aged twenty to fifty-five and black females aged twenty to forty-five, influenza mortality declined during the pandemic. This contradicted the perceptions of American medical authorities (and the colonial authorities elsewhere in the world) who had long held that non-whites were more susceptible to disease, particularly respiratory disease. However, it may be necessary to treat these figures with a degree of caution, as McBride counsels: 'the sharp jump in deaths among urban blacks shortly following the year of the influenza pandemic may have reflected recording errors in the early reporting on influenza mortality for blacks' (McBride 1991: 38). This is another variation in the mortality caused by the pandemic that displays a complicated pattern and there seems there is little consistency in the impact of race on the mortality experienced. Further, the variations in mortality by race seem more likely to have explanations other than simple biological or epidemiological ones. There may be behavioural, social and/or economic factors that play a role in determining these mortality experiences.

Gender

While it was the young adults who suffered the greatest mortality above all others, there has only been some reporting of any significant variation in mortality by gender. Different locations may have shown a slight difference between the sexes, but these appear not to be significant or consistent. A number of countries appear to report noticeably higher mortality in males than females, including the USA, Australia, New Zealand, Norway and South Africa, most particularly in the non-white populations of New Zealand and South Africa (Australia 1920; Crosby 1989; Mamelund 2006; Phillips 1990a; Rice 1988;). This may be due to recording problems with these data and the male mortality may be overstated relative to the female mortality. Further, in South Africa male mortality was already 'normally' significantly higher than female. This suggests two possibilities – males were dying at a higher rate in early twentieth century South Africa and/or that female mortality was being under-reported. It is quite plausible that both of these occurred. However, this apparent predominance of male mortality is not consistent. Other national figures suggest a more balanced sex ratio in influenza mortality or even a female predominance. Norwegian data suggests a relatively balanced distribution, as does the French, Spanish and Swedish data (Åman 1990; Echeverri 2003; Echeverri Dávila 1993; Norway 1919; Zylberman 2003). In some cases the balance can vary at different age groups, but the general distribution by age is very similar in both males and females.

In England and Wales slightly more female deaths were recorded than male. In the RG's re-calculation of pandemic mortality, some 100,000 female deaths were estimated along with 84,000 male deaths. This figure of approximately 184,000 total deaths was then rounded up to 200,000. Unfortunately, no rates are given for each sex, as the RG recognised that these figures only included civilian deaths and that the base populations for calculating rates, particularly of males, were much disturbed as so many British men were serving in the war effort (Registrar-General 1920: 3–7). This slight predominance of female mortality was also recorded in Scotland, where 52.2 per cent of recorded influenza deaths were of women. There the overall influenza death rate was 4.32 per 1,000, with the female rate being slightly higher at 4.37 per 1,000 and the male rate as 4.26 per 1,000. However, the Registrar-General for Scotland discounted this variation as being insignificant as the

> small observed difference between the male and female death-rates should not be accepted as a reliable indication of influenza having been in fact more fatal in the female population than in the male, for these rates depend on estimated populations, and at present time these estimations are not very reliable, their reliability being reduced by the long period which has now relapsed since the taking of the last census and also by the effect of war conditions on the population being unascertained . . . the two distributions are very similar.
>
> (Registrar-General for Scotland 1919: 10–11)

It has been suggested that in some locations the imbalance may be rather pronounced. For example, in Leicester 'female deaths outnumbered male in the ratio 3:2', but it was recognised that the 'toll of war and the number of men on active service had seriously curtailed the number of males in Leicester during the period in question so that the results are, to some extent, artificial.' While there are 'stories of men returning from the war finding that the brides they had married whilst on leave a few months previously had died in the epidemic', there were undoubtedly cases of men failing to return that were not due to battle mortality, but due to influenza (Wilshere 1986: iii).

It was the loss of so many men that actually attracted attention. In a column in *The Times* titled 'Survival of the unfit', the paper's medical correspondent linked influenza mortality with the losses sustained in the war and the concern for 'national efficiency' (Winter 1980). The influenza link largely stemmed from the impression that those young men dying were those of apparently better, stronger condition. Arguing that between them the war and the flu had killed 'some 18,000,000 young men' and 'rendered at least another 10,000,000 . . . incapable of earning a living, and so unable or unwilling to marry', these two events had 'gathered the flower of the world's young manhood'. The correspondent suggested that young women withstood the pandemic better, claiming that they had not been crowded together in camps, had 'not been exposed to the same hardships' and had 'fewer calls upon their powers of resistance' due to apparently being 'less exposed to infection'. Most of these are untenable assertions and the fact that more women died in Britain itself than men undermines these arguments. The article went on to conclude that the surviving men and, to a lesser extent, women are the 'poorer' specimens and they will only beget 'poor' children, and it is imperative that the nation care for the children of soldiers and sailors (24 February 1919: 10).

'Woe unto them that are with child'

This focus on male mortality, even where female mortality was actually higher, rather obscured an important component of the female mortality – the deaths of pregnant women. Influenza mortality levels can be considerably higher among pregnant women, often associated with abortion, miscarriage and/or stillbirth (Bourne 1922; Graham 1996; Kendal and Glezen 1998; MacKenzie and Houghton 1974; Phillips 1990a: 173–4; Stuart-Harris *et al.* 1985; Underwood 1984). Ed Kilbourne has argued that pregnant women may actually 'be peculiarly vulnerable to influenza' (Kilbourne 1987: 162–3), and the impact of pregnancy on the health of women in relation to influenza has been much debated (for example, Bourne 1922; Graham 1996; Kendal and Glezen 1998; MacKenzie and Houghton 1974). It was noted by various contemporaneous authors that there appeared to be high(er) levels of mortality among pregnant women, along with increased rates of abortion and miscarriage (Registrar-General 1920; Registrar-General for Scotland 1919), and pregnant women exhibited higher hospitalisation and mortality than non-pregnant women in the pandemics of 1957 and 1968. The mechanism for this is uncertain but it is suggested that 'susceptibility in pregnancy is related to hemodynamic changes' as the risk apparently increases as pregnancy proceeds. The increase in cardiac stroke volume as both blood volume and stroke volume increase during pregnancy may also play a role (Kilbourne 1987: 162–3). Other mechanisms may include reduced functional capacity of the lungs or PAIDS ('pregnancy associated immunodeficiency syndrome' – the immunosuppression necessary so as not to reject the foetus) (Reid 2005: 33).

Given this pandemic targeted young adults, the impact on pregnant women, who tend to be in those age groups, was potentially critical, and this vulnerability was recognised during the pandemic (Collier 1974; Kendal and Glezen 1998; Phillips 1990a; Starr 1976; Underwood 1984). The New South Wales Parliament heard that pregnant women admitted to the 'influenza hospitals in Sydney' had a 26.7 per cent mortality rate. The pregnant women hospitalised in Sydney also showed increases in premature births (forty-six of 224 cases with twenty-one deaths of the mother), and miscarriages (twenty-one with eight maternal deaths). Of the forty-one hospitalised women recorded as completing the full term of pregnancy, nine died with only twenty-nine of the babies surviving (New South Wales 1920). An item in the 'Annotations' column of *The Lancet* in October 1919 suggests that the situation in Sydney hospitals was not as bad as that experienced in Paris where, among pregnant women at the Paris Maternité Hôpitale, the mortality rate was 16 per cent. The mortality was even worse among the 73 per cent that developed pulmonary complications, with 58.4 per cent of those cases succumbing as opposed to only 5 per cent of those without pulmonary complications. In the pulmonary cases premature delivery occurred in 17 per cent of cases, with more than 50 per cent fatality. Miscarriages occurred in 6 per cent of the pulmonary cases with a 75 per cent fatality rate. As the item notes; '"Woe unto them that are with child," might have been written of this influenza epidemic' (*Lancet* 18 October 1919: 699). Similarly, Norway saw a 'significant increase . . . in both the spontaneous abortion rate . . . and the stillbirth rate' (Mamelund 2004: 244).

Bourne, writing just a few years after the pandemic, was convinced of the deleterious nature of the combination of pregnancy and influenza and noted that, in the epidemics of 1892 and 1918, 'pregnancy seriously prejudice[d] the prognosis and the influenza is a potent influence in causing abortion and premature labour' (Bourne 1922: 433). Pregnant women contracting influenza were apparently more likely to suffer a fatal outcome if they aborted or went into premature labour. Mortality due to influenza and pneumonia amongst pregnant women who did not abort or enter premature labour was still high. While influenza did not necessarily stimulate abortion or premature labour, Bourne considers the RG's figures 'afford positive evidence that evacuation of the uterus occurred very frequently in fatal influenza during the period . . . it seems that non-fatal influenza is by no means so frequently associated with abortion' (Bourne 1922: 436). This evacuation of the uterus was most notable in the 'cyanotic patient' (Bourne 1922: 437).

The deaths of more than 2,500 pregnant women were reported in Scotland, England and Wales, and these are only those deaths where the fact of pregnancy was recorded.[19] It is not possible to quantify the deaths of pregnant women who were not recorded as such. These could well be a significant number: as the RG noted, 'it seems probable that mention of pregnancy may have been omitted in many cases where the illness [influenza] was not complicated by confinement' (Registrar-General 1920: 36). Bourne suggests that under-recording of pregnancy in influenza cases would have been most common among those 'in early pregnancy, and when the patient has died without abortion' (Bourne 1922: 439–40). Somewhat contrarily, the RG also suggested that the largely unchanged mortality of premature infants and the only slightly lower than normal birth rate for 1918 indicated that a large number of births had not been lost (Registrar-General 1920: 37). At the same time, the RG had stated that puerperal mortality associated with the pandemic was far more likely to be attributed to abortion or 'other accidents of childbirth' than usual, and that these 'accidents' of pregnancy and childbirth were largely influenza. While recognising the limitations of the data and the very real likelihood that a proportion of pregnant women who died were not recorded as being pregnant, the RG has suggested that pregnant women may have had a death rate from influenza of 5.3–5.7 per 1,000 in England and Wales, only marginally higher than the rate for all women of the selected ages, of 4.9 per 1,000, and that 'pregnancy did not materially affect the risk of death from influenza, but fatal influenza led to abortion or premature delivery' (Registrar-General 1920: 36). In Scotland, the 266 recorded deaths of women from 'diseases and accidents of pregnancy and child-birth in association with influenza' constituted 2.9 per cent of the total recorded female influenza deaths at 'a death-rate of 13 per 100,000 of the female population' (Registrar-General for Scotland 1919: 11). However, this rate relates to the entire female population, not that of the 'population at risk' (the pregnant female population). It does not allow us to determine if influenza had a notably deleterious effect on pregnant women or if they perished in much the same proportion as the rest of the population.

Bourne, however, calculated that influenza had a major impact on the death rate from abortion. The death rate from spontaneous abortion in 1917 was 0.16 per 1,000 or 'one in 6,302 pregnancies' but during the pandemic 'the rate works out at one death from influenza-abortion in 624 pregnancies' or 1.60 per 1,000 and this is 'about ten times that of the death-rate from abortion in a normal year, and yet refers only to those cases of death from abortion plus influenza, omitting the deaths from abortion uncomplicated by influenza' (Bourne 1922: 437). As the RG conceded, such figures 'clearly demonstrate that fatal influenza very frequently led to abortion or miscarriage' (Registrar-General 1920: 36), yet this is not limited to fatal cases as it is likely that influenza would be responsible for a great many non-fatal spontaneous abortions (Reid 2005: 34), and 'it can be gathered what an enormous incidence of abortion there was due to influenza alone' (Bourne 1922: 437). Foetal loss and premature deliveries would have led to yet higher numbers of stillbirths and premature live births. So if women were not specifically at a greater risk from influenza than men, pregnant women and the children they were carrying certainly were.

Socio-economic dimensions

A number of the dimensions along which there may have been variations in mortality can be argued to have a socio-economic basis or component. For example, racial differences may be more an expression of socio-economic realities rather than biological ones. Those racial groups excluded from the mainstream of society are also excluded from the mainstream economic and social spheres, and exclusion from one sphere is compounded by exclusion from the others. Similarly, regional variations determined by hierarchies and networks may be a reflection of the social and economic structures that determine the nature of those hierarchies and networks. Better-off areas may have coped better with the pandemic. They may not have avoided the disease, and morbidity may have been relatively uniform, but due to their greater wealth they may have been better informed about the danger and/or healthcare opportunities, had better health resources, and survived at a positive differential. Additionally the existing state of health, housing and access to healthcare could be significant in determining the impact of an epidemic disease. In previous influenza epidemics there had been a recognition that there were such variations in mortality. For example, in 1847 the 'epidemic was much more fatal in some districts of London than in others . . . influenza killed twice as many people in the insalubrious parts of London as it did in those less unhealthy (Tenth *ARRG* 1847: xxix–xxx).

The relationship between socio-economic factors and disease has been a focus for much research, and a portion of this has been influenced by structuralist or ideological approaches. Such explanations have been applied to the 1918–19 influenza pandemic, for example Zhdanov *et al.* (1958). They presented a compelling, if ideologically driven, argument for the role and nature of society in determining the pattern of influenza epidemics. This position is based on accepting that at the end of the nineteenth century there was an 'essential change . . . in the character of the epidemic process' as the 1889 to 1890s pandemics were followed by an increase in influenza morbidity that persisted until 1918, apparently indicating that influenza was essentially endemic. This argument claimed that the 'new' form of 'epidemic process' became characteristic in 'all the countries with a temperate climate' as a direct consequence of what they regarded as the 'completion' of the 'development of the capitalistic economy'. This 'completion' brought with it the 'spread of railroads, the appearance of mechanized water transportation, the extension of international trade and the growth of the population in cities through the creation of large industrial centres' which all changed the 'form of communication between people and had a decisive influence on the spread of the influenzal infection' (Zhdanov *et al.* 1958, in translation, 1960: 650–2). This view could be interpreted as supporting the hierarchical hypothesis of influenza spread as the hierarchical nature of society and the connections between locations governed by the economic model upon which society is built, and the development of the (capitalist) economy with its railroads and urbanisation of population to drive the capitalist machinery, materially determined the spread of disease.

While some specific respiratory conditions (and respiratory infections in general) have been argued to have strong relationships with the social and economic setting, this has generally not been the case with influenza. Influenza is generally regarded as an egalitarian disease – classless and 'colour-blind'. One of the few opposing suggestions came in an examination of the 1976 'swine flu' scare in the USA where it was claimed that influenza is 'almost twice as common among poor adults as the affluent, and age-adjusted death rates for influenza and pneumonia are about 50 per cent higher among nonwhites than whites' (Dutton 1988: 298). Additionally, work on the role of children has shown their important role in the dissemination of the disease and that younger children from lower-income households displayed greater risk of infection than the pre-school children of middle-income families (Frank *et al.* 1983; Glezen 1980; Glezen *et al.* 1980; Schoenbaum 2003).

Thus there are some suggestions that influenza may exhibit some socio-economic variation. Was this true of the 1918–19 pandemic? Or was the level of infection so great that it overwhelmed any barrier to the disease? Tomkins is not alone in claiming that 'the epidemic was remarkably democratic in its victims' (Tomkins 1992a: 446). One commentator, writing in the 1920s, offered that it was 'a matter of common knowledge that the pandemic . . . affected all classes of the population irrespective of their social and economic status, or even of their personal vigour and physique', but wonders if any class suffered solely because of their economic status. However, he noted that researchers who had considered the 'social and industrial dislocations' caused by the war-time conditions were 'in some degree responsible' for the pandemic had concluded that there was no evidence to support the view that economic status materially affected the intensity of the pandemic (Gill 1928: 276). Considering Gill was advocating an environmentally deterministic view, it is not surprising that he enlisted the work of a number of MOHs that provided evidence suggesting there was no link with deprivation. Arguing that the number of persons per room 'affords an index of the economic condition of the occupants' (as well as of overcrowding), he stated that various investigations in Britain found that the 'attack rate, in tenements occupied by more than one person per room, was not appreciably greater than it was in houses in which there was less than one person per room' (Gill 1928: 277).[20] Mamelund has argued that, in the case of Kristiania (Oslo), not only did the working class exhibit higher mortality than the bourgeois and middle class, but also claims that social factors at the individual level, particularly as demonstrated by dwelling size, affects mortality (Mamelund 2006).

Socio-economic dimensions investigated in Britain, and found to show little association with influenza mortality, included over-crowding, including measurements of number of persons per dwelling, persons per room and other aspects of 'bad housing' (Ministry of Health 1920c: 164–72). Crowding may not have been such an issue as the virus was so virulent and infective that the 'necessary exposures and contacts of all persons living under urban conditions are sufficiently numerous to provide opportunities of transfer so effective that any increase above the average is relatively a factor of negligible order' (Ministry of Health 1920c: 171). While Crosby argued that, on occasion, there was a 'discernible correlation between flu, pneumonic complications, and crowded living conditions' with implications for the poor who live in more crowded housing than the more affluent, he concluded that in the pandemic 'the rich died as readily as the poor' (Crosby 1989: 228). Thus, if there is a socio-economic dimension to flu mortality it seems a minor contributory factor.

Certainly, in South Africa, the influence of poverty, hygiene and sanitation were regarded as important and much of the press coverage was given over to 'accounts of the dank, insanitary and over-crowded living conditions' (Phillips 1990a: 143) in the slums from where flu apparently was spread to the 'better' areas. Even the medical authorities considered that while the slums had not caused the pandemic, 'there was no doubt that they had materially assisted in its dissemination' (Phillips 1990a: 215). The British press certainly considered sanitation, both of the city and the individual, to be very important in the spread of the disease. In late October 1918, *The Times* claimed that it 'has frequently insisted upon the need for more thorough cleansing of our cities, the more efficient removal of refuse from houses and the more careful washing of streets. It has also demanded a pure milk supply', and claimed that if their warnings had been heeded and acted upon, then the situation would not have been so dire. However, it does not claim that these measures would have slowed the influenza, but rather that the 'influenza victims would not have been so liable to get additional infection.' Moreover, *The Times*' intent was to have a scapegoat as the 'real meaning of the present calamity is that steps must be taken to make somebody answerable for the nation's health. It will then be possible to bring home neglect and lack of foresight to those responsible for them' (28 October 1918: 6).[21]

The need for better sanitation and for some form of national health body were arguments that *The Times* returned to. A story on the influenza was the pretext for a story run with the sub-heading 'Danger of insanitary houses' which argued that inspections of dwellings were necessary for public health as an 'insanitary house is always dangerous' and, given the reduction in immunity allegedly caused by the influenza, they were now even more dangerous. This required 'a really competent sanitary survey of the country' that had to be performed by a national body so as to avoid local difficulties or failures. The medical correspondent for *The Times* argued that 'Sanitary science has become a branch, a most important branch, of preventive medicine', a position Newsholme at the LGB would almost certainly have endorsed (4 November 1918: 5).[22] As the second wave of the pandemic subsided, *The Times* argued that with more widespread use of masks and isolation along with better sanitation 'prevention . . . was no impossibility' and that if the authorities had warned people adequately they would have been happy to take these measures. This article claimed the pneumonias that killed so many were the consequence of poor sanitation and that the 'coming Ministry of Health should be given powers to deal with this matter' (19 December 1918: 5).

Sanitation was not just an issue for a future Ministry to contend with, but was also to be a personal issue. Reporting on a conference on 'Influenza and its Prevention', *The Times* noted that a speaker who advocated that 'persons who in an omnibus or tube coughed without putting up their hands, or sneezed without putting up their handkerchiefs, should be prosecuted for indecency' was greeted with laughter and cheers. Another speaker, Dr Hector MacKenzie, brought in not only the moralising attitudes but also the class dimension when he claimed that oral hygiene was important as he suggested that the 'great majority of the working people were wholly negligent of the hygiene of the mouth, and the men looked upon the use of the tooth-brush as effeminacy. Such neglect was responsible for an enormous amount of disease' (1 March 1919: 7). MacKenzie's attitude is actually rather unusual as influenza was so pervasive it could not so readily be attributed to individual failing, sin or other (mis)behaviour. Despite this, *The Times* was still looking for a role for sanitation in the influenza pandemic when reviewing the Ministry of Health's 1920 report on the subject. Noting that the report suggested that 'the war so altered conditions', particularly 'insalubrious' conditions that allowed for the modification of either the 'invading parasites' or of the 'natural resistance', it recognised that the Ministry was hedging its bets in also suggesting the disease 'manifested itself alike in crowded and insanitary areas and in districts where the conditions of life are normally favourable to health' (2 February 1919: 7 and 11).

An examination of the flu in a Canadian city attempted to establish if there was any relationship between the socio-economic status of the victims and the excessive mortality seen in the pandemic (Johnson 1998: 59–63, based on Johnson 1993) by raising questions such as whether those who died tended to come from any particular socio-economic class, and whether certain occupations and/or workplaces were more hazardous than others. Were the deceased spread evenly throughout the community or were certain groups or areas over-represented? There are many aspects of the human condition relating to socio-economics that could usefully be examined, including housing, occupation and income, but the limitations of existing data impinge heavily. Furthermore, could lifestyle have contributed to mortality? Could their occupations, their workplaces, their places of entertainment or their living conditions have contributed to their demise? While density, measured by population per lot, showed only a very weak association with mortality, the examination of occupations and the influenza mortality in the city of Kitchener, Ontario, was of particular interest as occupation is a major component in determining income, socio-economic status and social class. This led to questions of how occupations, particularly manufacturing-related positions, impacted upon influenza mortality. Were the factories prime locations for the contraction and transmission of the disease, thus leading to increased morbidity and mortality among manufacturing workers? Or did employee care programmes ameliorate the disease's impact and contribute to a lower than expected mortality experience for employees? The negative impact of the factories was obvious in the rolls of the dead, particularly in relation to their occupations, or the occupations of their immediate family, but the Kitchener manufacturers adopted a paternalistic attitude to their workforce, ensuring their workers' health to ensure the health of the company. This was achieved by providing home nursing care, offering to voluntarily suspend the operations of factories, and placing advertisements advising their employees what to do in case of illness and that they should only return to work when 'sufficiently recovered' (*Kitchener News-Record* 10 October 1918: 1). Comparing the known occupations of the victims or their spouse or parent(s) with that of the total labour force it is apparent that those employed in manufacturing may actually have died at a lesser rate than might be expected, as they comprised only 44.32% of deaths (where occupation was known) whereas manufacturing employed 57.0% of the 1921 workforce (Johnson 1998: 63). This may reflect the efficacy of the home nursing service, factory closures and delaying of the return to work that many of the factories in Kitchener adopted, thereby mitigating the possibly more deleterious effects of working in factories and less affluent urban life.

In Australia 'wealth offered no absolute protection' but there was a 'degree of social gradient to the epidemic', with the lower mortality levels among professional and commercial groups and higher rates in lower-status occupations, such as 'labourer'. The 'primary producers' on the farms actually recorded some of the lowest levels of mortality, again supporting the view that areas up the urban hierarchy may have suffered worst and that isolation had its benefits. While it is very difficult to identify the 'actual mechanisms by which occupational mortality differentials emerge', and in some instances these may be the result of direct 'on-the-job risk factors', in others it is a reflection of more general lifestyle and socio-economic factors that can be expressed through housing quality and density, nutritional status and general health status (McCracken and Curson 2003: 123–5).

While much of the analysis of the pandemic and socio-economic factors has been at best ambivalent, there were some commentators who argued that there was a variation in mortality based on socio-economic variations. The County Medical Officer and School Medical Officer for the County of London, William Hamer, certainly believed that 'total mortality . . . was conditioned by the social class of the population' (Hamer 1918: 8). However, the RG did not share Hamer's conviction. The RG's report into the pandemic examined the putative link between influenza mortality and both general health standards (as indicated by the average general death rate for 1911–14) and wealth (indicated by the proportion of indoor domestic servants in 1911) in the London Boroughs (Registrar-General 1920: 27–30). The Registrar-General's comparisons (Table 4.2), with the correlation coefficients, coefficients of determination and the Spearman rank correlation coefficients (and z-scores and alpha values) between these two factors and the annualised influenza death rate (Table 4.3), indicate only a moderate associ-

Table 4.2 Influenza mortality and health and wealth indicators, London

Epidemic death rate and health and wealth indicators			
Borough	*Health factor*	*Wealth factor*	*Epidemic death rate*
Kensington	13.6	15.74	3.4
City of London	15.1	5.83	3.8
Hampstead	11.1	16.06	3.9
Hammersmith	14.1	3.14	3.9
Lewisham	10.8	5.65	4.1
Stoke Newington	12.5	4.95	4.3
Wandsworth	11.2	5.55	4.4
Stepney	16.8	1.30	4.4
Lambeth	14.2	3.08	4.7
St Marylebone	14.8	11.64	4.7
Deptford	14.7	2.61	4.8
Paddington	13.2	9.70	4.9
Woolwich	13.2	2.76	4.9
Fulham	13.9	3.29	4.9
Hackney	13.7	2.91	5.0
Islington	14.6	2.44	5.0
Camberwell	13.6	2.63	5.1
Southwark	17.9	1.19	5.1
Westminster	13.5	12.24	5.2
Shoreditch	19.7	0.87	5.2
Greenwich	13.9	4.04	5.4
Poplar	17.1	1.16	5.4
Bethnal Green	16.9	0.75	5.5
Finsbury	18.9	1.21	5.5
Holborn	15.8	4.15	5.6
Bermondsey	17.8	0.94	5.6
Battersea	13.7	2.50	5.8
Chelsea	13.9	13.07	6.1
St Pancras	15.4	2.97	6.2

Source: Registrar-General 1920: 28–9, Tables XIII and XIV.

Table 4.3 Influenza mortality and health and wealth indicator correlations

	r	r^2	r_s	*z-score*	*α value*
Health factor	0.435	0.190	0.455	2.407	0.8%
Wealth factor	–0.367	0.135	–0.451	–2.388	0.9%

ation between the annualised influenza mortality rate and these 'health' and 'wealth' factors.[23]

The RG concluded that the 'mortality of the late epidemic fell almost alike on the sanitarily just and on the unjust' (Registrar-General 1920: 29), yet the correlation between wealthy/healthy places and low influenza mortality is distinct even though the direct effect accounts for an elevation of no more than a quarter of the rate of influenza mortality. It is noteworthy that while the two wealthiest boroughs, Hampstead and Kensington, had lower influenza mortality rates, the third wealthiest, Chelsea, is second only to St Pancras with an influenza death rate for the entire pandemic period of 6.1 per 1,000. A similar attempt to correlate existing health of the population, measured by the standard death rates for 1911–14, with the pandemic mortality (death rate for each wave) was made in the Ministry of Health's report into the pandemic, and also gave inconclusive results (Ministry of Health 1920c: 48–9). Patterns of flu mortality did not always mirror those of prevailing mortality or wealth. In London the associations were only moderate, whereas in France they were contradictory. In Nancy mortality and socio-economic status 'overlapped' as the flu 'attacked the poorer classes and neighbourhoods more aggressively' (Zylberman 2003: 198–9). Yet in Paris flu hit the affluent seventeenth *arrondissement* harder than the poorer and densely populated thirteenth. This has been attributed to the proportion of servant-keeping households in Paris and, while servants are an indicator of wealth, the servants, many of them single young women, lived in overcrowded poverty, dwelling in 'cramped, wretched rooms on the top of densely populated floors of bourgeois buildings'. Indeed, it is claimed that 'one-quarter of all women who died of the flu in Paris were maids' (Zylberman 2003: 199).

In order to investigate the possible relationship between pandemic mortality and socio-economic status in Britain, a database linking the annualised pandemic influenza mortality rate for 335 administrative areas in England and Wales to the infant mortality rates for 1911 and 1918, the demographic structure (male and female populations by age groups), and the occupational structure (male and female populations by occupational categories) along with an occupational environment classification developed by the University of Cambridge's Group for the History of Population and Social Structure (Garrett and Reid 1995; Garrett *et al.* 2001) was constructed. These data came from the Censuses of 1911 and 1921, *ARRG*s and the RG's report (Registrar-General 1920). Initial investigation of the 1911 and 1921 occupational data and the influenza mortality rates revealed only a small number of potentially important relationships and were the basis for selecting variables for further analysis (Johnson 2001: 285–8). For the 1921 data the Cambridge Group had categorised each administrative area into one of four 'environments': agricultural, light, staple or service, based on the predominant occupational categories in the census (Garrett and Reid 1995: 76). All the stronger positive correlations with flu mortality came from either the staple or light categories, with the staple category itself being among the stronger correlations (both for the male and total populations). Furthermore, the strongest negative correlation coefficients were with occupations classified as 'service' by the Cambridge Group. The following variables were selected for further analysis:

- percentage of the working male population in occupations classified as 'staple' in 1921.
- percentage of the working male population in occupations classified as 'service' in 1921.
- percentage of the working male population in occupations classified as 'ships and boats' in 1911.
- proportion of domestic servants per 1,000 households in 1911.
- infant mortality rate (1911).
- population density from the 1921 census.

These six variables can be said to act as indicators of factors such as social class (occupations and proportion of domestic staff), existing health conditions (IMR), crowding or risk of infection or even place in the national urban hierarchy (density), and proximity to points of entry of the disease (shipping). Placing the six variables in a linear regression analysis to test the contribution or relation to influenza mortality produced a correlation coefficient (r) of 0.5110 and a determination coefficient (r^2) of 0.2612. Thus the hypothesis that existing health standards, proximity to ports, and social class determine influenza mortality was not clearly demonstrated. However, there may be a role for these factors as they may influence the outcome to a degree. The analysis was then re-run, progressively removing the least significant variable at each stage. These suggested that the IMR and proportion of domestic servants contributed little or simply complemented other variables (possibly the service and staple occupational variables) (Table 4.4).

Examination of the outliers or residuals from the regression analysis saw a small number of centres emerge as outliers on more than one variable.[24] For example, when examining the results of regression of the service and staple variables with the influenza mortality rate, Hebburn, Jarrow and Tottenham emerge. It seems likely that these two variables (service and staple) are acting as different perspectives on the same dimensions. They have similar correlation levels but work in opposite directions. Hebburn and Jarrow are notable in that they recorded two of the highest influenza mortality rates, with annualised values of 11.94 (the highest recorded) and 8.77. They also have 'staple' values well above the mean (the mean being 27.29 and their values being 49.83 and 42.96 respectively, and the third quartile at 43.18) while the 'service' proportion of the male workforce is very low (mean 36.27, Hebburn 13.19 and Jarrow 20.05). Tottenham's values are almost exactly the reverse of these with influenza mortality at 4.64 (the mean being 4.86), 'staple' 10.98 and 'service'

Table 4.4 Regression analysis results

Variable removed (number of variables used)		r	r^2	*Reduction in* r^2
None	(6)	0.5110	0.2612	N/A
Proportion domestic servants	(5)	0.5046	0.2546	0.0066
IMR	(4)	0.5029	0.2529	0.0017
Density	(3)	0.4620	0.2135	0.0394
Service	(2)	0.4582	0.2100	0.0035
Staple	(1)	0.3704	0.1307	0.0713

45.45. The two Tyneside towns, Hebburn and Jarrow, not only recorded high influenza mortality levels, but they also have the highest proportion of the 1911 male workforce employed in 'ships and boats'.

Barnsley and Chesterfield emerge as outliers when examining the results of linear regression of the IMR and the 'ships and boats' variables with the influenza mortality rate. The shipping variable emerges as both of these have very low values for the proportion of the male workforce employed in that sector while having above-average influenza mortality (Barnsley 8.35 influenza rate and 0.01 shipping; Chesterfield 7.55, nil). With regard to IMR, both these centres returned high values, 206 and 177 respectively, while the mean IMR is 133.39, and the third quartile falls at 153.00. The other notable outlier on the IMR–influenza regression is Gainsborough where the influenza mortality was 8.19 (mean 4.86, third quartile 5.53) but the IMR was only 118 (mean 133.39).

The four centres identified in the examination of the proportion of domestic servants all have values above both the mean and the third quartile (161.59 and 206.50) while their influenza mortality figures vary quite markedly. They are (with the proportion of domestics and influenza mortality in brackets) Winchester (322, 2.5), Torquay (383, 4.18), Chelsea (544, 6.05) and Westminster (545, 5.24), with the two London boroughs recording both very high levels of servants and mortality (running counter to the regression line). But while these two urban boroughs showed up as unusual in that analysis, they did not do so when population density was examined. Indeed only one London borough (Stepney) emerged here, where the density was 78.50 (mean 22.57, third quartile 26.00) and influenza mortality was 6.20 (mean 4.86, third quartile 5.53). The other outliers (Taunton and Ilkeston) showed no such consistency with lower densities (16.70 and 12.80) paired with varying influenza mortality (2.72 and 6.33). Thus, there are no consistently emerging outliers and those that do emerge do so because of specific factors bearing on each variable.

One of the few variables to exhibit a stronger association with the annualised influenza mortality rate was the proportion of the 1911 male workforce in 'Ships and boats'. It was also noted that Hebburn and Jarrow had emerged as residuals from the analysis of other variables and these two locations had the highest proportion of the male workforce in this sector. Furthermore, it had been reported in Australia that one of the highest death rates was among those males employed in occupations classified 'Seas, Rivers, Harbours' (McCracken and Curson 2003: 124). To investigate this further in the data from England and Wales, the areas were separated into two groups, those with no male workers in the sector and those with. While in the group of areas where there were no males employed in this sector, the mean and median influenza mortality are slightly lower and the maximum and first quartile also lower than in the other group (areas with male employment in this sector), the minimum, third quartile and standard deviation are all higher (Table 4.5). The Mann–Whitney U-test was then used to determine whether these two groups differed significantly or if they essentially came from the same population and this indicated that, at a 95% confidence level, the two groups can be regarded as similar and that the presence or absence of shipping as a source of male employment did not materially influence the outcome of the influenza pandemic at the local level (Johnson 2004b).

So is there a socio-economic dimension to influenza mortality? While influenza mortality in the pandemic was spread across the entire community, it does appear that there may be an element of class differential in this mortality, but this is not a particularly strong association. As the RG's decennial supplement claimed, influenza varies 'definitely, though not greatly, with social class' (Registrar-General, 1921 Census, Part II. Occupational Mortality, Fertility, and Infant Mortality: xvii).[25]

While there may be an element of social variation in influenza mortality it has also been suggested that some occupations in particular experienced a mortality differential. For example, miners have been nominated as a group who suffered disproportionately high mortality (Andrews 1977: 24–5; Crosby 1989: 227).[26] Mamelund has suggested that not only were miners particularly hard-hit, but so too were fishermen and soldiers (Mamelund 1998b). However, it is notable that, in the analysis of occupations and

Table 4.5 Comparison of influenza mortality between groups

Influenza mortality values	*Male workforce in 'Ships and boats'*	*No male workers in 'Ships and boats'*
N	277	56
Minimum	1.880	2.093
Maximum	11.943	7.548
Mean	4.892	4.675
Standard deviation	1.217	1.339
1st quartile	4.061	3.707
Median	4.726	4.679
3rd quartile	5.530	5.584

mortality in England and Wales, fishing, defence and mining categories did not exhibit a strong correlation with influenza mortality (Johnson 2001). Categories that did emerge as having higher correlation with influenza mortality included those working with metals, and this coincides with what the RG found and reported in the *Decennial Supplement*. In suggesting that the highest rates are generally among those whose work involves 'exposure to dust or other respiratory risk', it was found that the highest figures came from 'cutlery grinders, brass foundry furnacemen and labourers, cotton strippers and grinders, iron miners underground, file cutters and slate masons'. Thus, people whose working life led to compromised or impaired respiratory systems as 'conditions lowering pulmonary resistance must increase . . . mortality' (Registrar-General, 1921 Census, Part II. Occupational Mortality, Fertility, and Infant Mortality: xvii). However, one must be careful not to overstate this coincidence as the comparison here is between 'ecological' correlations and class-specific death rates. The other occupations that were noted as suffering disproportionately were the medical ones, doctors and nurses. However, they do not emerge from the analysis of occupational categories as they were subsumed into the professional and service categories that actually bore a slightly reduced mortality. The RG's decennial supplement, in discussing influenza mortality for 1921–23, reported that the only 'Class I' occupation with a higher than average influenza mortality was that of medical practitioner, with the rather obvious conclusion that 'plainly influenza is a very definite occupational risk for the doctor' (Registrar-General, 1921 Census, Part II. Occupational Mortality, Fertility, and Infant Mortality: xvii).

But not all occupations conferred a penalty; indeed some were supposed to confer a degree of protection. Captain A. Gregor convinced the MRC that an investigation of his belief that workers exposed to gases and fumes actually seemed to benefit from an apparent disinfectant effect on the nasopharnyx was warranted (PRO FD 1 530 and FD 1 531).[27] Gregor claimed that it was an accepted medical fact that workers exposed to gaseous fumes 'consider themselves practically immune from nasal catarrh and respiratory diseases in general' and that in some parts of Britain it was customary to take children with whooping cough to gas works to expose them to the fumes given off by the 'oxide of iron purifiers during the process of cleansing' as this was considered to mitigate attacks. He then attempted to demonstrate the prophylactic powers of gases and fumes by comparing morbidity figures for a number of groups, including a navy patrol, an army battalion, nine gas works, the National Explosive Works and a tin works for July and autumn 1918 (Table 4.6). The National Explosive Works at Hayle was a cordite factory in which workers could be exposed to HNO_3 (nitric acid) or acetone fumes, while at the tin works those in the dressing plant were routinely exposed to SO_2 (sulphur dioxide) fumes. Gregor also claimed that even those living under the influence of the stack of the tin mine's burning house benefited as, of the twenty-seven inhabitants of seven cottages within 200 yards of the stack discharging the sulphur dioxide fumes,

Table 4.6 Reported influenza morbidity in various occupations

Group	*Population*	*Cases*	*Morbidity (percentage)*
Navy patrol	1,350	446	33.0
Army battalion	1,050	210	20.0
Gas workers (nine works)	148	10	6.7
National explosive works			
Not exposed	732	221	30.2
Full-time HNO_3 exposure	70	11	15.7
Part-time HNO_3 exposure	230	4	1.7
Any HNO_3 exposure	300	15	5.0
Acetone exposure	18	0	0.0
Any exposure	318	15	4.7
Tin works			
Underground workers	23	14	60.8
Dressing plant (SO_2)	27	3	11.1

Data source: PRO FD 1 531.

only one case of influenza was recorded, while a small village a quarter of a mile further away had 'numerous' cases.

There are a number of weaknesses in Gregor's argument. These include the fact that he is working solely with reported morbidity, which is prone to problems from the lack of diagnosis, under-reporting, and the unknown dimension of sub-clinical infection. Furthermore, we don't know how crowded the working conditions may have been. The small numbers of workers at the nine gas works and in the dressing plant suggest little crowding, and possibly little contact with others, whereas the army battalion, navy patrol and underground tin workers (miners) live and/or work in greater proximity to one another. However, as Gregor recognises, the figures from the cordite factory may indicate some benefit accruing to those exposed to fumes. Here was a group 'not only working but also living in their own homes under exactly similar conditions in every respect, except for the one fact that some are more or less exposed to fumes during their working hours, others are not.' These led him to conclude that 'certain chemical fumes must have some germicidal action'. This does not appear to have been found widely or subsequently.

Gregor's report does have another area of interest. He produces figures that are indicative of immunity being conferred on those who suffered during the summer, and other sources have also suggested a degree of immunity acquired in the first wave gave some protection in the later waves (Schoenbaum 2003: 212–13). In his navy patrol study group of 321 July cases, only two reported a second attack in the autumn. Similarly, in his army groups there were no cases of those who suffered in the summer being re-infected, and very few return attacks among the workers at the National

Explosive Works. This would have been one of the first reports to show some evidence of acquired immunity.

Discrete populations

Certain communities such as boarding schools, army camps or any 'enclosed communities with high mixing rates' can experience serious epidemics with high morbidity levels, even when the wider community may only be relatively mildly affected (Riordan 1986: 31). It has been speculated that it was in such enclosed communities that the pandemic strain of the virus arose: in military camps in one country or another. One suggestion has been the vast British camp at Etaples, France, with more than 100,000 men present on any given day along with flocks of poultry and masses of other livestock, with its outbreaks of 'purulent bronchitis' that so closely resembled the 1918 flu, may have seen an early outbreak of the pandemic strain (Oxford *et al.* 2002).

In Australia the inmates of a German internment camp were very worried about their prospects should influenza break out in the camp. It is worth remembering that Australia saw the disease delayed by quarantine and so even camp inmates knew of the dangers of the 'Spanish flu'. It was as early as 20 November 1918 (after the Armistice) that the inmates first wrote to the Camp Visitor, Justice Harvey, seeking release so as to support their families, especially in case of illness, and to avoid the danger of an outbreak within the camp. Justice Harvey forwarded the request to the Commonwealth Government who declined to release any internees but arrangements were made for inoculations, provision of inhalation chambers and face masks, and the consideration of hospital accommodation if necessary. When the disease did strike Australia, the internees felt compelled to write to the Camp Visitor on a number of occasions. The Camp Visitor and Swiss consul-in-charge (representing German interests) both raised the issue of camps with the government, with the consul specifically mentioning the conditions for prisoners of war. A 23 June 1919 letter to the Camp Visitor claimed that '[t]he influenza epidemic in the Holdsworthy Camp is assuming a serious aspect' as 'several hundred internees and a large number of guards have been attacked'. They were concerned that 'the plague seems to be spreading like wild fire' in the general community and that their families were already suffering. Complaining about the lack of or disruption to communications – due to the 'great delay owing to the disorganisation of the postal service' and difficulty in obtaining 'permission to send a telegram and [it being] almost impossible to use the telephone' – they warned it was 'sufficient to make any man desperate' and that the 'attitude of the Defence Department appears to be one of indifference'. They noted the reports of internees being paroled in South Africa and Britain and pleaded that they too should be paroled (NAA MP367/1 567/7/4467 held at PROV).

It was in such a camp that one of the first reports of large-scale influenza infection in Britain came from when, in July 1918, nearly 1,000 of 3,000

German prisoners of war interned at Bramley Camp, Hampshire, were reported to be ill (*The Times* 23 July 1918: 8). Towards the end of 1918, a further report mentioned that at Colchester Military hospital a further twenty-eight German prisoners had died, and at the Camp Hill Prison at Parkhurst on the Isle of Wight '[b]oth prisoners (preventive detention men) and the staff . . . are affected by an outbreak of influenza' (*The Times* 6 December 1918: 5). Once the disease entered the civilian population it was other 'enclosed' communities that reported high attack rates. Late in October 1918, *The Times* reported that the 'Metropolitan institutions in Essex are badly affected. Only two out of a staff of 30 nurses were available for duty yesterday at the Hackney Guardians' Institution, and many inmates, including *all* the children, were suffering from influenza' (29 October 1918: 7, my emphasis). Similarly when the epidemic took hold in Rochdale and the death rate was considered to be 'exceptionally high', it was noted that it 'has been worst at the workhouse' (*The Times* 29 November 1918: 3). Such patterns among closed communities may also account for the higher levels of morbidity and mortality reported among miners, fishermen and soldiers, as discussed previously, as many of these would have been groups concentrated in small spaces or compounds.

The Medical Superintendent at St Marylebone Infirmary, Dr Basil Hood, managed to find time to jot some notes on the pandemic into his notebook. In these pages he described the immense strain on the hospital, the loss of staff to illness and death (including his own collapse from exhaustion) and his recollection of the pandemic. The image he portrays is one of desperation and extreme fatigue. He wrote, 'We could hardly have been worse placed for dealing with an epidemic', before going on to detail how staff changes, staff shortages and having to deal with cases from other hospitals led to such a difficult battle with the pandemic that the 'labour and distress of that time especially was terrific. Indeed it hardly bears thinking about. Not only was there a great increase in cases, many critically ill with influenzal pneumonia but the staff also began to go down like ninepins'. This situation escalated until he 'collapsed completely in December . . . and returned in the middle of February' (CMAC GC/21 Volume 1: 93, 127–135A).

A more systematic study of the morbidity and mortality of the influenza on hospital staff was undertaken by Major D. Barty King at the County of London (Horton) War Hospital at Epsom. King monitored the health of the nursing and maid staff at the hospital during the second and third waves of the pandemic, with 'at least daily' inspections (King 1922: 68). King considers that this monitoring, particularly of the nursing staff, had a 'favourable influence' and kept mortality, if not morbidity, to a lower level than experienced elsewhere. Once diagnosed, nurses were removed from their ward duties, confined to bed and nursed by other nurses. The nursing staff that numbered 'on an average, 329 nurses' are reported as having suffered eighty-four cases (25.5 per cent) with only two deaths (2.4 per cent case fatality), while among the forty-nine resident maids, twenty-one were ill (42.8 per cent) and a single death occurred (4.8 per cent case fatality) (King 1922: 69, 75). The vast majority of cases were classified as 'slight' or 'moderate'. However, the dangers of the job were also apparent even here. King attributes four deaths and two further cases to contact with one acute case with 'broncho-pneumonia in Ward D (Ear, Nose and Throat Ward)'. Both nurses that died were considered to have contracted the disease when treating this patient, while another nurse endured a 'near-fatal case of severe influenza with acute broncho-pneumonia' and yet another had a 'moderate case'. In addition to the nurses infected (and killed), this patient's infection went on to kill the resident aural surgeon and the hospital chaplain who 'was also in contact with this acute case . . . throughout its course, contracted a severe type of influenza with acute broncho-pneumonia and died' (King 1922: 72).

Given the high rate of infection that can occur in groups and the important role children have in disseminating influenza (and other diseases) in the community, it is logical that the role of schools in epidemics should be debated (Glezen 1980; Glezen *et al.* 1980; Kendal 1987; Kendal and Glezen 1998; Schoenbaum 2003). The MRC certainly considered it useful to gain information on the nature of the pandemic and the efficacy of any preventive measures or responses applied in schools. This interest was, however, limited to writing to the school doctors or MOs at the 'chief Public Schools', and fifteen independent schools responded to this request.[28] The schools that responded reveal rather extreme morbidity experiences. While some schools reported no or few cases,[29] others reported quite severe outbreaks. One such case was Rossall School in Fleetwood, where 320 of the 444 boys (72.1 per cent) were infected, including fifty-seven out of the fifty-nine (96.6 per cent) in the Preparatory School.[30] Felsted School, Essex, reported somewhere between 143 and 162 cases among 'about 250 boys' (57.2–64.8 per cent).[31] Other schools that recorded high morbidity levels included Old Blundell's School in Tiverton, Devon, where 180 of 250 boarders (72 per cent) fell ill,[32] Cheltenham College who had 321 of their 480 Boarders (66.9 per cent) affected, along with five Masters,[33] and Wellington College where the spread was 'so rapid that it was not possible to keep records', but it appears that more than 90 per cent of the pupils contracted influenza.[34] Burnet and Clark gave figures for three English independent schools, which they considered might have had conditions similar to onboard ship, where morbidity rates for the summer and autumn waves were 35, 52 and 21 per cent in the summer and 22, 26.6 and 67 per cent in the autumn (Burnet and Clark 1942: 84).

A number of the letters to the MRC from the schools observed how maids and other staff were affected. In Cambridge so many of the maidservants fell ill at the Leys School that it 'prevented normal service of the School being carried on' and the decision was made to send the boys home and consequently only twenty boys were known to have been ill.[35] This is quite a different situation from that reported at the King's College School, Cambridge, where the Headmaster, Mr Jelf, considered that *all* of the boarders had been attacked by influenza in July 1918 and were immune during the later stages of the pandemic.[36] Across the county border in Essex, the Grammar School in Saffron Walden had nineteen of the thirty boys boarding attacked during the autumn wave, and the disease was also prevalent in the infants' school. First reports in the autumn wave from Cambridge schools came in late September with a number of cases at St Paul's Infants', Sturton Street Infants' and East Road Infants' schools. Few other cases were reported until 14 October 1918 when '63 children and two teachers were notified from Sturton Street Infants', two from St Philip's Infants', 79 from St Barnabas, and 144 from East Road Infants' schools. The epidemic had well and truly taken hold in the city's infants schools'.[37] The epidemic by no means spared the colleges and the university either. The MOH distributed 2,595 surveys to resident members of the university, of which 1,766 were completed and returned. Of these, 1,263 reported having suffered from the influenza (72 per cent of the returns). However, although widespread, the influenza took a remarkably light toll on the university where only four undergraduates and three resident graduates were known to have died, as well as a university lecturer, a fellow of King's College and the Librarian at Trinity College.[38] Examination of the spread of influenza in Cambridge concluded that it was 'based upon the intimate relationship between town and university' from its origins, believed to be brought into the town by naval cadets billeted into the colleges, and its subsequent passage through the various parishes of the town (Smallman-Raynor *et al.* 2002: 465).

Despite the large-scale outbreaks that occurred in some, if not most schools, there is little evidence of these leading to widespread disruption of the school year. In Britain there were few occasions when term dates or vacations were altered so as to reduce contact or to keep students in the apparently safer environment of the school. Nor does there seem to be any allowance for or re-scheduling of examinations. Did that year's students have to face their exams with less classroom time due to illness and the closure of schools? What allowances were made for this? What effect did it have on those completing final school or university exams?

While the isolated, discrete or 'enclosed' communities described so far could suffer greatly, there was another space that could be particularly dangerous. Being onboard ship was probably one of the worst places to experience the pandemic. On a ship, especially a crowded troopship with its rudimentary facilities for the masses jammed together, there would have been little escape and no way to avoid infection once it started to spread. Seeing one's fellow passengers fall ill so quickly and frequently exhibiting the shocking cyanosis that so often presaged death, and knowing that there was nowhere to hide from this infection as it spread throughout the ship, must have been a terrifying ordeal. The Ministry of Health certainly considered these to be among the 'most tragic events in the history of the recent influenzas, those witnessed on certain transports bringing great numbers of troops to Europe' (Ministry of Health 1920c: 170). One of the few times the influenza pandemic made it into the War Cabinet papers was in May 1918 when they were informed by the Deputy Chief of the Naval Staff that the Commodore of the Adriatic British Squadron had found it necessary to delay the docking of HMS *Weymouth* because of 211 influenza cases onboard. This outbreak was part of 'an epidemic of influenza not only in the squadron, but also at several naval bases' (PRO CAB 23 6 War Cabinet 413, 17 May 1918).

The Times considered what was happening on the trans-Atlantic shipping as particularly ominous and that it warranted stringent measures. In an October 1918 editorial under the headline, 'A Serious Epidemic', the paper painted the most pessimistic picture of the disease than it had at any time before, noting that this epidemic is 'by no means the simple matter we have been led to suppose'. Disavowing official optimism and noting how this 'most fatal type of septic pneumonia' was killing many in Britain and America as it penetrated to 'all sections of the community and to all places', the writer considered alarm was justified, as was the adoption of the 'most resolute measures'. Arguing that the question of inconvenience was irrelevant as 'inconvenience will be borne gladly enough if . . . the scourge can be stamped out' or at least controlled. The editorial argued that the issue of trans-Atlantic shipping was of prime importance and required the immediate provision of hospital staff and accommodation along with the examination of passengers prior to embarkation and the extensive cleaning of ships between voyages (*The Times* 26 October 1918: 7).[39]

But, as with the schools, the experience from one ship to another could vary markedly. In the Royal Navy there were cases such as the HMS *Africa* where of 779 personnel some 75 per cent had been attacked, with 9 per cent mortality, whereas the HMS *Newcastle* had been carrying 450, of whom 51 per cent fell ill but with no fatal cases at all. John Cumpston, Director of the Australian Quarantine Service, had compiled statistics on influenza on ships entering and within Australian waters (Cumpston 1919). Cumpston recorded observations on ninety-two vessels and while some recorded large outbreaks, thrity-four were reported to have had only a single influenza case. However, other vessels reported significant outbreaks (Table 4.7).

Harvey Cushing, later known as the 'father of neurosurgery' and winner of the 1925 Pulitzer Prize for his biography of William Osler, was a US forces surgeon in 1918 and recounted the experience of one of his colleagues, Bagley, and gave a vivid picture of the tribulations faced when an outbreak occurred.

> 15 October 1918 . . .
> Bagley turns up, after some three weeks in working his way by 'channels' to these H.Q. from Southampton, where they landed. The usual story. This time Transport 56 – i.e., the Olympic. He was ship Medical Officer. There had been no grippe in the States, but nine cases developed on the boat, with one death from pneumonia. They were held

Table 4.7 Influenza onboard ship

Vessel	*Total persons*	*Cases*	*Deaths*	*Incidence (%)*	*Case fatality (%)*
Barambah	997	800	25	80.3	3.1
H.M.S. *Africa*	775			75	9
Fantome	124	78	0	62.9	0
Atua	163	88	16	54.0	18.2
H.M.S. *Newcastle*	450		0	51	0
Boonah	1,095	470	18	42.9	3.8
Medic	989	313	22	31.6	7.0
Mataram	198	61	0	30.8	0
Meader case (unidentified)	5,951	1,668	317	28.0	19.0
Niagara	567	156	5	27.5	3.2
Makura	406	94	4	23.2	4.3
Charon	113	23	1	20.4	4.3
Nikko Maru	244	30	1	12.3	3.3
Sardinia	1,378	120	10	8.7	8.3
Devon	1,096	95	0	8.7	0
Marathon	1,041	89	4	8.5	4.5
Port Darwin	1,237	90	2	7.3	2.2
Neston	1,903	69	0	3.6	0
Malton	898	16	0	1.8	0
Saxon	1,603	25	1	1.6	4.0
Port Lyttleton	929	12	1	1.3	8.3

Sources: after Burnet and Clark 1942: 84, based on Cumpston 1919. Additional material from Thomas (1998: 2); Ministry of Health (1920c: 58) and Major Fred M. Meader's address to the Royal Society of Medicine's 'Discussion on Influenza' (Royal Society of Medicine 1918: 71–6).

> in Southampton Harbor 24 hours before disembarking, and 384 cases developed during this brief time – very severe – temperatures of 105° frequent in men at the very outset. People standing guard would fall in their tracks. They were sent to a rest camp near Southampton and in a week 1900 cases developed, with several hundred pneumonias and 119 deaths before he left. Of the 342 nurses who were left on shipboard after the troops disembarked, 134 developed influenza.
>
> (Cushing 1936: 472)

Shipping took the disease all around the world. Upon landing, the local transport networks, in particular the railways, facilitated its passage to all communities. It is these networks that connect and to an extent determine the hierarchies down which the disease cascaded and the movement of forces around the world was a factor in ensuring this outbreak became pandemic.[40] Many, many service personnel were struck, often with tragic results,[41] as in the case of Lieutenant Alan John Mawson of the Northern Fusiliers and Machine Gun Corps. Prior to the war he had worked as a clerk and a chemist's assistant. Having survived the war, Mawson died of influenza in the Military Hospital at Grantham on 4 December 1918, aged thirty-one. He had received his commission on 15 March 1915 and his mother claimed her right to his pension upon his death. The government attempted to determine her right to a pension based on how and when he had contracted the disease and died. This was complicated by the fact he had been home on leave just prior to returning to his base on 22 November 1918 where he was hospitalised four days later. His medical records track his decline and indicate that influenza was widespread among the troops with whom Mawson was stationed, a point his mother reminded the War Department of as 'the epidemic was at its height at that time and officers and men were dying in numbers daily'. Sometime after this she was awarded his pension, a payment that was made until her death in February 1945 (PRO PIN 26 22103).

Influenza was often not terminal, but the 'side-effects' could persist. For example, Nurse Nelly Stevenson claimed a military pension following 'double pneumonia' on account of her being infected while on nursing duties. Early in 1919 she was deemed '100 per cent disabled' and received a full pension. This was reduced following a 28 July 1919 Medical Board inspection that found a 'slight improvement' despite 'poor general condition. She is extremely nervous, shaky and debilitated – unfit for any duty' and was classified as 80 per cent disabled. A similar description on 13 October 1919 nonetheless saw a reduction of her assessed disability to 60 per cent. Less than a month later this was halved despite the fact that she 'is easily fatigued and not able to undergo prolonged exertion'. It is doubtful she could have earned her living as a nurse in the circumstances. The inconsistencies of the assessments continued as a January 1920 inspection left her disability at 30 per cent despite 'some improvement', while a February 1920 inspection assessed her as 50 per cent disabled in spite of a note of 'progress satisfactory' and the following month she was deemed fit for home service, including active duty with troops, preceding her discharge on 19 March 1920. However, this was overturned a month later when a Board assessed a 20 per cent disability, a level which was concurred with by Resurvey Boards in April 1921, 1922 and 1923. All told, Nelly Stevenson's suffering lasted more than five years (PRO PIN 26 20251).

The military authorities were not only burdened by the ill and the dead but also had the duty of notifying the next-of-kin. Sometimes this took more effort than was usual. In Sydney, Corporal William Medley died of 'pneumonic influenza'. Fair-haired and hazel-eyed this apparently unmarried labourer who had done four years' previous military service volunteered, and enlisted at Sydney's Victoria Barracks on 1 November 1915 when aged 36 years 8 months. On enlisting the slight (5'9½" and 146 lbs) Medley was told that his previous double hernia was 'not sufficient to cause rejection'. Serving for much of the war – and keeping out of trouble as his Regimental

Conduct Sheet has no entries – his death certificate states he died of 'A. Pneumonic Influenza. B. Broncho pneumonia. C. Cardiac failure'. However, Medley had actually been married and by 1923 the military authorities were trying to contact a Mrs M.E. Medley in Queensland asking to confirm if she had indeed been married to him so they could 'issue a Memorial Plaque and Scroll on account of his services . . . and in order to ensure that these mementos are disposed of in keeping with the regulations'. He had enlisted in 1915 as a single man but the military authorities thought otherwise and now sought evidence (NAA, MT1487/1 MEDLEY W – held at the PROV).

It is not only war records that document the scale of the problem. Will Pickles – who later commented in his renowned *Epidemiology in Country Practice* that epidemics of influenza with large numbers of deaths had been rare in Wensleydale over the previous 'few hundred years' and that 'there is nothing to compare with the entries in our own time during November and December 1918, the period of the great influenza pandemic' – battled the pandemic as he served as a Medical Officer in the Royal Navy (Pickles 1939: 11). His biographer records how over-worked Pickles and his fellow MOs were and that he had to have 'two houses adapted as extra sick bays. Men were stricken in their billets and he had to go round with stretcher bearers and have them carried out and taken to the emergency hospital. In many instances he knew the man he was helping was doomed as his face had turned the heliotrope hue which was soon recognised as a fatal sign' (Pemberton 1970: 83). Pickles' experience was by no means unique, in either civil or military practice, as this pandemic extracted an unparalleled toll.[42]

5 Impacts and responses

A major stumbling block in studying past episodes of many diseases, including influenza, is the lack of evidence on morbidity. Mortality data have their limitations but they are usually collected reasonably systematically, at least for the last couple of centuries. This is not the case for morbidity data, and this is particularly true of influenza. Where morbidity data are found, they are often simple and have a number of limitations. First, they are likely to be an under-estimation and, second, they usually have no temporal or spatial element – there is no detailed intelligence regarding where or when the cases occurred. Influenza is often self-diagnosed and self-treated, and only a small proportion of cases ever come into contact with the medical professions, and even then diagnosis is not certain. These problems are as true now as ever. Consequently, modern surveillance of influenza is often based on serological testing and pathology of a sample of the population. Little information relating to morbidity during the 1918–19 pandemic exists, and when it does it tends to be anecdotal.

Compulsory notification for influenza was a rarity at the time of the pandemic, a number of Scandinavian nations being notable exceptions. However, in some locations this was changed (at least for a while) following the pandemic. For example, 'influenzal pneumonia' was made notifiable in Britain for a number of years from early 1919 when the Local Government Board (LGB) issued a memorandum requiring notification (Local Government Board 1919a).[1] The British notification requirements were confirmed by a Ministry of Health circular – *Circular 85, Notification of Infectious Diseases* – dated 23 April 1920 (Ministry of Health 1920b) and the *Public Health (Infectious Diseases) Regulations, 1927*, before being revised by the Ministry of Health in 1935.[2]

This lack of notification around the pandemic is unfortunate for a number of reasons. The virologist Ed Kilbourne noted this lack and called on historians to come to the aid of the scientists as

> no precise figures on age-related *morbidity* in 1918 exist, in contrast to the reasonably reliable data on age-related mortality. In order to understand the relative sparing of the elderly from the high mortality of the

> young adults, we must know whether fewer elderly were *infected* or fewer had severe disease.
>
> (Kilbourne 1998: 11)

There have been some suggestions that during the pandemic young adults did not exhibit a higher morbidity rate than other age groups; however, their mortality rates were very much higher than all other age groups (Burnet and Clark 1942).

Consequently, what little morbidity information there is may not allow us to make particularly robust (statistical) statements about case fatality, etc., but it may afford some insight into the pandemic, including an understanding of the levels of social disruption it brought. Influenza can be exceptionally widespread, even in non-epidemic times. For example, it has been reported that 'even in unexceptional years [non-epidemic years] up to 20 per cent of people get flu' (Dillner 1995), and that influenza causes 'between three to five million cases of severe illness and between 250,000 and 500,000 deaths every year around the world' (WHO 2003). Pandemics are generally defined by unusually high rates of morbidity globally, and the 1918–19 epidemic was most certainly a pandemic. The increased morbidity is to be expected as the population had little or no immunological experience of the virus and thus little immunity, rendering the population exceptionally vulnerable. Modern serological testing reveals up to 90 per cent infection, including sub-clinical infections, in epidemics. Consequently, the estimate of a billion people infected in 1918–19 (half the global population) may actually be an under-estimate. Where morbidity data exist for the pandemic they are somewhat variable. This variability may be due to problems of diagnosis and reporting rather than varying levels of exposure and infection. Morbidity rates that have been reported range from 25 to 100 per cent of the population infected.[3]

Such a pervasive pestilence must have had a tremendous impact on life – the levels of illness, the lack of staff in businesses, the impairment of services, the sheer number of bodies could not have been ignored. However, it was an impact that was apparently soon forgotten. The first wave had little noted impact. The second wave certainly had an impact with its massive surge in fatalities. The third wave attracted attention as is evident in the increased coverage of influenza in the newspapers and the medical journals, the increased advertising of flu remedies and increased pharmacy sales during this stage of the pandemic.

Britons may have become somewhat used to the strain of life in a nation at war, but the influenza was to bring great disruption – to transport, communications, emergency services and every other aspect of life. Bus and train services were curtailed, schools, hospitals, chemists, post offices, bakeries and laundries were short of staff, police and fire services were similarly affected, undertakers were unable to make enough coffins, dig enough graves or bury the bodies quickly enough. Some undertakers had to decline requests, while in some areas the cemeteries were opened longer hours to allow for more interments, and many locations saw local authority or military personnel brought in to help deal with the piles of bodies. The Postmaster General was driven to ask people to only make necessary phone calls as the telephone services had been 'interfered with' as many operators failed to take their places.[4] Sandra Tomkins noted that 'Particular concern was voiced over the impact of absenteeism on war-related industries such as mining and munitions, but all services, employers and institutions were affected' (Tomkins 1992a: 441).

In Reading, a nurse lamented:

> It happened so suddenly. In the morning we received an order to open up a new unit for flu and by night we'd moved into a converted convent. Almost before the desks were out the stretchers were in – 60–80 to a classroom. We could hardly squeeze between the cots and oh, they were so sick!
>
> (Morton 1973, cited in Kilbourne 1987: 15)

Not so far to the east, the Chelsea Health Society and School for Mothers Annual Report noted that 'attendances during the last year have been steady, save during the influenza epidemic', an epidemic they noted contributed to the fact that deaths had outnumbered births 1,114 to 790 in the borough during 1918.[5] Gladys Wauchope, the first female student at the 'London' (Royal London Hospital), recalled as a student seeing 'patients with lilac faces being wheeled in the receiving room', a 'surgical ward was transformed into an influenza ward', and the loss of one of her fellow medical students as 'Thompson, was playing Rugger for the hospital on Saturday and was dead on Monday' (Wauchope 1963: 40–1).[6] Over at St Bartholomew's the staff were infected: Geoffrey Bourne recorded that the 'two most brilliant aspirants to permanent staff rank, Stansfield, a physician, and Blakeway, a surgeon, each died after a few days' illness'. Later at the Evelina Children's Hospital, Bourne found 'the menace of the still rampant influenza' where a nine-year-old girl who was 'terribly ill, coughing and blue with the fatal heliotrope tinge' coughed in his face. Less than two days later he was 'seized with headache, malaise, muscle pains and fever' (Bourne 1963: 165), and his condition was to worsen as he wrote:

> I felt poisoned and miserable. I then knew I was facing a serious situation. That night I was delirious and . . . [in] a semi-conscious dozing condition. . . . I appreciated the literally mortal danger of the attack, but the worse I grew the more I seemed to achieve a detached state of mildly interested resignation. I had vague illusions of place, time and actuality. There was little suffering or distress from difficulties of breathing. . . . I still remember the feeling of, as it were, gritting my teeth and fighting for fighting's sake. The whole experience may have been just a trick of the mind, but I still think that I was very near death.
>
> (Bourne 1963: 166–8)

But even when faced with a massive wave of disease there were still lighter moments in the lives of the struggling doctors. In Aberdeen, Dr Mackie recalled:

> It happened to me one day. I was in one street visiting the urgent cases, when a woman asked me to visit her house. When I got to the kitchen she informed me that a tame starling, she had in a cage, had broken its leg, would I attend it? Oh, yes, I attended the wee birdie, and was glad it hadn't Flu.
>
> (Mackie 1949: 44)

So great was the disruption that the politicians noticed. Despite the fact that the pandemic was not mentioned in parliament until the end of October 1918, it did curtail their activities on occasions.[7] In Sunderland the influenza prevalence led to the candidates' decision to abandon 'house-to-house canvassing during the election campaign and not to convey electors in carriages on the polling day' (*The Times* 28 November 1918: 3).

An outbreak of disease that afflicts billions and kills millions in less than a year must have impacts beyond those of morbidity and mortality. The disruption and dislocation of society had to be immense. Much of the power of the disease to disrupt life came from the sheer scale and rapidity of the pandemic. Social systems and logistical networks all failed due to the sheer weight of numbers. The logistics of disease and death on such a scale overwhelmed the medical profession, the funeral industry and disrupted all forms of activity. These disruptions were more-or-less universal – issues of adequate medical care, the use of masks, the imposition of quarantine, the lack of coffins and people to bury the dead, massive absenteeism from all industries and services were all concerns that virtually every society and community came to face. Naturally the British experienced many of the same privations and tribulations endured elsewhere. Throughout the literature there are recurring images of massive disruption of normal life with transport networks, communications (for example, telephone exchanges unable to cope due to absenteeism, the mail undelivered) and all forms of social and economic activity interrupted, impaired or stopped due to the spectacular levels of both illness and death. This is true of both belligerent and neutral nations, Western and non-Western. These impacts ranged from the strains put on systems such as hospitals, public transport, telephony and mail through to impairment of industry, including those important to the war effort in a number of countries through to social impacts. The latter included the closing of public entertainments, racecourses, hairdressers, schools, churches and even the cancellation of socially important events ranging from the debate as to whether to cancel Carnival in Cadiz (Rodriguez 1996) to the cancellation of the Centennial Royal Easter Show in Sydney (McQueen 1976: 137) and the abandonment of professional ice hockey's Stanley Cup play-offs in North America (the only time prior to the industrial dispute of 2005 in which the Stanley Cup was not awarded).

A number of debates raged around the influenza. One major source of contention was the use of masks. In some locations the wearing of masks was made compulsory, often with varying levels of enforcement and resistance.[8] This led to some of the few enduring images of the pandemic: masked policemen in Seattle, masked medical personnel, volunteer nurses, Post Office and bank staff in Sydney (Figure 5.1) and masked Chicago street sweepers. In Australia the wearing of masks is one of the most clearly remembered aspects of the pandemic (Curby 1998; Taksa 1994). In Britain the use of masks was not made compulsory, despite some encouragement to do so, but the British response was very much a decentralised one, the LGB giving little specific direction and leaving decisions on school closures, quarantine, masks, and what sort of assistance (if any) was offered to the local authorities and/or their MOH.[9]

This was an event that brought much suffering but elicited little public reaction.[10] There was little objection or resistance to the action (or inaction) of authorities other than the relatively isolated cases of disquiet stemming from closures of churches, schools and/or public entertainments, while other crowded places, such as public transport, remained open. Arguments put against the closing of churches included that in this time of crisis people should be turning to religion, not excluded from it. This lack of unrest is drawn out in the WHO *Influenza Pandemic Plan* (1999d, 2005c) where there is explicit reference to the maintenance of law and order and the minimisation of public disorder in the face of a pandemic. Obviously, modern healthcare planners anticipate the possibility of large-scale public anger or action in the event of a pandemic, perhaps particularly if the authorities are perceived as having failed to warn people or as neglecting their responsibilities and duty of care to the people. The WHO plan regards the worst-case scenario as being a rapidly spreading pandemic without anything ameliorating the morbidity and mortality resulting in over-strained health services weakened by a reduction in staff and facing a greatly increased workload. The consequences of these could then be that the 'national economy is seriously affected. Public fear and protest are likely. Possible disruption of civil order' (WHO 1999d: 25). For these reasons the plan also suggests that the military and law enforcement authorities should be part of the planning process for each nation's pandemic preparation. Furthermore, it suggests that countries may want to consider what laws and regulations may be needed to regulate public gatherings (WHO 1999d: 26–8). It is useful to consider why there was so little civil unrest or panic at a time when death and disease were so prevalent. The association with the war may be playing a role in that by conflating the two it was considered inevitable and something about which little could be done. Being 'only' influenza may have led to people downplaying their own experiences and negating the scale of the pandemic. The emphasis placed on these issues is starkest in the conclusion to the WHO's 1999 plan. The *only* highlighted paragraph in the conclusion read:

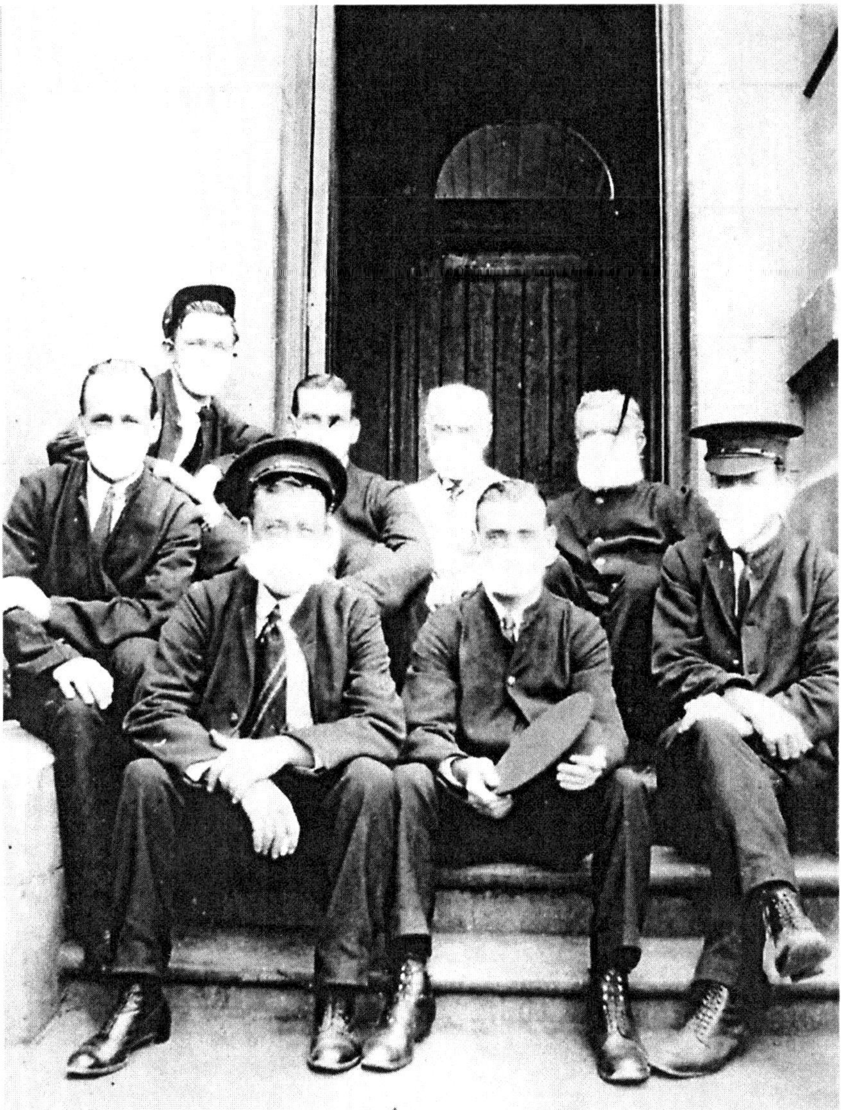

Figure 5.1 Masked Post Office staff, Balmain, Sydney, 1919 (image courtesy of National Archives of Australia: C4076, HN558).

> Management of risk does not imply an ability to prevent a pandemic, but rather to make best use of available resources to reduce the extent of disease, reduce the impact of secondary catastrophes, and to prevent panic from occurring in the population.
>
> (WHO 1999d: 31)

Quarantine and regulation

Quarantine was one response that was widely considered at both local and national scales. With a disease that is so freely transmitted as influenza, quarantine is rarely likely to be successful. National quarantines were rarely imposed as they were seen as impractical and unsuccessful. The most commonly cited national quarantines were those of American Samoa (in contrast to Western Samoa) and Australia. However, it was at the local level that quarantining was most commonly debated and enacted, ranging from the closing of an entire settlement to all incoming traffic (rarely implemented and even more rarely successful) through to the closing or curtailing of certain places or activities. Localised quarantine often meant not so much the isolation of a settlement from the outside world as the restriction or enforced closure of certain activities or premises, and included the closing of public entertainments, such as bars, theatres, music halls and cinemas, or hairdressers, schools, Sunday schools and churches. Such moves were often very controversial as they could become moral issues for the communities involved. Restrictions inevitably led to disquiet, and these arose in many contexts, sometimes from the uneven application of such controls, in other cases because certain activities were halted while others were not. Such closures often reveal prejudices or other biases of the elite. One area of comment was the overcrowding of public transport – people were no longer permitted to take part in various social activities but they were generally still expected to work and to be crowded together as they went to and from their workplace.

There are very few parts of the world that did not endure the passage of the influenza. Those lucky few that did escape tended to be more remote islands, including St Helena (South Atlantic) and a number of South Pacific island groups.[11] Most of these appear to have escaped due to their relative isolation and lack of contact with infected people, rather than through the imposition of quarantine,[12] though it has been suggested that those in the south-western Pacific that were unscathed had most of their trade with Australia and 'their escape can reasonably be ascribed to the strict outward quarantine enforced by Australia' (Burnet and Clark 1942: 74). In sharp contrast were those south-western Pacific islands that can trace the arrival of the pandemic to ships coming from New Zealand (Edwards 1986; Herda 1998; Rice 1988, 1989; Tomkins 1992b).[13]

Australia is one of the few nations that achieved any measure of success with the imposition of a national quarantine (Cumpston 1919). Obviously being a remote island, albeit an extremely large island, made maritime quarantine feasible. The remoteness may have helped ensure that any outbreak on board ships bound for Australia may have subsided before arrival and led to the *Medical Journal of Australia* to (prematurely) claim that 'the Federal Quarantine Service will be in the proud position of having achieved the greatest triumph of its kind in the history of epidemiology' (*MJA*, 30

November 1918: 455). Ships were forced to wait before disembarkation or had passengers disembark at quarantine stations to stay for a period of days before being allowed to enter the country. This delay frustrated many of the returning forces – having been to war and having survived, they were now detained when they were so close to home and to being reunited with all they had left behind. Indeed, soldiers 'escaping' from quarantine have been blamed for the eventual penetration of the influenza into the Australian community (Hyslop 1984, 1995, 1998a, 1998b; McQueen 1976; Mihaly 1998; Thomas 1998).[14]

While Australia saw quarantine eventually breached, American Samoa successfully maintained theirs as the American Governor (John M. Poyer) mobilised the indigenous population to ensure its success. This was all the more notable when compared with their neighbour, Western Samoa. Western Samoa was ravaged by the flu to an extent unseen elsewhere, with an estimated 22 per cent of the total population dying, whereas American Samoa apparently had no cases at all (Boyd 1980; Crosby 1989: 232–40; Herda 1998; Tomkins 1992b). Poyer's actions were recognised with the awarding of the Navy Cross, for which the citation read:

> for exceptionally meritorious service in a duty of great responsibility as governor of American Samoa, for wise and successful administration of his office and especially for the extraordinarily successful measures by which American Samoa was kept absolutely immune from the epidemic of influenza at a time when in the neighbouring islands of the Samoan group more than 10,000 deaths occurred, and when the percentage of deaths throughout the Polynesian Islands as a group, is reported to have ranged from 30 to 40 per cent of the population.[15]

The South African government had been well aware of the dangers of the virus being transported by ship and went to some lengths to warn those countries where shipping routinely travelled between them and South Africa, but was unconvinced of the merits of quarantine. The South African Influenza Epidemic Commission concluded that the

> evidence . . . is so decidedly against the effectiveness of maritime quarantine in a disease of the nature of Epidemic Influenza that, although giving full credit to the experience of Australia, the Commission is not prepared to state that maritime quarantine should have been enforced [in South Africa]. Neither is the Commission of the opinion that even the timely enforcement of maritime quarantine would have necessarily prevented an outbreak of Epidemic Influenza in South Africa.
>
> (Union of South Africa 1919: 9)

Writing on the epidemic in Senegal, Echenberg agreed that 'even the most diligent actions of public health authorities would have failed to arrest the epidemic' as the air-borne virus is nigh on 'impossible to stop by quarantine measures' (Echenberg 1998: 6). In Australia, 'great stress [was] laid on the value of measures of quarantine taken in that country' (PRO MH 113 51)[16] but some argued that quarantine was a waste of time. Some of this criticism was based on the inability of preventing the entry of an undetectable organism, the need to maintain activity due to the war, and so on. Other criticism stemmed from quite different arguments. Gill argued that, in fact, 'the drastic quarantine regulations imposed by the Federal Government on October 17, 1918' had nothing whatsoever to do with the delay of the pandemic in Australia, arguing that it was in fact the Australian climate that determined the timing of the pandemic (Gill 1928: 292–5).[17]

While quarantine was being enforced in Australia and American Samoa, it was not widely employed elsewhere. In Britain where reports of the influenza's impact elsewhere were appearing in the newspapers, there were some calls for controls. For example, *The Times* in late October 1918 noted the increasing number of cases and called for 'the most resolute measures' (26 October 1918: 7). At the LGB Newsholme saw things rather differently and resisted all forms of quarantine, either national maritime or at the local level. Opening the Royal Society of Medicine's 'Discussion' on influenza on 13 November 1918 he discussed the 'difficulty of preventive measures in war time', arguing for the need to 'carry on' and that 'the relentless needs of warfare justified incurring this risk of spreading infection' (Royal Society of Medicine 1918: 12–13). After the pandemic another LGB officer, Carnwath, specifically addressed the question as to why quarantine was not imposed when he told the Royal Institute of Public Health that it was

> not considered practicable . . . mainly on account of the large numbers of unrecognizable cases. It must be borne in mind that the disease was introduced into this country in a mild, unrecognizable form some time about May . . . and that the autumn epidemic was . . . a recrudescence of the disease already imported.
>
> (Carnwath 1919: 149).

This view of the impossibility and impracticability of quarantining influenza was reiterated in the 1927 revision of the *Memorandum on Influenza*, which stated that the 'question of the prevention by quarantine of the importation of influenza from abroad has been considered and may be dismissed as impracticable' (Ministry of Health 1927: 11)[18] – given the highly transmissible nature of the disease, it is probably appropriate not to waste resources on attempting to enforce quarantine for influenza and instead direct those resources to other areas, such as influenza vaccine development, public health information and vaccination campaigns.

While quarantine was only rarely imposed at the larger scale there were many local actions, particularly preventive measures, restrictions and controls that were attempted. These included the compulsory wearing of masks, restriction or closure of some forms of commercial and social activity and even isolation of communities in some cases. The control and regulation of various public and semi-public spaces such as the closure of schools, churches and public entertainments (cinemas, theatres, bars, etc.) were quite common, as was the wearing of masks. The efficacy of such measures has been much questioned, and generally it is considered that quarantine and closures failed to have any significant impact upon the disease. For example, on 7 October 1918, the Board of Health in the city of Kitchener, Ontario, issued a pronouncement that they 'deem it to be in the interest of the public health to close schools, churches and theatres, and also all public gatherings, until further notice',[19] this being later expanded to take in all places of entertainment. Examination of the progress of the epidemic there, through maps of influenza mortality and the epidemic mortality curve, show no interruption or discontinuities following this decree. It is apparent that the quarantine imposed upon Kitchener was such a permeable barrier that it had a negligible effect and the disease ran its course, waning only when the susceptible population was too small to support its continued spread (Johnson 1993: 150–1; 1998).

While local restrictions appear to have been relatively commonplace (and ineffectual), some communities adopted stronger measures. Richard Collier noted some of the more extreme examples, including the Naval Training Station on Yerba Buena Island at San Francisco which 'clamped down a nine-week quarantine on 4,000 souls – forbidding all liberty, sterilising drinking fountains hourly with blow torches, compelling new trainees to exist twenty feet apart from one another'. But such restrictions are rarely possible or acceptable outside a martial setting. One of the few exceptions was the New Zealand village of Coromandel that 'cut itself off from the outer world through a roster of vigilantes armed with shotguns', and apparently successfully kept influenza at bay (Collier 1974: 144–5). But even such extreme measures were not always a guarantee of success. Lee Reay was a young boy in Meadow, Utah, USA, at the time and recounted that, as the town realised the disease was approaching them, his

> father was selected as the health officer. We had never had a health officer in our town before, but we felt now that we needed one and so Dad went out to the city limits signs (I went with him), and we put a sign that said, THIS TOWN IS QUARANTINED – DO NOT STOP. So we had purposely isolated ourselves. But it wasn't enough, the disease came anyway – the mailman brought it.
>
> (Channel 4/WGBH 1998)

The danger of the mailman was recognised in Canberra, Australia. Regulations had been issued enforcing a four-day quarantine on people arriving from 'infected areas' but the authorities were unsure as to what to do with a mail coach driver.[20] In South Africa similar measures were taken on individual farms and properties and in some remote villages, where not only was incoming traffic prevented, but all movement was halted. Again, varying levels of success were experienced as quarantine is all too easily breached by such an easily transmitted virus, and one where those without symptoms can be infective (Phillips 1990a: 135–6).

Within a nation it was not just the local communities and authorities that attempted to implement controls. In some countries there were attempts to contain the disease to particular cities or parts of the country, examples of this include Iceland, Spain and Australia. Once the influenza had been introduced into Iceland, the disease was generally contained to the south-west by isolating the Reykjavík region, but only 'by the imposition of the most draconian quarantine measures'. However, there were instances when these 'communication bans' were evaded, for example by mailboats or a group of Reykjavík youths attending a dance in another town (Cliff *et al.* 1986: 148–50). Similar controls were employed in Spain, where quarantine was adopted, particularly in the Canary Islands, and sanitary cordons established at railway stations where 'passengers were disembarked, examined and those who showed symptoms of the flu were put on quarantine. Those allowed to proceed with their trip were generously sprayed with foul smelling disinfectants' (Echeverri 2003: 180). Such controls were later expanded to include closing the national borders with Portugal and France. However, the regulations imposed on railway travellers seem to have done little to stem the disease. The maritime quarantine restrictions played a role in restraining mortality in the Canary Islands, largely due to the smaller numbers involved (Echeverri 2003: 181). The imposition of such quarantines often led to dispute. In the port city of Cadiz, for example, these included not just the protests of those being quarantined, but also those of the local citizens who objected to where those being quarantined were to be housed in the city (Rodriguez 1996), just as in Sydney, Australia, where questions were asked in state Parliament as to whether the quarantine station at Manly was too close to the city's growing population.

In Australia, once the national maritime quarantine had been breached, interstate quarantine assumed greater importance. This too was soon to fail and the disease spread throughout the nation. This failure of interstate controls rapidly became a source of acrimony among the states as they apportioned the blame upon their neighbours.[21] The Australian experience is illuminating in that despite strenuous efforts to maintain both national and local quarantines they were ultimately unsuccessful and Australians still died in large numbers. These examples demonstrate the all-but-universal failure of quarantine and restrictions with the very few exceptions where there was total exclusion. Such control is, in the vast majority of cases, impractical, if not impossible.

In addition to the British aversion to the imposition of a national maritime quarantine, there was no desire by the national authorities to apply any controls to prevent the spread of influenza. Any such measures were left largely to the whims and discretion of local authorities. While the use of masks and other controls were debated in the press and in meetings such as the Royal Society of Medicine's 'Discussion', the LGB took little action and left all such decisions in the hands of local authorities.[22] The notable exception to this was the cinemas, as they became the only closely regulated public space for the duration of the pandemic. Here the LGB published regulations that limited the duration of performances and prescribed ventilation practices that had to be followed. These measures were more a reflection of the 'anti-vice concerns regarding the perceived immorality of cinemas rather than sound public health' (Tomkins 1992a: 443). They are also an indication of the medical establishment's deep loathing of the 'kinema', a dislike driven by class as much as anything else (Lawrence 1999). Whereas the South African authorities had regarded the cinema as a way of educating the masses about influenza, the British authorities had a more ambivalent response. The LGB did make an educational film on influenza available to MOHs, but also regarded cinemas as most unsavoury spaces. The medical historian Chris Lawrence has noted how the patrician medical elite regarded 'Mass consumption and entertainment (notably cinema going, an object of particular contempt . . .) . . . enervating.' He quotes Crookshank,[23] who described 'kinema' as 'the "greatest enemy of the epoch to intellectual culture", specifically associating the lower stages of evolution with the "shiftiness of the monkey, the film star and the imbecile."' (Lawrence 1999: 7–8; original citation is Crookshank 1931: 107, 179). In the light of such views it is not surprising that cinemas became a target for regulation.

The LGB was moved towards these controls by debates elsewhere, for example in the press. It was also asked by some local authorities and MOHs for advice on what they could do about places they perceived as sources of infection. It was reported that the Portsmouth Health Committee had requested the LGB's permission to close public entertainments in late October 1918. Other centres, including Edinburgh, Grimsby, Liverpool, Leicester and Newcastle also debated the issue and instituted some restrictions. It was reported on 28 October 1918 that in Portsmouth the military authorities had issued an Order of the Day placing all theatres and cinema houses in the garrison out of bounds for troops, and suggesting that all commanding officers should encourage outdoor sports for their men.[24] Under this pressure the LGB considered the issue and, on 4 November 1918, issued a letter to all Sanitary Authorities regarding 'the closure of places of public entertainment, especially of picture palaces'. As ever, the LGB made no unequivocal statement and left it to the local authorities in advising that the 'point should be carefully considered by the Medical Officer of Health in the light of local knowledge as to the relative importance of these places as likely sources of infection'. The LGB suggested that, in addition to closure, actions such as longer intervals with greater ventilation with the 'hall being thoroughly flushed with fresh air in the intervals' may be considered. Such suggestions became a major element in the Regulations that quickly followed (PRO MH 10 83, 184~18, 4 November 1918 letter to Sanitary Authorities).

But the pressure intensified on the LGB and within weeks they proclaimed regulations specifically setting out controls on cinemas. While recognising that many cinema proprietors had adopted changes to operating practices (hours and ventilation), the LGB issued *The Public Health (Influenza) Regulations, 1918*, requiring that public entertainments were not to be conducted for more than three consecutive hours, there was to be an interval of at least thirty minutes between performances and during that time the premises were to be thoroughly ventilated. While the definition of 'place of public entertainment means a building used as a theatre, music hall, place for public singing, dancing, or music, place for cinematograph exhibition, or other place of entertainment or amusement, to which the public are admitted by ticket or by payment', the emphasis and target of these regulations was very much the cinemas (PRO MH 10 83, 197–18).[25] Such an emphasis was explicitly declared by Deptford Borough Council's Public Health and Housing Committee, who reported that 'although we are alive to the possibility that a certain amount of infection is spread through theatres, music-halls, churches, and chapels, we consider that a great deal more of the risk of infection is to be ascribed to the cinemas' (*The Times* 5 November 1918: 3). The cinema proprietors were not slow to react; in fact, the day after the pronouncement, the advertisement in *The Times* for Dally's in Leicester Square carried the strapline: 'THE BEST VENTILATED THEATRE IN LONDON WITHOUT DRAUGHTS' (5 November 1918: 3).

The Regulations obviously did not go far enough, for only two days later the LGB issued an amended Regulation, *The Public Health (Influenza) Regulations (No. 2), 1918*. The LGB issued 'an Order amending in certain particulars the Public Health (Influenza) Regulations, 1918, so far as they apply to places for cinematograph exhibition'. These amendments actually allowed for an increase in the duration permitted before an interval was required. However, they also restricted who was allowed to enter the premises by prohibiting the admission of children to cinemas in any district where any school had been closed 'on account of the prevalence of Influenza' for as long as the school closure lasted (PRO MH 10 83, 202–18).[26] Naturally the cinema operators resented being singled out and even mounted demonstrations and legal challenges. The proprietors of the Majestic Cinema, Clapham, unsuccessfully defended a prosecution for 'conducting an entertainment for more than four hours consecutively without an interval'. They were fined £5 and ordered to pay costs at the South-western Police Court. The sense of injustice was probably heightened as some authorities largely ignored the regulations while other enforced them rigorously (Tomkins 1989: 141–2).[27] The LGB eventually rescinded the Regulations in May 1919 (PRO MH 10 83, 53~19).[28] The British approach to cinema and theatre contrasts with that of the Australians. There, an MHR, William

Henry Kelly,[29] asked the Minister for Trade and Customs whether the lack of airspace and the sanitary conditions backstage could be 'a focus of the influenza outbreak' and whether they should be regulated. The Minister consulted the State governments and reported that all states had no concerns with theatres as they were not 'special foci of infection' (NAA A2 1919/2930).

Great discussion was given over to the issue of schools and whether to close them or not. In Britain this was a decision that central government again left to the local authorities. Closures became widespread, with the major exception of London, where closure only happened if staff absenteeism made it impossible to keep the school open. The closure of schools was actually one of the most commonly reported aspects of the pandemic in Britain, with closures as long as three weeks quite commonly reported.[30] The controversy over school closure usually revolved around the question of whether the children were better off at school and where they would be if not in school, and such arguments were by no means limited to Britain.[31] Subsequently it has become appreciated how important school-age children are in the dissemination of influenza as households with school age children tend to be involved prior to those without. However, the role of children in spreading the disease is not limited to school-to-home transmission, as unvaccinated children appear to act as a large, susceptible population within a community (Cate 1987; Schoenbaum 2003). Indeed, in the event of future pandemics the WHO suggests consideration be given to the closing of schools (WHO 1999d: 27).

From the newspaper reports it is readily apparent that closures were widespread in Britain, at least outside London. This pattern is true of all three waves of the epidemic, including the milder first wave. In London, the Chief Medical Officer of the London County Council was later reported as saying that

> We do not close schools in London as a matter of routine on account of influenza, but instructions have been issued as to the precautionary steps that should be taken when symptoms of the disease appear among teachers and scholars. There is undoubtedly a good deal of it about still, and we are hearing of schools with half the scholars away.
>
> (*The Times* 21 October 1918: 5)

Only two days after this, the press were reporting large numbers of school closures elsewhere in the country but noted that in the capital the 'medical authorities being of opinion that such action would simply release the children and allow them to congregate in places where the danger of infection is greater' and so had refused to take such measures (*The Times* 23 October 1918: 3). At least one school in England adopted the reverse approach and, rather than closing the school, they closed off the outside world. In a report to the MRC, the Cheltenham College school doctor wrote that the Boys'

School had avoided infection as 'None of the boys, staff or domestics were allowed to go near the town, and on my advice, even the daughter of the Headmaster, who taught at the Ladies College, where influenza was prevailing was not allowed to go there until the malady had ceased' (PRO FD 1 537, Report received by the MRC on 5 February 1919).

Before the end of October 1918, the issue of schools and whether they should be closed had become a Parliamentary matter. H.A.L. Fisher MP, as President of the Board of Education, replied to a colleague's question (Mr Rowntree MP, York, L.) on the closure of schools or the exclusion from school of children, setting out that while 'appropriate directions' had been supplied by the Board of Education, 'in conjunction with' the LGB, the decision to close or exclude was purely a matter for the local body (either the local authority or the school governors), as he claimed it was largely dependent on local circumstances. Circumstances 'upon which it is, of course, impossible for the Board to pronounce', he suggested, could include 'degree of prevalence and severity of the disease, as well as the home or other alternative circumstances of the children thus excluded from school'. However, any children exhibiting 'catarrhal symptoms, feverishness or other illness' should be excluded immediately. Having absolved the national authorities of responsibility, he conceded that many schools might be closed due to flu. He concluded by observing that school closure was more effective in rural areas, and that playgrounds should also be closed if schools were closed (*The Times* 31 October 1918: 8). But in London the LCC continued to follow Hamer's advice as he considered that closing schools would have negligible effect on the spread of the disease (*The Times* 6 November 1918: 3).[32]

Official (in)action

Being in the frontline of the pandemic put enormous strain on the world's medical practitioners. In those countries bound up in the war this was a pressure they were often poorly placed to bear when many of their fellow medical personnel were already committed to the war effort at home and abroad. Many were linked to the military establishment at home, caring for the returned wounded or inspecting potential recruits or other military medical tasks. The practical consequence of this was the widespread shortage of personnel and facilities. All in addition to facing a disease for which they had no cure and could offer little more than to try to ease the suffering. One Canadian doctor recalled how impotent he was: 'Keep 'em in bed, that was all. Protect them from getting more exposure. That was about all you could do' (Hagmeier 1981). In the face of this overwhelming and, to some extent unknown, enemy the frontline role was often taken by volunteers.[33] In Britain, the organising of such volunteers was one of the few successful actions taken by local authorities (Tomkins 1989, 1992a). Without these volunteers, it is quite possible that the medical systems of many localities may well have failed to cope at all. Failure of the healthcare systems (or

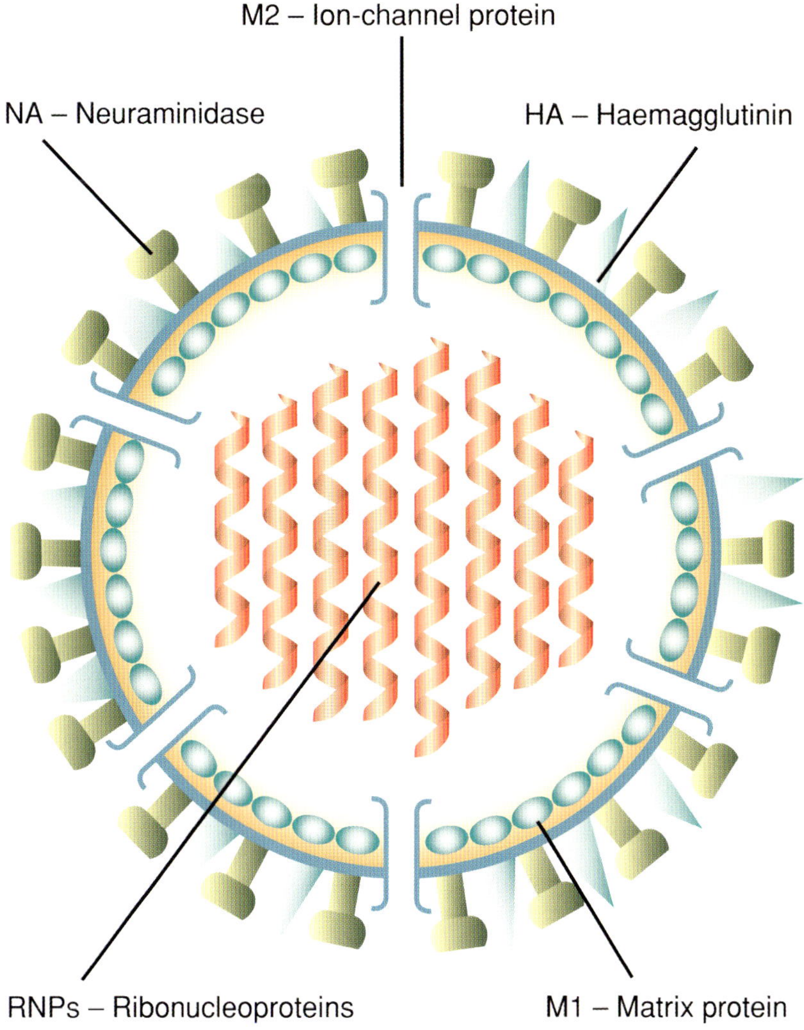

Plate 1 Influenza virus schematic (image courtesty of C.W. Broughton).

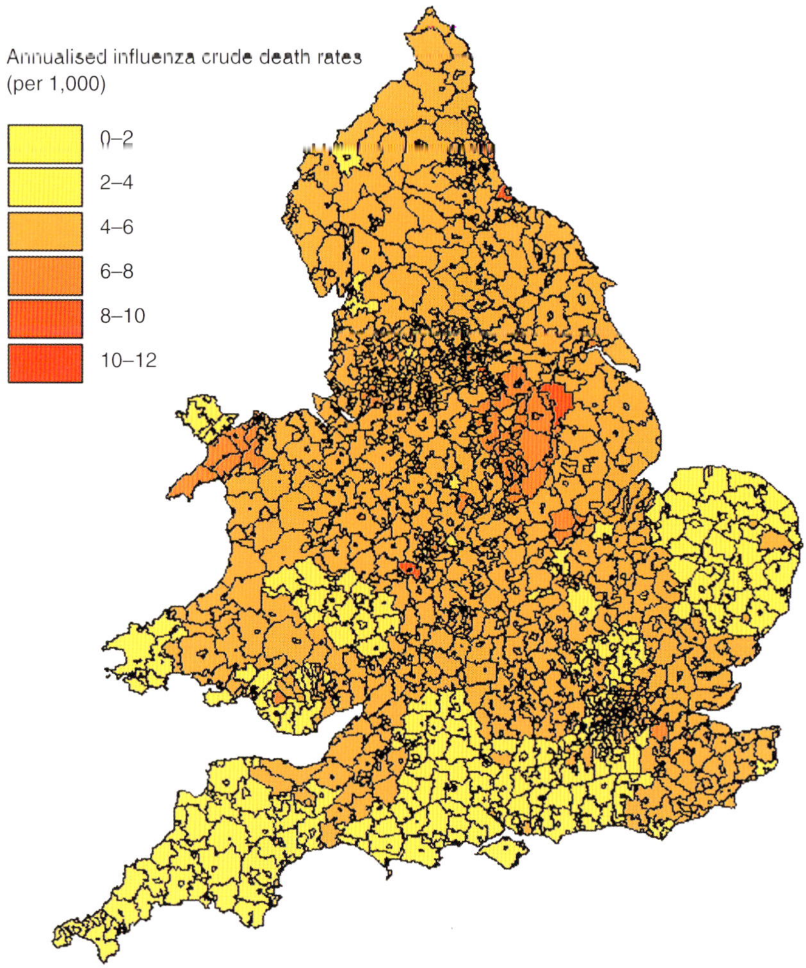

Plate 2 Pandemic influenza mortality 1918–19, England and Wales.

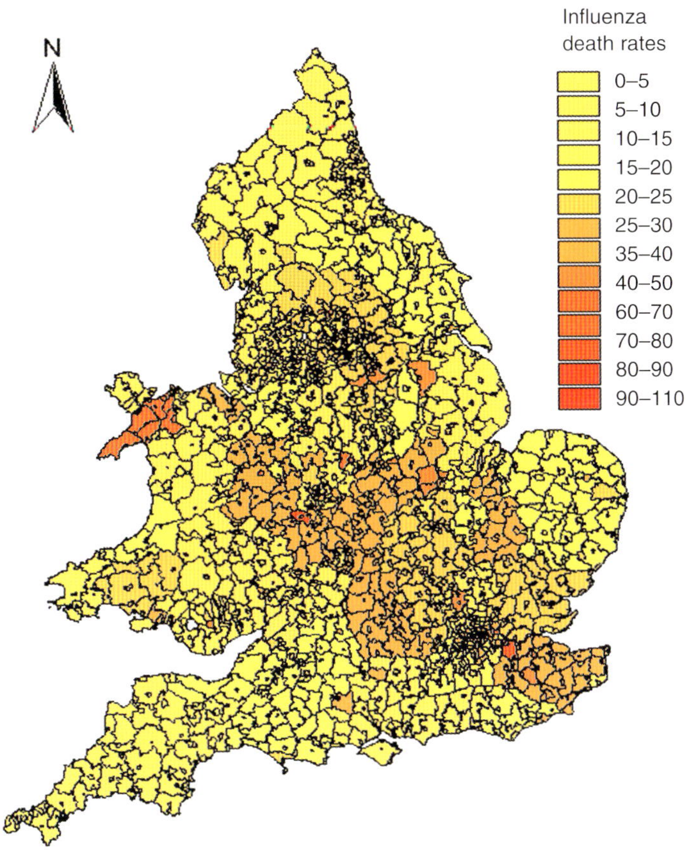

Plate 3 Influenza mortality, week ending 9 November 1918.

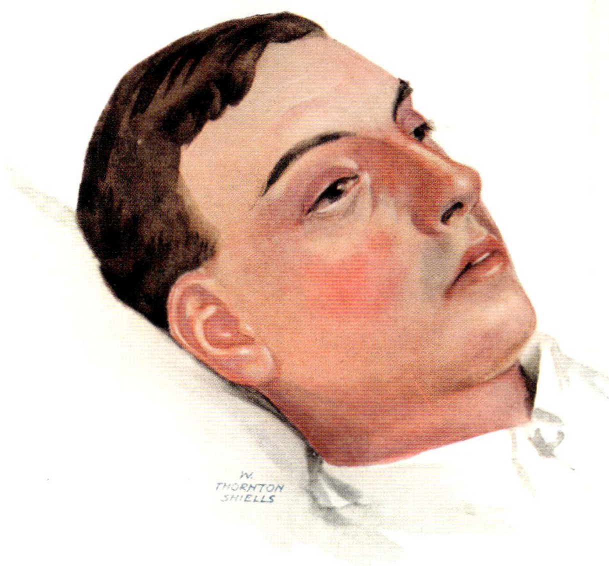

Plate 4 Heliotrope cyanosis – early case (source: Ministry of Health 1920c; by permission of the Syndics of Cambridge University Library).

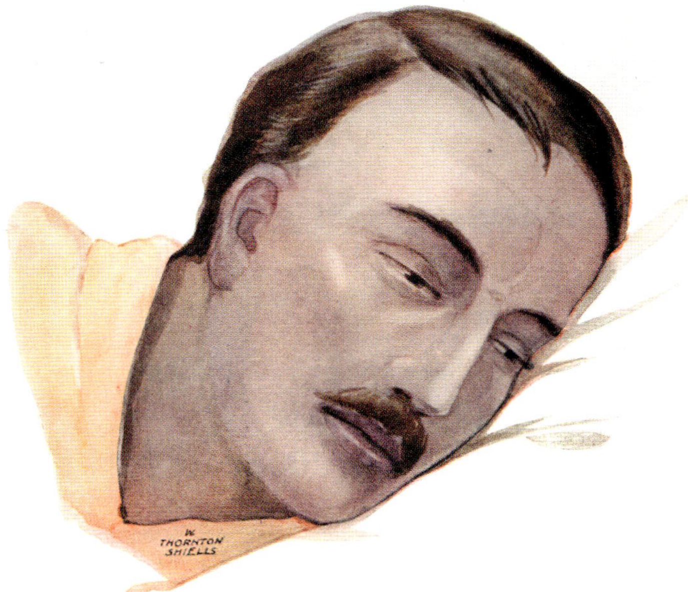

Plate 5 Heliotrope cyanosis – diffused cyanosis (source: Ministry of Health 1920c; by permission of the Syndics of Cambridge University Library).

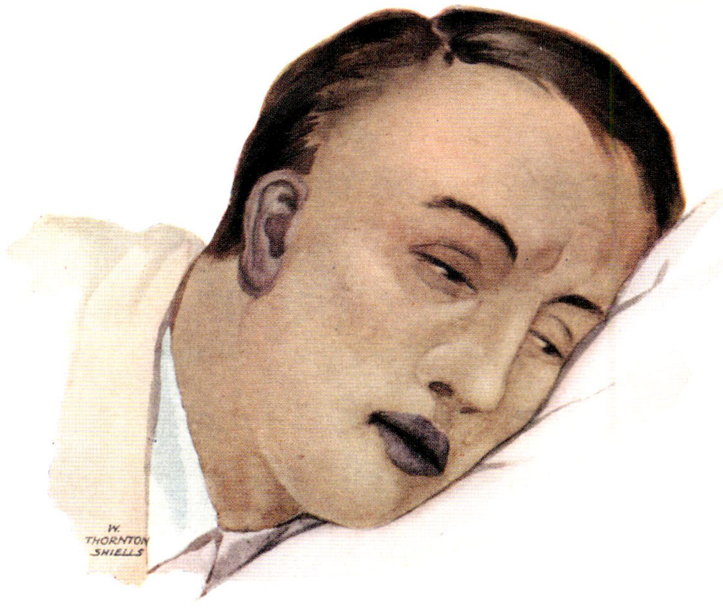

Plate 6 Heliotrope cyanosis with general pallor (source: Ministry of Health 1920c; by permission of the Syndics of Cambridge University Library).

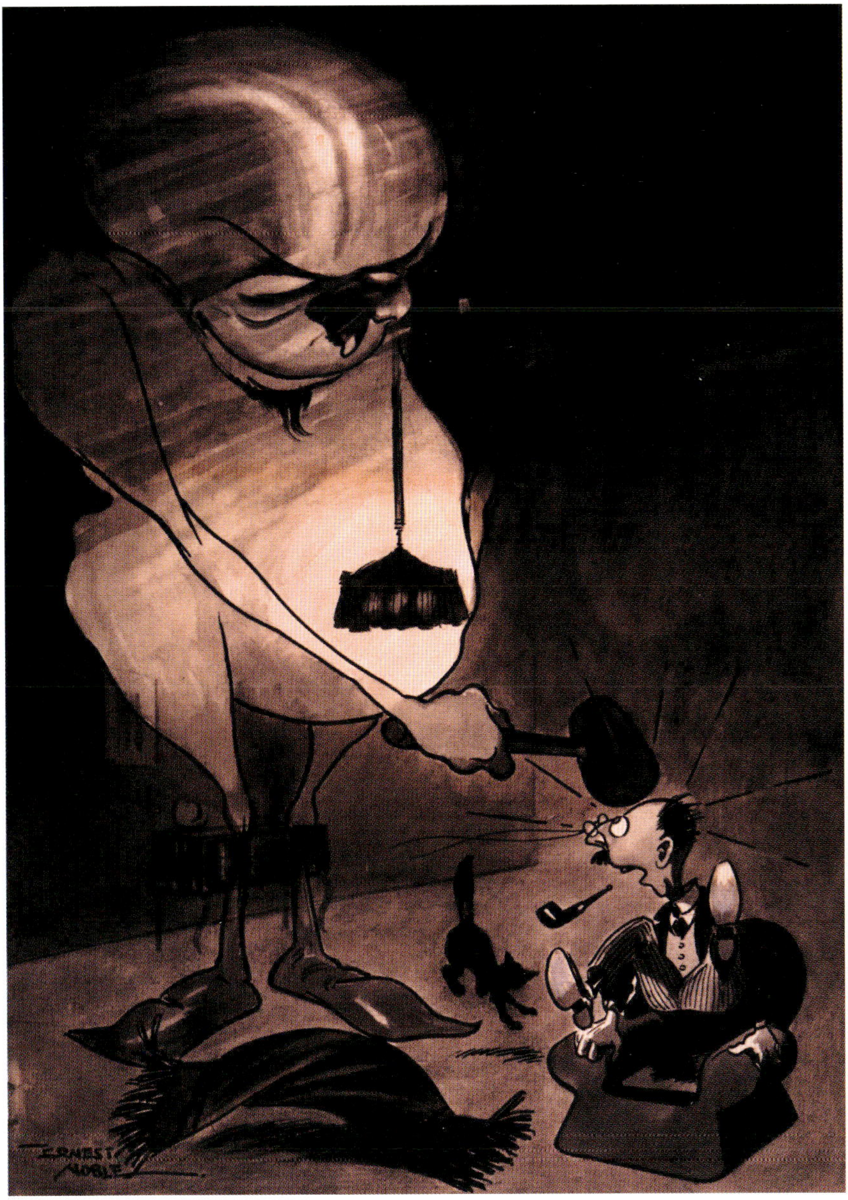

Plate 7 Ernest Noble, 'A-TICH-OO!! Good evening. I'm the new influenza' (source: Wellcome Icongraphic Collection, Wellcome Library for the History and Understanding of Medicine, Item 16001; image courtesy of the Wellcome Trust).

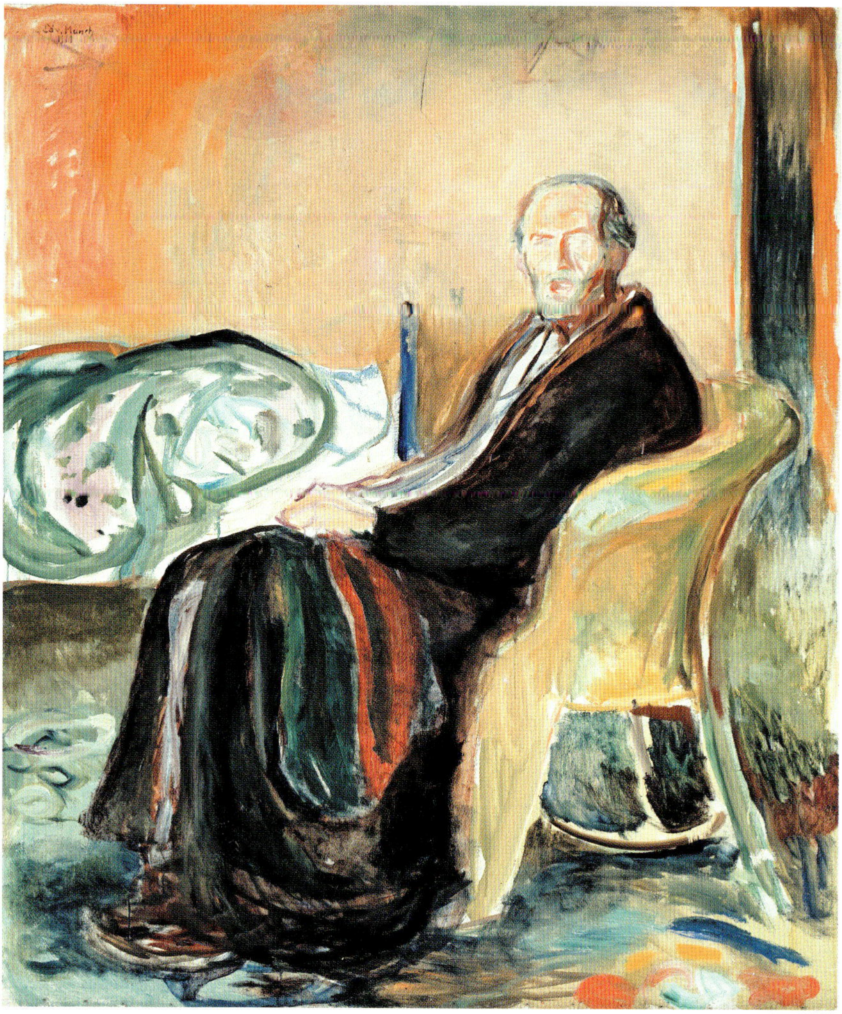

Plate 8 Eduard Munch: self-portrait, Spanish influenza (1919) (150 × 131 cm; oil on canvas; photographer: K.Ø. Nredrum; © National Gallery, Norway (Viscopy)).

rather the lack of them) became an issue in a number of countries, and this led to the creation or major revision of some national healthcare systems.

But while this disease was killing thousands, what were the various levels of British government doing? Not very much, it would seem. The response of government and the medical establishment has been characterised by Tomkins as a 'failure of expertise' in spite of having one of the most highly developed public health establishments of the period (Tomkins 1992a). In 1918, the British central government department charged with responsibility for public health in Britain was the LGB. It was to take quite a low profile in the pandemic, issuing the occasional 'Memorandum' (Local Government Board 1918, 1919a, 1919b) with advice on avoiding and treating influenza, distributing a film about influenza prevention, and generally leaving the local authorities and their MOHs to work it out for themselves.

It was only in late October 1918 that the LGB issued its nine-page *Memorandum on Epidemic Catarrhs and Influenza* (Local Government Board 1918) to local authorities with a covering letter suggesting that MOHs 'consider whether it would not be desirable ... to prepare ... some precautionary instructions'. Some weeks prior to this, the LGB had been communicating with the MRC about the origins of the disease, the periodicity of influenza and how epidemics came in waves (PRO FD 1 535). This was followed by a 3 November letter requesting that the local authorities collect detailed information on the 'present extremely fatal epidemic' as the LGB did not have enough staff to collect such data. The following day the LGB reminded local authorities of the recently circulated Memorandum, granting them the power to provide further 'medical (including nursing) assistance within their district', and urging consideration of using isolation hospitals or obtaining a building for such a purpose. This letter also carried one of the first indications that cinemas were to be targeted (PRO MH 10 83 letters 171~18 and 184~18).

Opening the Royal Society of Medicine's 'Discussion' on influenza on 13 November 1918, Sir Arthur Newsholme (Medical Officer of the LGB) adopted a rather defensive posture, arguing that they could not have predicted the epidemic, and even if they had, they could not have done much about it (Royal Society of Medicine 1918). The first point is debatable given the widely reported outbreaks elsewhere; the second may be fair comment. At the time of this 'Discussion', the pandemic had peaked in London and only then was the LGB doing much about communicating with the medical profession and the local authorities. On 18 November, after the pandemic had peaked, the LGB sent copies of its Memorandum to the Royal College of Surgeons and reminded them and their members of the LGB's desire that they collect data on the disease, suggesting that the LGB were receiving only partial information. Two days later, the LGB had obviously been piqued into action, moving against the cinemas and issuing the *Public Health (Influenza) Regulations, 1918*, enforcing greater intervals and ventilation. A further two days later, the LGB informed of an amendment to those regulations (*Public Health (Influenza) Regulations (No. 2), 1918*), changing the maximum duration of events and banning children from such venues once a school had been closed in the area (PRO MH 10 83 letters 197~18 and 202~18).

In mid-December, the LGB informed local authorities of the existence of the fifteen-minute film, *Dr Wise on Influenza*, in which the audience was lectured on 'the precautions to be adopted by a person suffering from influenza in the patient's own interest as well as in the interest of those he comes in contact with'. The lecturing or 'exhortations of the doctor' were 'emphasised by cinematograph pictures in a popular vein designed with the intention of leaving a marked impression on the audience'. To give the film greater authority, it was 'prefaced by an appeal from Sir Auckland Geddes [then President of the LGB[34]] to the public to assist the health officials by adopting the precautions indicated'. The LGB had a number of copies of the film that they were willing to lend to the MOHs for 'exhibition purposes'. However, to borrow this film, which was only permitted for a very short period as 'demand . . . may exceed the number of films', the local authority had to complete an application form and a 'statement of the extent of prevalence of influenza'. Thus, it would seem that the areas that managed to have this film screened were those that had already experienced much illness, rather than providing some form of advance warning (PRO MH 10 83).

Early in 1919, the LGB issued a Memorandum to MOHs regarding their annual reports for 1918, in which the LGB specifically requested that they provide more detail than usual on influenza, referring to Newsholme's 'circular letter of 3rd November last on epidemic influenza' for what information was sought (PRO MH 10 84 5~19). The LGB also issued a short *Memorandum on Pneumonia*, obviously prompted by the high proportion of influenza mortality associated with pneumonic complications (Local Government Board 1919a). The lack of apparent activity on the LGB's part prompted *Punch* magazine to make one of its customary pointed remarks: '"Our chief hope of control of influenza," writes Sir Arthur Newsholme of the Local Government, "lies in further investigation." Persons who insist upon having influenza between now and Easter will do so at their own risk' (*Punch* 22 January 1919, 156: 53).

In February 1919, during the third wave of the pandemic, the LGB published an amended version of its October Memorandum, this time with the title *Memorandum on Prevention of Influenza* (Local Government Board 1919b). Recognising the scale of the problem faced in 1918, particularly its impact on young adults, this version noted how little could be done about influenza and advocated a number of preventive measures, concentrating on the individual:

1 The golden rule is to keep fit, and avoid infection as much as possible.
2 The way to keep fit is to cultivate healthy and regular habits, to eat

good food, and to avoid fatigue, chill and alcoholism. Healthy living does not of itself ensure against attack, but it makes the patient better able to withstand the complications which kill . . .

4 It is not always possible to avoid infection, but the risks can be lessened by–

a healthy living;
b working and sleeping in well-ventilated rooms;
c avoiding crowded gatherings and close, ill-ventilated rooms;
d wearing warm clothing;
e gargling the throat and washing out the nostrils;
f by wearing a mask and glasses when nursing or in attendance on a person suffering from influenza.

(Local Government Board 1919b: 3)

These and other suggestions on what to do if attacked were followed by observations on influenza and further advice on what the individual should do. Part III of the Memorandum briefly discussed what Sanitary Authorities could do, which largely amounted to education campaigns and informing the public how to apply to their local authority for assistance with home nursing or domestic help, what local arrangements were available in the way of crèches, public kitchens, ambulances, medical practitioners and hospitals. Once again, the onus was very much on the local authorities and medical professionals to deal with the pandemic. Such actions are exemplified in the sections detailing the actions taken in Manchester and Birmingham, contributed by the respective MOHs, James Niven and John Robertson (Local Government Board 1919b).

The LGB memoranda were requested by and circulated not only to the domestic local authorities but also to the dominions and colonies. In many of these locations the advice was repeated or other similar advice was given in public notices and handbills, such as the Victorian Board of Health notices published in November 1918 (Figures 5.2 and 5.3).[35] Because the British reaction was a devolved or decentralised one, it rather precluded larger actions. Whereas in Melbourne, Australia, for example, the Exhibition Building was converted into a massive temporary hospital (more than 4,000 patients passed through), and in both Sydney and Melbourne military hospitals were used as emergency civilian hospitals (SRNSW 4/7776; Hyslop 1996). These were not without their own problems, including sectarian disputes as to whether the staff from Catholic hospitals should serve and disputes between the state and national governments that ran for some years concerning who was to pay for what and whether military-attached medical personnel should be paid 'quarantine' (double) pay rates for the extra work.[36] Relief efforts and the provision of assistance in Britain tended to be at the local authority level whereas in Melbourne it was across the entire city.[37] In Sydney the state premier reported to the state Parliament

BOARD OF PUBLIC HEALTH, VICTORIA.

"SPANISH" INFLUENZA.

"Spanish" influenza is ordinary influenza associated with germs which cause pneumonia.

Symptoms.—The onset is generally sudden, beginning with a chill or a shivering fit and high fever. Headache and backache ensue, followed by a general aching of the body, and extreme weakness. Sometimes the disease begins with reddening and running of the eyes, coughing, sneezing, and sore throat.

Occasionally the attack is ushered in by—

(*a*) Vomiting and diarrhœa, accompanied by severe abdominal pains; or
(*b*) A sudden faint; or
(*c*) An epileptiform fit; or
(*d*) Symptoms of acute mania; or
(*e*) Delirium tremens.

Complications.—The most important and the most dangerous complication of influenza is pneumonia. The presence of pneumonia is revealed by high fever, flushed face, cough, increased frequency and difficulty of breathing, and sharp pains in the chest.

Treatment.—Bed should be sought at the onset of symptoms. Complete rest is the best way to prevent complications. Plenty of food and water should be taken. Quinine, salicylates, acetylsalicylic acid, and phenacetin have proved to be the most useful drugs in relieving symptoms. They do not, however, prevent or cure influenza. Air and light should freely enter the room. Owing to the dangerous complications that may follow even a mild case of influenza, medical advice should be obtained early.

How influenza is spread.—The infecting organisms are contained in the discharges from mouth and nose; hence the disease is spread by the transmission of these germs from the infected to the healthy. The commonest way in which the disease is contracted is by inhaling small particles of infected sputum or nasal mucus expelled in the act of coughing or sneezing. Infection is also acquired by medium of common towels, cups, glasses, and any other article soiled with infected discharges.

Prevention.—

(1) Isolation of patients and contacts.
(2) Disinfection of discharges from mouth and nose of patients and contacts.
(3) Disinfection of nose and mouth cavities by douches, mouth washes, sprays, and inhalations.

H.226/11.18.—18207.—20M. [OVER.

Figure 5.2 Board of Public Health, Victoria, 'Spanish' influenza notice (front).

(4) Attendants on patients and contacts should wear a gauze mask or suitable respirator.

(5) Avoid crowds; be in the open air as much as possible. Allow sunshine and air to freely enter all living, sleeping, and working rooms. Avoid fatigue, and beware of the cougher and sneezer.

(6) Evidence from South Africa shows that the special vaccine prevents serious complications, if not the disease itself. This vaccine is supplied by the Health Department to Councils, to which application should be made for inoculation.

Disinfection of nose and mouth.—

Douche—A flat teaspoonful of salt, baking soda, and boric acid dissolved in a quart of warm water.

Sprays—Permanganate of potash, 1 in 1500, or 2 % solution of hydrogen peroxide. These may also be used as mouth washes.

Inhalant—Eucalyptus oil, 7 parts; terebene, 2 parts; and menthol, 1 part.

The above have been found satisfactory, but many others are available. Medical advice should be sought as to what is best to use under the circumstances.

Legal obligations.—

(1) Every householder shall immediately send a report, in writing, to the Council of every case of influenza, or any illness resembling influenza, which occurs in the house, and such report shall include the name, age, and sex of the patient, and the exact location of the house.

(2) Every person who suffers from symptoms of influenza shall immediately inform the occupier of the house wherein he resides of his condition.

(3) Every person who has been in contact with a case of influenza shall immediately send a report to the Council, and such report shall include such person's name and address.

(4) No contact and no person suffering from symptoms of influenza shall enter any public building or place where persons are congregated.

(5) Any person who fails to comply with the foregoing regulations, or is guilty of any neglect or disobedience thereof, is liable to a penalty of **£20.**

By order,

MELBOURNE, 23rd *November*, 1918.

T. W. H. HOLMES,
Secretary.

By Authority: H. J. GREEN, Acting Government Printer, Melbourne.

Figure 5.3 Board of Public Health, Victoria, 'Spanish' influenza notice (rear).

that the government 'issued food orders to the value of £100,000, the value of rent grants was £9,000, and we paid £12,900 for board and lodging' as well as establishing 'no less than seventy-nine emergency hospitals throughout the State' and '109 relief depôts'.[38]

Other actions eventually taken at the national level in Britain include the regulation of quinine, the slight relaxation of alcohol controls (for medicinal purposes, of course), declining to increase the meat ration and the eventual release of some doctors from military service to resume civil practice and help in the battle against flu, joining those doctors who were freed from their military-related medical board duties. The last year of the war had seen military recruitment examinations being conducted by civilian doctors and thus the bulk of British doctors 'not in uniform were occupied in the difficult and time-consuming task of determining the fitness for military service of over 2,500,000 men' (Winter 1982: 724). This diversion of medical personnel led to warnings, during the pandemic, that the civilian health was endangered; petitions and implorings came from many areas – local authorities, especially rural ones, were desperate for assistance, requesting the return of their doctors and drawing others out of retirement or facing being left with no medical assistance. While difficult to quantify, it can be concluded that 'levels of medical intervention throughout Britain were significantly reduced' (Winter 1982: 724).[39]

The LGB and its successor, the Ministry of Health, took more action after the pandemic when they finally appreciated how serious it could be. Not long after the establishment of the Ministry of Health, George Newman[40] produced a new version of the *Memorandum on Prevention of Influenza* (Ministry of Health 1919b). Issued in December 1919 with fears of another epidemic occurring that winter, it updated the previous Memoranda by recalling the scale of the pandemic. Much was retained from the previous editions and the emphasis on personal preventive measures still dominated. However, there was now specific discussion of measures such as the closure of schools, cinemas and other 'centres of overcrowding' along with consideration of measures that could be taken for the 'organisation of domiciliary medical and nursing service' and the 'provision of institutional treatment', but these still placed the onus on the local authorities. Newman also authorised the release of a three-page notice on vaccines that informed MOHs of the Ministry's fear of an epidemic and that, in the light of this, the Ministry was preparing a stock of anti-influenza vaccine, while recognising that until the 'causal organism . . . has been isolated with certainty . . . we cannot hope to prepare a vaccine which can be guaranteed to ward off an attack of the disease' (Ministry of Health 1919a). This meant various 'recipes' of vaccines would be used with the hope that they contained something that may help. This rush to distribute unproven vaccines caused some disquiet at the MRC where its head, Walter Fletcher, was moved to record his concern over this and a number of other issues (PRO FD 1 535).

The Ministry's detailed report into the pandemic and the RG's Supplement to the *ARRG* for 1918 that solely concerned itself with the pandemic in England and Wales were published in 1920 (Ministry of Health 1920c; Registrar-General 1920). Whereas a number of countries or states instituted enquiries or Royal Commissions into the episode, there was no such enquiry in Britain, nor calls for one.[41] It seemed it was considered that the newly-established Ministry of Health would address such problems. At the time the national authorities were overwhelmingly concerned and occupied with the prosecution of the war above all else. Consequently they left coping with the influenza to the local authorities (Tomkins 1989, 1992a). Evidence that indicates how little the national authorities regarded the influenza include the decision not to bother with any form of quarantine (due to the necessity of the war), the need to 'carry on', and the difficulty in getting doctors and nurses released from military service back to civil practice, even once the Armistice had been signed. Is it possible that this lack of action, both during and subsequently, was related to the short duration of each peak of influenza activity? Could it be that such a fast-acting disease mitigated against central action and central planning? Would the short duration make the organisation, preparation and delivery of resources and care seem largely pointless? This would then place the onus for planning and delivery on the local authority as they would be the only level of government 'close' enough to deliver anything that might assist in such a circumstance. Did the local authorities have the resources to provide assistance, especially at the end of the war? Once more, the shadow of the Great War falls heavily across the pandemic; long years of a brutal war could make the rapid passages of influenza, just a couple of weeks in each wave, seem insignificant.

Before action can be taken the existence of a problem has to be recognised and a need for action has to be perceived or created, and it was at the local level that this need was most acutely felt.[42] This seems not to have occurred in Britain in 1918; that is, no problem addressable at the national scale was perceived and, consequently, no action was taken by central government. Tomkins argues that it was the local authorities who acted as that was the level at which a problem was 'visualised' and encountered. Influenza is a much less 'visible' condition, with its lower mortality and its frequent visitations. Even when a disease is (finally) recognised as a problem, there can be obstacles to an effective response. For example, in discussing the 'Russian' flu of the 1890s, Smith suggested:

> Once influenza joined other communicable diseases formerly thought to be atmospheric and occult, like cholera, it behoved authorities to enforce isolation and quarantine. But government action was precluded by the uncertainties in early diagnosis and the cost and the resistance to official meddling with everyday business to contain what the public regarded as a minor illness.
>
> (Smith 1995: 64)

A couple of decades later, many of the same obstacles were to play a role in the response to the pandemic. Many of these relate to the nature of medicine, the profession and the role of government at the time.

Some of the changes in the profession and governance of medicine had been allied with shifting views of disease, changes that 'redirected the eyes of the local health authorities from environmental sanitation to the control of infectious patients' (Eyler 1992: 276). These were often more about control of the individual (as seen in the preventive measures proposed during the pandemic) than the control of disease per se. This control came from and contributed to notification, home visits, epidemiological tracing of antecedent cases and contacts, isolation of individuals and the construction of isolation hospitals. The political climate of the time was one in which individual rights were considered important and the role of central government was to be curbed. As part of this, the treatment of those at the bottom of society improved. For example, local authorities were beginning to provide treatment and other services to the diseased and their families, in addition to the 'older police and regulatory functions implicit in sanitary reform', and by the second decade of the twentieth century, 'beginning with infants, local authorities were offering personal services to both the sick and the well in the hope of preventing future disease or disability' (Eyler 1992: 276). Such changes came most rapidly under the Liberal government between 1906 and 1914, as old-age pensions, national health insurance, unemployment insurance, school medical service, free school meals, infant and maternal welfare services, and national systems of treatment for tuberculosis and venereal disease were all introduced (Eyler 1992: 277). In 1918 alone the Education Act raised the school leaving age, extended school medical inspections, and allowed treatment for defects found at inspection, while the Maternity and Child Welfare Act required local authorities to appoint a maternity and child welfare committee, and the Building Construction of Dwellings for the Working Classes committee recommended greater minimum standards for housing. The change of focus from the punitive to the provident, aided by arguments about national efficiency (in light of both the South African and First World Wars) that included elements of poverty, nutrition and health was accompanied by the rise of scientific medical professionalism (Lees 1998: 317–18).

These changes accompanied a shift in how the poor were perceived. Under the Poor Laws, the receipt of welfare was regarded as 'a sign of personal failing and character defect. To receive relief was not only to lose some of one's civil rights and sometimes one's freedom, but to be morally stigmatized' (Eyler 1992: 277). The changed welfare environment of the early twentieth century now regarded some provision of services as an entitlement with far less penalty. However, such changes in policy do not necessarily produce rapid changes in the systems and people delivering those policies, as it takes time to change the mindsets and attitudes of people delivering and using the systems. Eyler considers Newsholme a very good case study in how these changes in British public health came about and were expressed, as Newsholme's career ran in parallel with many of these changes.[43] For many years, Newsholme 'wrestled' with the themes of a individualistic and moralistic healthcare that promoted the power of doctors with an attendant rejection of environmentalism and an extension of the commodification of healthcare in his writings on public health. Kearns illustrated this in examining Newsholme's writings on tuberculosis, and demonstrated how public health at this time was conceived of in terms of the needs of National Efficiency and the need for a population ready for imperial combat (Kearns 1995; Winter 1980). Social diseases at this time could be defined as those complaints resulting from personal failings and which reduced national efficiency. Thus, influenza, as a social disease can be linked to sanitation, and the connection between the pandemic, sanitation, national efficiency and the 'fitness' of the population was certainly being discussed.[44] Sanitation was regarded as critical – much of the LGB's advice was about sanitation and many of the newspaper reports, particularly *The Times*' medical correspondent's comments, focused on sanitation, either for the individual or as a primary target for a new Ministry of Health. Personal cleanliness and morality were also invoked when it came to the regulation of the cinemas, over and above all other public gatherings. This was rather undermined when the RG concluded that the 'mortality of the late epidemic fell almost alike on the sanitarily just and on the unjust' (Registrar-General 1920: 29).

In her study of George Newman, Margaret Hammer barely raised the issue of the pandemic, even though it occurred at the height of the battle between Newman and Newsholme over the forthcoming Ministry of Health (Hammer 1995). She recognised Newman's long-standing disdain for Newsholme, epitomised in Newman's 29 October 1918 diary entry after a conference at the LGB (to discuss influenza) that described Newsholme as 'weak, vacillating, incompetent, untrustworthy, and vain' (PRO MH 139 3).[45] This antipathy dated back to their differences in opinion over child and maternal welfare and the activities of Newman's Medical Department at the Board of Education. The two held quite differing opinions on what constituted 'preventive' medicine. Newman regarded it as an issue of education and social condition whereas Newsholme's conception was a more environmental approach to preventing disease (Hammer 1995: 217–18, 260–1). These differences about the role of public health and of any future ministry were not confined to these two. While the LGB was regarded by many as 'the logical nucleus for any kind of future Ministry' this was at odds with Newman's 'rather contemptuous attitude . . . towards the administrative inefficiencies of the LGB [which] only exacerbated the situation' between the two (Hammer 1995: 213). Newsholme's earlier appointment to the LGB had been seen as a step forward by those pushing for a Ministry, but his subsequent failure to move the LGB in that direction and have it take a more active role in health administration was held against him, despite the fact that he (Newsholme) had 'remained committed to the idea of a national health service based around the LGB' (Hammer 1995: 214). Hammer considered the battle for the heralded Ministry as being centred around issues of child and maternal welfare, the conceptions of preventive medicine, and whether the medical profession or government should control health policy rather than about any thing as prosaic as a single epidemic (Hammer 1995: Chapter 6, 187–272, particularly 259–67). It is arguable that these conflicts played a role in dragging the process out,[46] and ensuring there was no Ministry when the pandemic struck. It could be said that a vacuum existed at the peak of British health administration at the time and thus further ensured that any responsibility for dealing with the pandemic fell to the local authorities. However, there was a role for influenza in the battle between the two men. As the Ministry became an inevitability, Newman replaced Newsholme at the LGB, which was to become the core of the new Ministry, and Hammer considered that 'Newsholme's departure . . . was not entirely unexpected in view of his "incompetent" handling of the influenza epidemic' (Hammer 1995: 274).[47]

With the LGB's activity limited to the provision of advice, it was the local authorities that took any direct action. The responses of the London boroughs to the pandemic have been categorised into three levels (Tomkins 1992a, 1989) ranging from little or no response, through to those who acted on the LGB's recommendations and passed out information, to those boroughs that focused on dealing with the effects of the epidemic, including home nursing, domestic help, hospital and burial services.[48] Essentially these were really the only actions that were of any practical use in the face of the epidemic, but were often difficult to deliver. As Carnwath (Medical Inspector, LGB) noted, the

> great difficulty . . . was to secure early and adequate . . . treatment. . . . Many doctors had been called to colours, and consequently the burden thrown on those remaining in civil practice was very great. . . . The shortage of nurses we felt even more. Some authorities eked out the supply by using each trained nurse round which a service of more or less trained voluntary helpers was gathered . . . local authorities were ultimately impelled to suspend temporarily their maternity and child welfare work, and to liberate their health visitors for domiciliary nursing . . . much was done in the way of providing home assistance. Some authorities even set up emergency hospitals, crèches, kitchens, bed linen supplies and subsidised district nursing association activities.
>
> (Carnwath 1919: 154–5)

Unlike in many other cities around the world, London's response was decentralised and fell to the local authorities, as it did all across the UK. The continued prosecution of the war took precedence over domestic health issues and, with the disease being seen as beyond the capabilities of the medical profession, a profession already hamstrung by the large proportion of medical personnel diverted into the military effort, the responses were varied, ranging from inaction to the mobilisation of nurses, many volunteers, provision of food, including baby foods, and house-to-house inspections. In Manchester, the MOH Niven (Niven 1923) mounted one of the most active responses. Indeed it has been pondered if the bottle of Glaxo that the young Anthony Burgess was enjoying when his father returned to find his wife and daughter dead of flu but the baby Anthony 'chuckling in my cot' when he 'should have been howling for food' and the neighbour 'who had herself just been stricken had provided ... a bottle of Glaxo' (Burgess 1987: 18) had actually come from the provision of emergency aid as nearly half the value of the emergency aid given in Manchester for flu victims between 4 December 1918 and 11 January 1919 was in the form of Glaxo, the dried baby milk (Reid 2005: 53–4).

Did the British state and medical profession fail? Were there structural limitations or failings at the LGB? The pandemic struck a society aware of the disease but blasé about the dangers. Appreciation of how grave a danger there was did not come until the second and third waves. But Britain's pandemic mortality is not particularly different from that experienced elsewhere, and by this measure the response to the pandemic cannot necessarily be deemed a failure. The medical and public health professions everywhere were hampered by the lack of knowledge, and this was often made more difficult by a lack of resources due to the war. Given the emergence of an entirely novel influenza virus to which there was no immunity initially, millions were doomed to be infected, with many of those succumbing. It could be argued that the LGB, being more a regulatory and advisory body than a service delivery one, was structurally incapable of dealing with the pandemic, and therefore their response could be nothing more than a muted one. However, with a pandemic that peaked and fell as rapidly as the flu did, whether a large, centralised authority could have reduced the toll or perhaps have mitigated the impact somewhat is contestable. To have combated the pandemic with any degree of success would have required a large, well-resourced medical workforce distributed at the local level, and even that would have been hard-pressed to do much more than alleviate some of the suffering. Nearly a century later, the medical profession fears a flu pandemic would overrun their capabilities, and consequently advocates detailed planning and preparation, not so much as to stop a pandemic, but to attempt to manage its impact. Thus while the LGB's role, and the nature of public health at the time – with the local authorities and MOHs essentially responsible for whatever action was taken – may have contributed to the variety of responses to the pandemic, ranging from neglect to generous provisions of nursing assistance and other aid, it is unlikely that any other ordering of public health responsibilities would have had a markedly different outcome.

The medical profession

Many of the issues surrounding the changes in the administration of welfare and public health in Britain also affected the medical profession itself.

Medicine had been undergoing profound changes as it moved from being 'an uncertain kind of knowledge' (Foucault 1976: 96) towards regarding itself as an objective, scientific and professional discipline. The establishment of the primacy of the hierarchical, professional and scientific medicine was still underway in early twentieth-century Britain and could be regarded as one of the sources of the 'failure' of the British medical profession to respond to the pandemic (Tomkins 1989, 1992a). But while the profession was trying to establish itself in British society, this society was itself undergoing major change. Britain was moving from the golden age of Victorian Britain, when it was the superpower of its day, presiding over the largest empire in history (Colinvaux 1983: 186–96), to one having to adjust to the loss of that status, the shocks of the South African war and the trauma of the Great War. Moves towards a scientific, objective medicine were aided by the changes in how disease was perceived, the rise of the bacteriological paradigm, the change from ideas of 'disease attacking life . . . replaced by the much denser notion of pathological life' (Foucault 1976: 152) as diseases 'lived' and took on an existence independent of the body. Indeed, it is arguable that the bacteriological view hampered how influenza could be conceptualised and delayed the discovery of the virus.[49] Changes in disease conception led to a greater concentration on these organisms and the 'body's response to the growth and reproduction of specific microbes' which along with

> research on the transmission of such specific living agents provided a biological explanation for the results of epidemiological studies, which, since mid-century, had suggested that epidemic diseases were contagious and had suggested vehicles, such as food and water, for their transmission.
>
> (Eyler 1992: 276)

These permitted the interventionist approaches advocated by some for the LGB, the Ministry of Health, local authorities and the medical profession.

However, the early twentieth century was not a time for unalloyed celebration of 'scientific progress' and agreement on how to solve various medical and health issues. This has already been demonstrated in the tension between Newsholme and Newman. Lawrence has described early twentieth-century British medicine as being led by a patrician elite that harked back to an imagined 'Great Tradition' in British (specifically English), medicine. Both the linking to history and an apparent tradition and the harnessing of 'science' can be regarded as ways the British medical establishment took to secure their position in twentieth-century Britain. By applying both historical and modernising beliefs, they could build alliances and arguments that legitimised the profession. However, Lawrence argues that these

> Élite doctors . . . summoned up organic ideals of the body, emphasized the importance of the healing power of nature and warned of the

> dangers of the unrestricted proliferation of laboratory science. The latter was seen by some of them as an embodiment of the division of labour, the destroyer of an individualism that, clinicians held, was the bedrock of sound medical practice.
>
> (Lawrence 1999: 1)

In the pandemic, scientific medicine and scientific research were not able to offer any solutions, but nor was the individual bedside practitioner in a position to do much to stem the disease.

Lawrence argues that one of the underlying 'motifs' for this medical elite was the 'perceived peculiarity [superiority] of the English mind' in medical matters and the belief that this helped in giving 'English medicine its natural historical turn and its down-to-earth, commonsensical quality. This quality was contrasted with the theoretical tendency of continental medicine that, in some way, was part of a frame of mind that gave rise to dangerous things such as Fascism and communism' (Lawrence 1999: 1–2). Could it be that, given such a mindset and the fact that the influenza was a global phenomenon, it did not fit this view and was therefore excluded from the gaze of English/British medicine? Furthermore, could this complement what could be regarded as an Imperialist or racist element – that the disease affected 'lower' races?[50] Given the lack of attention that seems to have been paid to the reports of large-scale influenza morbidity and mortality occurring in various countries that were appearing in the newspapers, this seems a reasonable suggestion.

This was a medical profession that was unsure what it was battling – a bacillus or a 'filter-passing' virus. Nor could the profession agree on remedies. Consequently a vast array were suggested and argued over, with alcohol being both the most popular and the most controversial. Remedies, treatments and vaccines were debated at length. One doctor or authority would advocate one action, shortly followed by another contradicting the former. Issues such as nasal douching and masks were hotly discussed, but none as much so as alcohol. Tomkins suggests this debate indicates a secure profession, one that can withstand open debate (Tomkins 1992a). Could it also be interpreted as being the response of a profession that does not know what to do, but is not short on opinion? A more favourable interpretation could be a secure and confident profession but one lacking the knowledge to cope. Carnwath certainly regarded it as most unfortunate. He regarded masks as being of great value but noted that it would 'be hopeless to attempt to enforce . . . unless we have with us an educated and intelligent acquiescence on the part of the public, and agreement amongst medical men themselves on its protective value' (Carnwath 1919: 152). There were even debates about how to protect themselves, with a report in the *Medical Journal of Australia* from a Resident Medical Officer listing the precautions they had adopted:

1 A close fitting mask, consisting of from four to eight thicknesses of gauze.
2 A hood of four layers of gauze, which covers the first mask and the whole head, neck and face, except the eyes.
3 Motor goggles.
4 Rubber gloves.
5 Gown.
6 Goloshes or sandshoes.
7 When any of the medical or nursing staff is attending a patient, the nose and mouth of the patient is also covered with gauze.

(*MJA*, 1 February 1919: 393)

Those who advocated the role of scientific medicine, especially those who had successfully negotiated the debates over vaccination during the nineteenth century, expected the laboratories to rapidly identify the causal organism and produce a vaccine shortly afterwards. In Britain the MRC, under Walter Fletcher, had drawn up a list of influenza research aims and a survey of what work was 'already arranged for investigation' by Armistice Day. The research was to investigate the clinical and bacteriological features of both acute uncomplicated influenza and complicated cases, along with the pathological anatomy of these complicated cases and investigations of the transmission of the disease. Fletcher was also fully aware of the need to obtain 'results quickly while the opportunity lasts, both as to the epidemic and as to the personnel. But I am sure I need not emphasise that' (PRO FD 1 529).[51] The recipient of Fletcher's words, Major Gibson, succumbed to the disease himself shortly afterwards. His death, along with those of two other colleagues, shocked Fletcher as they were 'all bowled over with this beastly thing' (PRO FD 1 529).[52] Further correspondence to and from Fletcher indicates that many in the research community came down with the flu or their establishments were greatly inconvenienced by absenteeism due to it (PRO FD 1 529; FD 1 534) – a toll also seen in their colleagues delivering medical assistance. Fletcher's biography noted his concern and the consequences of this concern as 'he was terrible concerned about it, and from then on he initiated a real attack . . . [including] the starting of the Field Laboratories up at Mill Hill where the vast Laboratory of the Medical Research Council was to be built' (Fletcher 1957: 143). Mill Hill was where the human influenza virus was isolated in 1933 (Smith *et al.* 1933), so 'scientific' medicine did eventually produce results.[53] Not that the isolation of the virus led to the rapid development of a vaccine, but that is due more to the virus' capacity for change than anything else.

As ever, research did not always go according to plan. In one case the object of examination proved most uncooperative. A monkey intended for research into the transmission of influenza sought freedom from one of the research laboratories and effected an escape. Fletcher recounted to Cummins that the

> next day he was seen in New Scotland Yard, presumably about to report himself to the police. Chased by a policeman he crossed Whitehall, and was run over by a motor-bus. When they tried to pick up the dead body, he came to life and ran up the façade of the Home Office, to the great delight of a large crowd. He was found dead at the top of the Home Office that evening, dead, but not dishonoured.
>
> (PRO FD 1 529)[54]

One of the major aims of the research was the development of a vaccine. Many attempts at creating a vaccine were made in many countries, with little or no idea of the causative organism. Many of these were at best useless as they were based on Pfeiffer's bacillus, streptococcus or pneumococcus. The composition and efficacy of vaccines was much debated, in Britain as elsewhere. These debates took place on the pages of the medical journals and the newspapers, at meetings such as the Royal Society of Medicine's 'Discussion' on influenza in November 1918 or that of the Royal Institute of Public Health in February 1919, and even between the LGB/Ministry of Health and the MRC. The LGB made a number of alternative vaccines available, but uptake was apparently mixed due to the lack of specificity.[55] The published proceedings of the Royal Society of Medicine 'Discussion' actually carried an advertisement on the inside rear cover advertising Parke, Davis and Company's 'Vaccine Therapy in Influenza' which consisted of six different vaccines. These would appear to be more of the 'shopping list' or 'recipe' vaccines in which a number of organisms have been included in the hope that some good will come of it all; a South African doctor termed this a 'bigger blunderbuss' approach in which the vaccine contains many different antibodies (Phillips 1990a: 120). Any positive outcomes would then seem to have come more of good fortune than good design.

Fletcher's caution, and moves to quell Newman's enthusiasm for these vaccines, echoed that of the South African Influenza Epidemic Commission. After gathering evidence on vaccines and their efficacy, they concluded that it was not possible to make any definite recommendation due to the controversial nature of the evidence and 'no public recommendation should be issued by the Government to use vaccines the utility, or at least harmlessness, of which has not been thoroughly and scientifically established' (Union of South Africa 1919, quoted in Phillips 1990a: 119). Even where there is an effective vaccine there is a requirement for a great deal to be available, especially in times of epidemic, even if there is an expectation of a herd immunity effect. The creation, holding and timely delivery of sufficient stocks is a major logistic problem, both then and now, and is one that the modern WHO influenza pandemic plan discusses at some length (WHO 1999d: 22–4, 28, 46–53; 2005c).

The response of the British medical profession to the pandemic has been termed a failure and the suggestion made that the mortality of the pandemic in Britain was higher than it should have been (Tomkins 1992a). This claim may be a trifle harsh as comparing British mortality with that elsewhere suggests that British mortality was much in line with that of many other nations, and well below that of some. However, if one wishes to examine other measures of 'failure', then the British medical profession may not fare so well. In attempting to tend to the British public, the medical professionals bore a heavy toll. Carnwath noted in a public lecture shortly after the pandemic that 'One of the most tragic features of the epidemic has been the heavy sickness rates and the high mortality amongst hospital and ambulance staffs' (Carnwath 1919: 151). Obviously such losses, to illness and death, would only exacerbate a difficult situation. In Britain this only compounded the problem of a very real shortage of doctors and nurses. A very substantial proportion of all British medical staff were committed to the war effort. These included not just those actually in attendance on or near the battlefields but also large numbers working in hospitals, medical examination boards and so on at home. As the pandemic struck, especially at the peaks of mortality, the national authorities were being implored by local authorities and the press to release or loan personnel to aid the civilian population.[56] Eventually these calls led to changes in recruiting and examination boards, particularly as the war ended, with some medical personnel being released, and with the National Service Department sending a telegram to 'All Regions' on 29 October 1918:

> In view of Influenza epidemic all outstanding 3509 and 3491 are being cancelled until further orders. . . . Please arrange to liberate medical Practitioners from Recruiting Boards in your Region to assist in civilian work where necessary. . . . This does not apply to Pension Boards or Discharge Centre Boards.
>
> (PRO NATS 1 797)

These changes to Army Medical Boards also came following criticism about how those inspections were being handled, including men being forced to wait undressed for hours on occasion in cold, draughty conditions before being inspected, and this at a time when influenza was rife. As the epidemic worsened, more local authorities beseeched the national authorities for medical assistance or the release of their own local medical people who were on national duty. In the face of such demands, and with the cessation of war, more of these requests appear to have been granted. However, it is worth remembering that the war overshadowed everything in Britain, at least in terms of official business. An epidemic was still very much a lower priority.

If the British medical profession did fail, it was a failure to appreciate that an influenza epidemic was coming and the scale of it when it did arrive. What contributed to what has been seen as the failure of British medicine? There may be many reasons as to why the gravity of the situation was not appreciated. These included issues such as the perception of disease, the fact that it was 'only' influenza, the relatively mild nature of the first wave in the spring of 1918, Imperialist or racist views and the 'superiority' of the English, the confidence in scientific medicine to find a vaccine, the quest for professional status of the profession, the power of 'scientific' medicine prevailing over preventive, and the rejection of state intervention. Many of these contributed to a delay in the reaction and recognition of the existence of a problem, particularly when the second wave arrived in the autumn of 1918; this was a fatal delay in the circumstances of such a fast-moving epidemic. This lack of recognition meant it was an epidemic that essentially escaped the view of much of the government. Whereas it became an issue for the very highest levels in other countries,[57] the pandemic is almost totally absent from the comparable British records.

Britain had the infrastructure, the co-ordination of hospitals and volunteers and was also considered well-versed in dealing with epidemic disease (Tomkins 1992a). This last position was certainly one that was attacked in the press during and after the epidemic. Rather, it was felt that the medical profession, particularly in teaching, had neglected infectious disease and accorded it lesser importance than surgery and chronic conditions (*The Times* 24 December 1918: 3; 17 February 1919: 7). Another failure could be that of the LGB who may have been able to do little more, due to their size and role, thereby being forced to devolve all responsibility and action to local authorities. In a way this is similar to the current role of the WHO with regard to nation states; their role was to suggest and to encourage actions they had neither the power nor the resources to demand or to undertake themselves. Furthermore, the fact that the LGB was already a doomed body, with the planned Ministry of Health due to assume its functions, may have contributed to its inactivity. This transitional period coinciding with the epidemic was probably an unfortunate coincidence. But given the limited role of the LGB, could it have been much different? The criticism that was meted out to public health administrations elsewhere was absent in Britain, perhaps because the LGB was by then defunct, and attacking the nascent Ministry served little purpose.

It was not only bodies that could be criticised, but also individual practitioners – and criticised they were. The National Health Insurance Committee for the County of London noted that 'claims dealt with during November, 1918, show an increase of 26 percent over the number dealt with in the corresponding month of last year. The increase for the month of December is 72 percent' (PRO MH 65 3 January 1919 report). The records of the Insurance Committees show this increase in complaints and it is obvious that many of these stem from influenza cases. These records also indicate how the pandemic put strains on the institutions in addition to the individual medical practitioners. For example, it was noted that the 'recent epidemic of influenza has interfered considerably with the admission of the Committee's [Insurance Committee for the County of London] patients to the Downs Sanatorium, the Hospital for Consumption, Brompton, and the Victoria Park Hospital' (PRO MH 65 2 November 1918 report). The overworked doctors trying to deal with a disease whose true cause was unknown, and for which they had little to offer, even in the way of reducing symptoms, let alone curing, were not always able to offer what patients and their families wanted and expected. The Insurance Committee heard cases where doctors failed to attend their own patients who later died, cases where misdiagnoses were made and cases where pharmacists failed to supply the required drugs. In a number of these cases, the defence of overwork due to the pandemic was used, and frequently accepted by the Committee (PRO MH 65 3).[58]

One of the most tragic cases had seen a patient's family attempt to get a doctor to attend her on seven occasions, contacting four different doctors and a nurse. She was never seen by a medical professional and died of 'influenzal pneumonia'. Her own doctor, the defendant of their complaint, faced other complaints at the time and had been complained about on a number of occasions. This time he successfully evaded sanction as the Committee paid 'regard to the doctor's own health and to the pressure of work due to the influenza epidemic' (PRO MH 65 3. Case M. 19/17, quotation from the July 1919 report: 14). However, the influenza was not always such a successful defence. In November 1918, Marylebone Police Court heard a rather unusual defence when two men, Sidney H. Birkbeck and Frank A. Dyton, were remanded on a charge of attempting to steal a 'commercial motor car'. Dyton's mother presented a doctor's certificate suggesting his behaviour was due to the after-effects of influenza! As *The Times* reported, 'The magistrate remarked that it seemed rather a serious development of the disease' (12 November 1918: 5).

Despite the efforts of the medical profession and the volunteers, millions died. Frequently it was the rapidity in which the cases and the corpses mounted (often literally) that caused so many difficulties. While the pandemic's various waves may have been played out over as much as a year, the actual peaks of the waves, and the vast bulk of the deaths, often occurred in quite short periods of time.[59] A lack of ambulances, morgue space, coffins, gravediggers and graveyard space (and time to bury) were recurring themes. The WHO's *Influenza Pandemic Plan* makes explicit reference to the potential logistical problem of corpse disposal in any future epidemic. In a document that sets out what might be done in the event of a pandemic, and suggests what national authorities could do, it states that one question national pandemic plans must address is: 'In case of high mortality how would corpses be stored, transported and buried or cremated?' (WHO 1999d: 28). The rapid and hygienic collection and disposal of corpses is seen as a very important step in a successful response to a pandemic, both in terms of public confidence and in prevention of further disease.

Further dimensions

Any large-scale epidemic that incapacitates so many has a vast economic impact. Influenza and the common cold cost the British economy millions of pounds every year, and as much as 10 per cent of absenteeism is thought to be due to influenza. The cost to the US economy of an average flu year is estimated to be US$71–167 billion (WHO 2003). The sheer scale of the 1918 pandemic means it must have had a commensurately large impact. A full economic costing of the pandemic is probably impossible due to the problem of separating the impact of the influenza from that other global disaster – the First World War. However, a number of specific economic consequences are known. These include concerns about massive levels of absenteeism, particularly where it was seen as a threat to the war effort, changes in economic and social structures as a consequence of the pandemic, and the massive impact the pandemic had on the insurance industry (although in some countries the insurance industry made great use of the pandemic in writing new business, particularly in the areas of health and life insurance). For example, in Nigeria, the influenza pandemic caused major changes to the agricultural, economic and societal structures as the shortage of labour due to the pandemic forced the replacement of yam as the staple crop with cassava as it is a less labour-intensive crop (Ohadike 1981). Certainly the pandemic had a major impact on the South African economy for a number of years with severe disruption of the agricultural economy and of gold and diamond extraction, it also contributed significantly to famine in some areas in the following years due to the lack of planting as people were either too ill to tend the fields or there was a lack of people available to work (Phillips 1990a: 191–2; see also Phimister 1973).

Analysis of the economic consequences on the American economy, booming due to the war, saw an initial contraction due to the massive loss of life followed by growth. But it was calculated that each extra death per thousand in the death rate then gave an average annual increase in the economic growth rate over the next ten years of at least 6.2 per cent. Flu deaths among 'prime-age adults' were a 'significant predictor of business failures in 1919 and 1920' and the implication drawn is that one reason for the positive association between flu deaths and later economic growth is that the flu deaths led to business failures that in turn drove the economy to being below the economic trend for 1919–1921 and the growth following the epidemic was a return to the prevailing trend after the 'large temporary shock' (Brainerd and Siegler 2003). In Britain as well, the sharp social impacts of the influenza brought allied economic impacts. It was reported that, whereas normally the number of people in 'receipt of relief' (the number of paupers) fell to a minimum at the end of October before rising slowly through the winter, 1918 saw an increase in numbers in October – more people were being impoverished because of the flu. Another impact was that felt by the insurance companies. For example, the Prudential's exposure to influenza claims was noted in the City pages of *The Times* and the City reporters speculated whether the annual reports of the life assurance companies would list the influenza-caused losses, as they had done with war-related claims. On 11 January 1919, *The Times* reported that:

> In eight weeks the Prudential is known to have paid as much as £620,000 in claims attributed to influenza, which compared with

> £279,000 paid on account of direct war losses in the same time, the latter amount itself being the largest paid during any similar period of the war.

The Prudential's annual meeting later revealed that in the two months between 2 November and the end of the year some £650,000 had been paid out 'in the industrial Branch alone in consequence of the epidemic' (*The Times* 7 March 1919: 7).

There were a number of religious dimensions to the pandemic, including religious explanations for the pandemic, people turning to religion as a refuge or salvation from the disease, and the emergence of new religions or an increase in missionary work taking advantage of the perceived failure of the existing religions. In examining the explanations put forward for the pandemic, the South African historian Howard Phillips recognised several forms of religious explanation (Phillips 1990a). These included the pandemic as unintended consequence of the fighting in Europe, as the direct action of malevolent individuals or groups, as being due to human neglect of social conditions, and the action of God (or gods) as either punishment or as part of a divine purpose. In attempting to discern a deity's actions, most explanations then concentrate on sin. What sins could have brought this calamity or this retribution? Such views of sin are revealing about society. What acts and/or people are sinful? The answers suggested provide those in (moral) authority with an opportunity to denounce and control people and practices.

A number of scholars have discussed the influenza in terms of being an 'imperial' disease. It could be argued that one form of imperialism that saw the pandemic as an opportunity were the Christian missionaries. With faith in traditional belief systems undermined, the missionaries saw their chance. But then again, the failure of the 'imperial' colonial life to protect indigenous peoples may have led to questioning the new set of beliefs, encouraging a return to older beliefs and lifestyles. In South Africa, some black Christians in the Transkei were so disillusioned by the religion's inability to protect and comfort them that they turned their backs on Christianity completely and either returned to their previous beliefs or looked elsewhere. But the same forces could provoke the opposite reaction, and for some South Africans a similar disillusionment led them to question their existing belief systems and be more receptive to the words of the missionaries. A history of the London Missionary Society noted that in Central Africa the influenza epidemic was 'very severe and caused terrible suffering in the churches, and heavy losses by death; but it gave the medical missionary an opportunity which was well used, and there is now a wide open door in Central Africa for medical work' (James 1923: 105).

But it was not only Christian missionaries to whom the masses turned. It was also an opportunity for local religious and spiritual leaders to emerge, promoting both existing religions and new alternatives. As the influenza reached those areas that had no experience or living memory of the disease, it did sometimes pose a serious 'challenge to the existing social system and to social patterns of reaction to diseases'. Consequently it is not surprising that, if traditional healers and chiefs could not explain such extreme levels of sickness and death, that people would question their authority and authenticity and seek out protection and assistance from others. Consequently many people were more open to witchcraft, 'millenarism and charismatic prophets' and that a number of 'spiritual churches in Africa with healing as a liturgical element see the Spanish influenza as a source of their foundation' (Mueller 1995).[60]

Another form of religious response occurred in both South Africa and Australia. In both nations the Governor-General or Prime Minister received requests, bordering on demands, for a national day of prayer or humiliation or atonement. In South Africa, Izak Bosman of Sterkstroom wrote, in Afrikaans, suggesting that a day be set aside for 'humiliation and prayer in view of the Spanish influenza.' The demand the Australian Acting Prime Minister (Watt) received from William Short in Sydney was more ambitious:

> Pneumonic-Influenza Plague
>
> I am now writing to suggest at least a week's Humiliation and Prayer to God to stay the ravages of the Pneumonic-Influenza Plague. You have done well, and should be commended for closing Theatres, Picture Shows, Racecourses, and even Churches, so as to minimise the danger, but you have left one of the greatest plagues and curses (the Devil's gin palaces) open to dispense their death-dealing spirits, and to be an ever open plague spot. If you did well in closing all other places of public resort, you did ill in leaving the Public-Houses open. Close them at once, and so remove a plague-spot.
>
> (NAA A2 1919/887 Part 2)

But their demands were not met. However, these demands echo some earlier events in Britain, including the declaration of 21 March 1832 as a Fast Day in response to the cholera. Then moral turpitude, corruption and a decline in religious observance were seen as the stimulus for God's wrath and thus a Fast Day, a day of atonement and repentance, was required (Durey 1979). By the time of the flu pandemic, the British churches were similar to the 'modernist' churches of South Africa and Australia in that they did not see God as having a direct role in the pandemic and they were trying to reconcile modern views of science and medicine with religion. In Britain the public discussion of the pandemic played out in the newspapers was almost devoid of any religious dimension or contribution. Modern professional scientific medicine and the bacteriological paradigm had established a secure grip on the discussion of medicine in both specialised and general circles and, with a disease such as influenza that has little or no element of taboo or sin involved (unlike sexually transmitted diseases), there was little need or scope for apportioning blame to the morally suspect.

6 Cultural dimensions

An outbreak of an infectious disease such as the flu pandemic is not just a biomedical phenomenon, it is also a social one. The propagation and transmission of the disease are channelled by human activities and interactions, our social structures and behaviours. There are social aspects to the spread of the disease, the responses to it and its impacts. A disease that claims so many millions of lives has an impact that extends beyond the simple and terrible roll calls of the dead. Some of those impacts can resonate over centuries, such as the plague song that is the nursery rhyme *Ring-a-ring O' Roses*. This chapter examines some of the social and cultural dimensions of the 1918–19 influenza pandemic, including naming of disease, diseases and metaphors, and representations and recollections of the pandemic.

'Othering' of disease – blame and guilt

There has been a long history of the 'othering' of disease. This has largely been the blaming of outsiders, either those not of the mainstream population, of foreigners residing in the community, or foreigners in general. These are all forms of what Farmer terms 'the geography of blame' as we attribute danger to places that we perceive have the ability to hurt us, or to be the sources of danger (Farmer 1992). This externalising or projecting of blame or guilt can be related to religious conceptions of disease connected to sin or simply the desire to find an explanation or a scapegoat for a scourge afflicting a community. Sontag could be interpreted as suggesting that this projection is quite natural when she writes 'there is a link between imagining disease and imagining foreignness. It lies perhaps in the very concept with wrong, which is archaically identical with the non-us, the alien' (Sontag 1988: 48). What is wrong or unnatural cannot be of us, but must be of the 'other'. One of the most obvious expressions of such externalising of blame is when a geographical name becomes attached to a disease. The name suggests both disease origin and blame. Frequently these tend to be countries inhabited by people of another race[1] or countries that have a history of conflict.[2] Crookshank found several readily came to mind as he wrote 'many diseases have received geographical designations: syphilis, the "Morbus

Gallicus," is a case in point, while the "Morbus Hungaricus," which may have been typhus: and the "Pestis Britannica" (or "Sudor Anglicorum")' (Crookshank 1922: 70).

Arguably one of the most extreme examples of a religious dimension in the reaction to disease was that directed by the Christian majorities on the Jewish populations in Aragon, Catalonia, Provence, Switzerland, southern Germany and the Rhineland as Black Death swept Europe in the mid-fourteenth century. The majority accused the minority, the Jews, of poisoning springs and wells to spread the plague. For this they were persecuted, and hundreds of Jewish communities were eradicated, the people exiled or burned en masse, or imprisoned and tortured, with all their possessions confiscated. The 'destruction was enough to shift the centre of gravity of the entire European Jewish population significantly eastward'. Nor was this scapegoating entirely unprecedented as previous epidemics had 'provoked similar accusations against lepers, foreigners and beggars as well as Jews; however, the violence of the popular reaction was extraordinary, in some places resisted and in some places abetted by rulers and municipal government' (Park 1993: 614).

This externalisation of blame, reflected in the naming of disease, has been especially true of the sexually transmitted diseases. These, obviously, carry so much opprobrium. In order to excuse one's affliction, someone else has to be blamed, particularly their 'dirty' behaviour. There are many examples, one of the best known being that of syphilis: the French and the English blamed each other for centuries (French and Arrizabalaga 1998), while another example is that of the Spanish regarding syphilis as 'the sickness of Hispaniola, believing it to have come from what is now Haiti when Columbus returned from his voyage' (Sabatier 1988: 42). Some of the more extreme examples of blaming related to sexually transmitted diseases come from modernity, from the continuing scapegoating of syphilis through to the emergence of HIV/AIDS in the late twentieth century. Earlier in the twentieth century, syphilis was largely viewed as a 'black disease' as white doctors 'saw blacks as "diseased, debilitated and debauched," the victims of their own uncontrolled or uncontrollable sexual instincts and impulses' (Fee 1988: 127). This demonstrates the conjunction of racist, sexual/sinful and victim blaming, including the belief that the disease is the victim's fault and due to their failings of behaviour, hygiene, poverty or education. Such views of syphilis amongst the African-American population made possible the excesses of the 'Tuskegee Experiment' (Jones 1981).[3] These images of syphilis make a vivid contrast with the images associated with tuberculosis at much the same time as TB was seen as a pitiful disease of the white middle and 'artistic' classes. Its victims, white females particularly, were regarded as unfortunately being martyred by 'consumption', while the existence of black victims was effectively denied (Ott 1996).

More recently there has been the emergence of HIV/AIDS – quite possibly the most image-laden disease of all. Farmer examined how Haiti came to be blamed, and how being Haitian came to be classified as being in a 'risk category'.[4] Blaming Haiti and Haitians for HIV/AIDS arose from a context of imaginary geographies and racism. These were constructed upon voodoo imagery and perceptions of Haiti as the most backward of nations, and suggestions of other deviant practices such as cannibalism. These perceived deviances were repeated in depictions of the African origins of HIV/AIDS in which imaginary geographies of 'others': black, 'jungle-dwelling' peoples whose cultural and sexual practices had seen this disease more easily spread after being carried across the species barrier from primates, also apparently due to practices such as consumption of monkeys and bestiality. In the Haitian case this was overlaid with the idea of Haiti as the source of contagion, and not a 'simple' one but a contagion 'most foul' – transmitted sexually, particularly by 'deviant' sexual practices or by other deviant practices (Farmer 1992). Racism is certainly a component of why Haitians were seen as the source of HIV/AIDS. Haitian-Americans presented 'characteristics of an already non-normative character. They are black, tend to be poor, are recent immigrants, and the association of Haiti with cult-religious practices fuel[ed] the current tendency to see deviance in groups at-risk for AIDS' (Albert 1986: 174–5, cited in Farmer 1992: 221). Haitians fitted an expectation of deviance, and the existing imaginings of Haitians by American society were sufficiently disapproving to easily marry with the negative imagery surrounding HIV/AIDS.[5]

Once Haitians were named as a 'risk group', this inevitably led to a 'calculus of blame that surprised few Haitians, the disease was said to have *come from* Haiti' (Farmer 1992: 212). Although Spain was seen as the origin of the 1918–19 pandemic, the Spanish were not seen as a 'risk group'. Rather, the risk was accepted as being universal as the disease was influenza – long-known and widespread in time and space. However, even now some Spaniards resent the use of the term 'Spanish influenza' as they perceive their nation is being blamed and strenuously point out the other possible origins.[6] While the Spaniards were considered the source of the influenza, as they were a European/Caucasian nation the racist element was not substantially attached to this pandemic in the West. This is rather different to a number of other epidemics where often Asia, and particularly China, have been viewed as the offender. It is probable that this blaming of Spain was a manifestation of the blaming of the victim. However, this blaming soon lost its power as the entire population was soon suffering, and as the whole world became enmeshed in the pandemic all these forms of blaming were thus diluted as the disease was no longer to restricted to 'Others'.

The disease we now recognise as influenza has a long history of afflicting humanity, and in that time it has gone under various names. Some of these have reflected this trend of blaming outsiders or locations, whereas others have reflected suspected causation. Names that were used in Britain have included the medieval Latin *tussis* or *cough*, followed by the fifteenth-century *mure* or *murre*. The Tudor period saw the use of the terms *hot ague*, *new burning ague* (1558), *new acquaintance* (1562) and the *gentle correction* (1580). The designation of 'new', suggesting a prevailing epidemic was of a new disease, continued to be used in the seventeenth century with the names the *new disease*, *new ague*, the *strange fever* and *new delight*, while another seventeenth-century name was the *jolly rant*. Eighteenth-century names included *catarrh* or *catarrhal fever* and Horace Walpole's 'blue plagues'. But it was in the eighteenth century that the name *influenza* came to the fore (Creighton 1965: 305). Many sources repeat the Italian origin of the name, claiming it was originally attributed to the influence of the stars, later changing to the influence of wind, particularly cold winter winds, thereby reflecting the usual seasonality of the disease. Léon gave an additional alternative explanation:

> As early as the year 1554 the Venetian Ambassador in London called the sweating sickness of 1551 an influsso, which is the Italian form of influxio, the latter being the correct classical term for a humour, catarrh, or defluxion, the Latin defluxio itself having a more special limited meaning.
>
> (Léon 1921: 3–4)

Léon did, however, return to the conventional view in noting that the 'Italian chronicles describe it as *una influenza di freddo*' (Léon 1921: 3–4). Mueller (1998) claimed that the oldest references speaking of 'influenza' as a connotation for the disease we recognise date from 1504 when 'A[n] Italian writer described an epidemic of fever and coughing in Florence'. This epidemic coincided with an unusual astronomical occurrence as, in October 1503 and again in January and February 1504, the planets of Jupiter, Saturn and Mars formed a 'great equilateral triangle in the night sky. This was a significant event' (Mueller 1998: 2). Apparently, once every twenty years, Jupiter 'passes' Saturn, and on occasion Mars may also be visible. Checking the Jupiter passages of Saturn and the Mars passages of Jupiter and Saturn between 1400 and 1610, it was only in 1504 that these happened in opposition to the sun and were therefore visible for the whole (Italian) night. Further, there were no other 'equilateral triangles' of the major planets in the sky for at least a hundred years before. Consequently, if there was a major epidemic of influenza in the winter of 1503–04 in northern Italy, it would have been quite logical to connect this disease with such an unusual event. It has been suggested that it was only with the epidemic of 1743, when Italy was apparently an important source for the spread of the disease elsewhere, that the name influenza was exported from Italy and established itself in other languages as a specific name for the disease (Mueller 1998: 2). It was in 1743 that the word first appeared in print in the English language, appearing in *The London Magazine and Monthly Chronologer*.[7] Not until 1762 did the term become widely adopted, entering more general use in 1782, the same year it was 'formally adopted by the College of Physicians' (Creighton 1965: 362).

While the term influenza has become widespread, it is by no means universal. One of the other relatively common words for the disease, *grippe*, came into currency at the same time when 'In the accounts of this epidemic [1742–43] we find for the first time the designations "Influenza" and "La grippe," designations which the disease has retained' (Léon 1921: 3). It has been argued that the name grippe, 'introduced by Sauvage in 1743', may stem from the 'Polish word "chrypy" or "chrypki"' and could be connected to the 'stay of the Polish king Stanislau Leszczinski at Nancy in 1738' (Zhadanov *et al.* 1958: 3). Apparently the Polish and Czech terms (chripka) 'have a common Slavic root "khrip" (to speak hoarsely)' (Zhadanov *et al.* 1958: 3) and *grippe* has wide usage across France, Germany and the Slavic nations, including Russia.

In 1922 it was asserted that 'no epidemic disease has been ascribed so frequently, in respect of particular prevalences, to neighbouring, or antipathetic regions as influenza' (Crookshank 1922: 70). This may be more a function of the disease's long affinity with humanity than an indicator of how people regard the disease itself. Crookshank observed that the 'Chinese are said to have spoken of some visitations as Russian . . . they have called others Japanese', while the Russians have considered some epidemics as 'Chinese Fever' and 'on many occasions (notably in 1889–90) Germans, Italians, French, and English have written of the Russian Influenza'. The terms bandied around Western Europe indicate the long-standing rivalries between the major powers. Since the sixteenth century, the Italians and the French have spoken of Spanish Fever or catarrh, and the Spanish and French have at other times described 'that which they have deemed Italian'. The Germans have exchanged similar 'amenities (such as Nordische Ziep, Spanische Ziep, etc.) with their neighbours and enemies: the Dutch were not slow to retaliate on the Germans'. In 1709 Britons spoke of the 'Calais Sweat and the Dunkirk Rant and later American doctors distinguished "Influenza Europæa"' and there were also references to the 1803 epidemic of 'French influenza' (Crookshank 1922: 70–1). The flu epidemic that struck Western Europe prior to the 1918–19 pandemic was first reported in Moscow (as had the epidemic of 1830–31) and 'almost simultaneously in St Petersburg, Courland, Poland and Finland'. From this it was popularly known as the 'Russian Influenza' as it spread across Europe during 1889–94 (Léon 1921: 4; see also Burnet and Clark 1942: 61). Obviously such a tradition made geographical attribution of the next pandemic virtually inevitable.

The term influenza has become standard nomenclature. This fixing of the term dates from the development of the nosologies of disease that became more secure as the medical world became professionalised and established. However, while the basic term has been essentially fixed, there have been some outbreaks that were given popular names indicating apparent (geographical) origin. These names were not only popular but have sometimes formed part of the official nomenclature used to distinguish different strains of the influenza virus. These have included the Asian and Hong Kong flus of the 1950s and 1960s. As new strains are identified part of their official designation is the location where they are first isolated. For example, the strain that struck the northern hemisphere in the winter of 1998–99 was a 'Sydney' strain and the vaccine composed for the 2005 southern hemisphere flu season was targeted against an A/New Caledonia/20/99 (H1N1)-like virus, an A/Wellington/1/2004 (H3N2)-like virus and a B/Shanghai/361/2002-like virus.

Not all the names that have been attached to influenza relate to geography or attaching blame to a place or a group of people. Some of them reflect other perceptions or conceptions of the disease. Some of the names can reflect views on the mechanism of the disease or the physical sensation it gives the sufferer (Table 6.1) Recent work on this pandemic has brought to our attention names attached to the pandemic, particularly by indigenous

Table 6.1 Mechanistic names

Location or people	*Name*	*Meaning*
Hong Kong	'too much inside sickness'	
Germany	*blitz katarrh*	lightning cold
Persia/Iran	*nâkhushuî i bâd*	illness of the wind
Switzerland	The Coquette	(due to way it spread its 'favours' so freely)
Siam	*Kai Wat Yai*	Great Cold Fever
Hungary	The Black Whip	
Cuba and Philippines	*trancazo*	A blow from a heavy stick
South Africa	*ifeva* and *isibetho*	that which smites
	mbethalala and *sbhatalala*	the thing that strikes you down and sends you to sleep
	dreidagsieke	From the Afrikaans for 'patients who survived for three days would recover'
Nyasaland (Yao speakers)	*chipindupindu*	the new disease bringing on momentous changes as a result of seeking profit from the wartime service
Southern Rhodesia (Ndebele speakers)	*malibuzwe*	let enquiries be made concerning it
Indonesia	*pagi sakit, sore meninggal; sore sakit, pagi meninggal*	sick in the morning, dead by evening; sick in the evening, dead in the morning

Sources: Afkhami 2003; Brown 1987; Collier 1974; Mueller 1998; Page 1998; Pettigrew 1983; Phillips 1990a.

populations. In some of these examples, these names have persisted for all subsequent influenza outbreaks, whereas in other locations they were attached specifically to that one pandemic. Some, as the Yao peoples did, place the occurrence in their own linguistic context, whereas others used influenza (from the colonial language) or corruptions of it (Echenberg 2003; Ellison 2003; Mueller 1998; Musambachime 1998; Page 1998). Table 6.2 lists names used that came from other diseases or epidemics and Table 6.3 lists a number of corruptions of influenza that have been documented.

Examination of the pandemic in South Africa reveals a variety of names that were used. Some of these reflected doubt as to whether the disease was actually influenza. Such doubts were openly expressed, for example when an exasperated reader of *The Star* demanded '"In God's name, when are you going to cease talking piffle about 'influenza'? . . . Influenza does not turn a corpse black but pneumonic plague does"' (Phillips 1990a: 130–1). Many Afrikaners shared this conclusion, calling the disease *longpest*. Others employed more general terms: plague, black plague and pestilence were freely used, while among indigenous peoples, *ifeva*, *isibetho* ('that which

Table 6.2 Names from other diseases and epidemics

Location or people	*Name*	*Meaning*
Nyasaland, Tanzania	*ikigwaja*	a generalised plague
Nyasaland (Yao speakers)	*chipindupindu*	came to mean any epidemic of a new disease or a series of deaths from any unknown cause
Australia	plague bubonic plague	
South Africa	longpest plague black plague pestilence	
Zambia (Bemba speakers)	*ichinkunka*	epidemic
Southern Rhodesia (Gwanad district)	*umlenka*	formerly used for the 1890s rinderpest epidemics
Freetown, Sierra Leone	cholera	
	Man Big Daddy	formerly used for a serious form of smallpox
Zimbabwe (Shona speakers)	*mukondombera*	previously meaning 'war and battle'. Over time this word came to later be the general word for plague and more recently one of the local names for HIV/AIDS.

Sources: Ellison 2003; Mueller 1998; Page 1998; Phillips 1988; Taksa 1994.

Table 6.3 Corruptions of influenza

Location	*Name*
Nyasaland	*'fluenza*
Northern Rhodesia and Nyasaland	*furwenza* *fulwenza* *fuluensa* *falunyense*
Zulu speakers	*influwenza*
Zimbabwe	*ifulenza*
Shona speakers	*fluenza, fruenza*
Igboland, Nigeria	*ifelunza*

Sources: Mueller 1998; Musambachime 1998; Page 1998.

smites'), *mbethalala* ('the thing that strikes you down and sends you to sleep') or *sbhatalala* (possibly a variant of *mbethalala*), *lerôbôrôbô* ('the epidemic'), *semagamaga* ('the epidemic', also used in eastern Botswana) and *driedagsiekte* were common labels, the latter presumably taken from local Afrikaners. In one area where indigenous people were the first victims, the accusatory term *Kaffersiekte* was coined; in another district, where the position was reversed, the compliment was returned with 'White man's sickness' (Phillips 1990a: 131).

Studies of the pandemic among Canadian First Nations peoples and Pacific Islanders suggest that those peoples did not develop terms from their own existing vocabularies. Rather they tended to have used the colonial language, usually English (Herda 1999; Kelm 1999). These may have been adopted as a coded form of dealing with disease by indicating that it had come from the world of the colonisers, thus being another form of blaming of a people or place. By adopting the name the colonisers used, the native peoples could have been expressing their understanding of the disease as being external to them and blaming the colonisers for its presence.

In the contemporary reports there is little sense of a strong blaming or attacking of the Spanish. This is an epidemic that is largely downplayed in all senses, and that includes blaming. It seems to be generally accepted, and therefore resisting and blaming were pointless. The term 'Spanish flu' is common but is applied more as an indicator of supposed geographic origin rather than a term of abuse aimed at the Spanish. Indeed, in those occasions where any individual or group of persons is blamed in the pandemic, it seems to be most commonly those who have been identified as bringing the disease into an area, and not the actual 'origin' of the illness. For example, in examining the epidemic experience of Norwood, Fanning (1995) re-iterates the local authorities' claim that new immigrants were responsible for bringing the disease. Another localised incidence of blaming occurred in Dakar,

Senegal. Here a whole series of people were blamed for either bringing the disease or for not stopping it elsewhere:

> At first labelled 'Brazilian' flu after a fleet of the Brazilian Navy which imported the disease to Dakar from Freetown, Sierra Leone, influenza spread from the Brazilian sailors in Dakar harbour to the over-crowded city and the surrounding districts.
>
> (Echenberg 1998: 4–6)

> French officials were quick to blame the Brazilians and especially British officials in Freetown . . . for not having alerted them earlier.
>
> (Echenberg 2003: 232)

This pandemic was in many ways to live up to the claim that 'in every country and in every age, the popular names for influenza have been of the same types; sometimes geographical: sometimes zoological: sometimes derisive or jocular: sometimes descriptive' (Crookshank 1922: 78). A selection of names that indicate blaming or causation attributed to geographical location or certain people is given in Table 6.4.

In Ghana, one of the first names adopted was the result not of blaming a group, but actually commemorated an individual as it was termed *Mowure*

Table 6.4 Geographical or group names

Location/people	*Name*
British troops	Flanders Grippe
Ceylon	Bombay Fever
Dakar, Senegal	Brazilian flu
France	Swiss wave (second wave)
Germany	Russian pest
Ghana	*Mowure Kodwo*
Italy	German disease
Japan	American influenza
Japan	Wrestlers' fever
Kenya	Nairobi Throat
Northern Rhodesia	White Man's Flu
Penang	Singapore Fever
Poland	Bolshevik Disease
Portugal	Soldier of Naples
Russia	Chinese Disease
South Africa	White Man's Sickness
	Kaffersiekte (blacks' disease)
Spain	Naples Soldier

Sources: Dowdle and LaPatra 1983; Echeverri 2003; Mueller 1998; Pettigrew 1983; Phillips 1988; Zylberman 2003.

Kodwo, after a Mr Kodwo from Mouri Moree, a village east of Cape Coast, who was the first to succumb (Mueller 1998: 4). There are also a number of cases where it was not the people that named the influenza, but the influenza that named the people. For example, in 'Igbugo and other Igbo towns of eastern Nigeria, so powerful was the impact of influenza that all men and women born between 1919 and 1921 named their age set the Ogbo Ifelunza, or "Influenza Age Group"' (Echenberg 2003: 236). This naming of 'age sets' is also recorded in Kenya where age-set names during or after the pandemic experience included *Mesiawa* ('I am OK, I have survived') and *Kimiri* ('to crush, to squeeze' as the disease had crushed the people 'with heart and chest pains leading to fatal pneumonia') (Mueller 1998: 8–9).

Metaphors

Another aspect of language and disease is that of metaphor. Metaphors of disease have attracted a degree of academic interest in recent times, much of it due to Susan Sontag's work, and this in turn has fed into and off examinations of the social construction of disease. Much of this interest has focused on the metaphors surrounding HIV/AIDS and many of these metaphors are recognisable from mainstream media and popular conceptions of HIV/AIDS, and include terms such as 'holocaust', 'war' and 'firestorm'. These are very strong metaphors attached to what is seen as a very serious threat to human health, one that has extreme social and cultural dimensions. The social and emotional 'baggage' attached to our perceptions of some diseases, particularly those that are principally transmitted sexually, can lead to extreme and prejudicial names and these same processes lead also to strong metaphors. However, influenza, for various reasons, has not seen the emergence of popular, sustained names that attach blame. Nor has it seen the emergence of particularly sustained metaphors for the disease, nor is influenza itself used as a common metaphor. Flu is too common and too banal to work effectively as a metaphor; even when the pandemic was at its height, it was rarely invoked as a metaphor. The only regular use we have for the term is to exaggerate how bad our 'common' colds are. Perhaps the only recent exceptions to this lack of metaphor and imagery have been the bird flu scares. These outbreaks of what may have the potential to be a pandemic strain of influenza have seen images of teams of 'detectives' or 'Ghostbusters' hunting a mutant or evolving 'Frankenstein' virus being evoked (Brown 2003; Gladwell 1997; Kolata 1999; Larson 1998).

Epidemic diseases have been used as metaphors of social disorder and the horror of disease has been transposed through metaphor to political events. For example, the developments leading to the American Revolution were equated to the spread of cancer or smallpox, the French Revolution was likened to a palsy and Stalinism was referred to as being akin to cholera, syphilis and a cancer (Taksa 1994: 87). In the American revolutionary years, which coincided with a widespread epidemic of smallpox – the war is considered to have facilitated the spread of the dreaded pox – contemporaries 'wrote of republicanism itself spreading "l[ike a Contagion"'. A not dissimilar example from 1919 was a pamphlet entitled *The two plagues: influenza and bolshevism* that bemoaned the fact that 'at the same moment that this mysterious physical poison of influenza issued from its semi-dormancy and struck the world with its virus, there emerged with equal suddenness a vast deluge of moral and mental poison, under the name of Bolshevism' and that 'they are both a deadly aftermath of the wickedest war in history'. Indeed Bolshevism was not only 'distinguished from its fellow plague' as a 'moral, mental and spiritual infection' but was indeed claimed to be 'a graver danger than the Influenza plague' (Hoare 1919: 2–3, 10). But influenza is in many ways quite different from a number of other epidemic diseases. Its low fatality rate and relative frequency render it an impotent force in metaphoric terms. The same factors that seem to make it so easily lost from our collective memory, as shall be seen, also seem to ensure it has no power as a metaphor and that few or no metaphors are applied to it, even in epidemic and pandemic form.

Media, memory and medicine: representations, remedies and recollection

Faced with the vast 'increase in cases, many critically ill with influenzal pneumonia' overwhelming his hospital and seeing his staff 'go down like ninepins' under the onslaught, the superintendent of a London hospital grabbed a precious moment to scribble in his notebook.[8] He considered that 'We could hardly have been worse placed for dealing with an epidemic'. Indeed, the strain was not just upon his hospital: his own health failed under the pressure and he 'collapsed completely in December' and was not to return to work until the middle of February 1919. His brief notes of the pandemic are among the very few memories and commentaries that we do have from Britain. This was a pandemic that infected most of the world's population, killed millions and yet left little trace in our collective memory. In Chris Marker's 1982 film, *Sans Soleil*, the narrator tells us that 'I will have spent my life trying to understand the function of remembering, which is not the opposite of forgetting, but rather its lining. We do not remember, we rewrite memory much as history is rewritten' – a statement that in itself recalls an observation in Marker's earlier film, *La Jetée*: 'Nothing sorts out memories from ordinary moments. Later on they do claim remembrance when they show their scars.' How was society scarred by the pandemic – and why do scars not always form?

The 1918–19 flu pandemic is one of the three largest mortality events in human history. But while this was perhaps the greatest medical disaster of the twentieth century, it was one that was not trapped in the collective memory. But how do we know if it was appreciated as such and then forgotten or if it was simply never known, or never had a chance to lodge in the collective memory? One route to understanding what happened is to see how the pandemic was presented and represented in a range of media, from the short-term view of the daily press to the longer-term cultural record, including literature, memoirs, art and music. For an outbreak that had such a massive impact there is a decided paucity of material relating to the pandemic. Here we have one of the three most devastating epidemics in history, and it occurred in living memory (just), yet what do we have to show for it? In the local and national histories, in the national archives and in our collective memory, it has slipped away, leaving the merest of traces. Yet, if we start to scratch the surface of our own family histories, we often find it.

Representation

The lack of material is reflected in the scant attention paid to influenza domestically in the British newspapers and the medical press. Here, interest was largely restricted to the foreign (mostly 'Imperial') reports before being piqued by the high mortality of the second wave, an interest that seems to have been rather disappointed by the relative mildness of the third wave of the pandemic. The role of the newspapers and the way the pandemic was reported around the world was extremely variable. As Fincher recognised, 'partly to avoid panic, mainly because it was overshadowed by the war, some newspapers tended to downplay the epidemic, just as the country would at first downplay the spread of AIDS' (Fincher 1989: 137–8).[9] There are instances of newspapers negating the importance of the disease, others reporting massive mortality, and others acting as public health advocates and condemning the (in)actions of public health authorities. Indeed such contradictory messages could appear in the same newspaper, in a single issue and even on a single front page. For example, the front page of Kitchener, Ontario's *Daily Telegraph* on 17 October 1918 carried headlines reading 'Toll of deaths is decreasing' and 'Flu epidemic still unchecked'.

In America the major newspapers tended to focus their coverage on the domestic experience with little reporting of the foreign experience of the pandemic (Jenkins 1998). This approach contrasts with the coverage in Britain where the domestic dimension of the disease was understated, particularly in the earlier months of the pandemic. While many stories of the pandemic abroad were printed, they tended to be very short reports, often single-line entries in the 'Imperial and Foreign News' columns. *The Times* carried few reports of influenza before July 1918, with only occasional stories appearing in late June 1918. From the first week of July there were almost daily reports, mostly from abroad, and this pattern lasted several weeks before subsiding. However, the spring upturn in reporting was dwarfed by that seen in the fourth quarter, particularly from November onwards.

Domestic stories of the influenza tend to be briefer and less frequent than those from abroad. Some of the longer stories are about South Africa where it was reported as the 'worst epidemic' as early as 12 October 1918 (*The*

Times 12 October 1918: 5). It may be that the scale of mortality elsewhere made the impact in Britain seem trivial. The scale of loss and deprivation caused by the Great War may also have made all other trials pale into insignificance. Little connection was made between the pandemic elsewhere and that in the UK, the two were largely treated as quite unrelated and almost merely coincidental. This could be another manifestation of the need to 'carry on' in the face of the war. The scale of the epidemic abroad was apparent before it became established in Britain. Reports of more than 100,000 cases in Spain, 70,000 in the Ukraine, 100,000 in Argentina and Norway, one million in the Dutch East Indies and 350,000 dead in the USA date from as early as October 1918. For many nations, October saw the greatest number of deaths, whereas November brought the peak in Britain. As Christmas 1918 (the first peacetime Christmas in years), approached, *The Times* realised that 'Never since the Black Death has such a plague swept over the face of the world; never, perhaps, has a plague been more stoically accepted' (*The Times* 18 December 1918: 5).

Much of the domestic coverage concerned the efficacy or otherwise of vaccines and various remedies. Reporting of local disruptions such as school closures and absenteeism was common in the second wave, but there was little indication of the scale of the problem in terms of either numbers sick or dying. The only notable exception to this was the tracking of absenteeism and deaths among the members of the Metropolitan Police and the London Fire Brigade. The reportage seems to suggest that, while the influenza was an inconvenience, it was not seen as particularly serious, certainly not as serious as elsewhere as the reporting of the disease abroad gave ample evidence that this was indeed a tremendous killer. *The Times*' Tangiers correspondent made rather a feature of the impact of the influenza there and heavily criticised the actions and responses of the local authorities, lambasting the 'European authorities' for the 'scandal' of their 'official indifference'.[10]

In the USA, coverage of the pandemic peaked in October, as the mortality of the second wave peaked there, and was followed by a slightly lower level of coverage in the lower-magnitude third wave (Jenkins 1998). A similar pattern occurred in Britain, peaking in the second wave. This pattern was not restricted to the newspapers. The number of influenza articles in the premier British medical journals, *The Lancet* and the *British Medical Journal*, displayed much the same pattern but with a slight lag into the first quarter of 1919. Again, from a base of negligible numbers of influenza-related items prior to the pandemic, the number of articles rose extremely rapidly (a rapid onset – much like the flu itself). From only one 'influenza' entry in the *BMJ* index in the first half of 1918, this rose to sixty-eight in the second half of 1918, and eighty-nine for the first half of 1919. *The Lancet* recorded almost identical figures – zero, seventy and eighty-eight respectively. This rapid rise was followed by an almost equally rapid fall, each journal dropping to thirty-eight influenza entries in the second half of 1919. Over the remainder of the 1920s, the vast majority of influenza references in these two journals appeared in the first half of the year (following the northern hemisphere winter) and numbers of entries jump markedly in those years where any suggestion of an epidemic occurred, including 1920 and 1927.

The first wave of the pandemic was unregarded and relatively unremarkable, so when the second wave came, despite the reports from abroad, it was not viewed with any great trepidation. However, once it became apparent how serious it was, it seems reasonable to suggest that the British were terrified when the third wave arose. Thus there was a greater awareness of the disease and the threat it could pose when the third wave came.[11] This greater awareness is reflected in renewed newspaper coverage of the pandemic, the greater discussion of influenza in the medical journals, elevated pharmacy sales and increased newspaper advertising of remedies. All of these reinforced one another and thus might have ensured there was an ongoing memory of the event. However, the lesser magnitude of the third wave compared with the second undermined the committing of the pandemic to the memory. It can be argued that the 'great' plague is always the last one experienced as we remember more clearly a recent trauma rather than an older one, the newest scars mask the older. Thus, as the third wave of the influenza pandemic did not attain the heights of the pandemic as a whole, then the retained image of the pandemic was of a lesser threat or of one that failed to live up to its billing.

Remedies

A vast array of products were claimed to have curative or preventative powers against the flu. These included Lifebuoy soap, Oxo, incandescent gas burners, aspirin, quinine, opium, ammonia, camphor, eucalyptus, iodine, salicylate of soda, blood serum, permanganate of potash, mercury perchloride, colloidal silver, creosote, turpentine, snuff, cinnamon, salt water, tobacco, beef tea, cocoa and disinfectant. But the most debated, and almost certainly the most desired, 'medicine' was alcohol.[12] The only thing that was as contentious as alcohol was the question of vaccines.

The Medical Research Council surveyed a number of schools in order to obtain 'definite information upon the incidence and varieties of this disease and its complications in the chief Public Schools'. The doctor at Repton School attributed the lack of cases there to the preventative properties of snuff and spraying the throats of the boys with potassium permanganate solution. This same solution proved quite useless at Rossall School in Fleetwood where 320 of the 444 boys were infected, including fifty-seven out of the fifty-nine in the Prep School. Similarly, Felsted School, Essex, found the solution did not prevent between 143 and 162 cases breaking out among the 250 boys.[13]

A government Memorandum advised people stricken with flu to 'stay at home for a few days' where a 'thorough washing and cleansing of rooms and their contents and washing of articles of bedding or apparel is desirable'.

The irrigation of the nose and throat with 'boracic and weak saline solution' was recommended as was gargling with a weak permanganate and 'common salt' solution twice daily, followed by the unpleasantness of snuffling this solution into the nose and then spitting it out. People should also 'avoid scattering infection in sneezing and coughing' by using a handkerchief and the handkerchief should be boiled or burnt (if paper) while 'expectoration should be received in a special receptacle' to be disinfected or burnt. Other advice included greater ventilation, warm clothing, avoiding prolonged mental strain or 'over-fatigue', avoiding 'indiscriminate expectoration', the avoidance of overcrowding, especially in unventilated spaces and the 'aggregation of large numbers of persons in one room, especially for sleeping', and avoiding 'dirtiness' or dusty conditions (LGB 1918). In many respects this advice differs little from that given in the 1892 *Provisional Memorandum on Precautions* that advised that sufferers should 'stay in bed, keep warm, drink brandy, and take quinine and opium, and disinfect bedding and clothes'.

Such suggestions were also the order of the day in South Africa where the Public Health Department recommended 'quinine and aspirin and purgatives such as Epsom salts and castor oil' and later distributed a number of the unproven and largely useless vaccines (Phillips 1990a: 112). Other than providing basic nursing and preventing dehydration, there was little the medical profession could do. As a consequence, many people turned to patent medicines, alternative medicines and treatments. In many countries a wide range of alternatives were used. These included traditional folk medicines, including indigenous medicine, or alternatives such as naturopathy. In South Africa the use of folk medicines is considered to have been widespread, including herbal remedies and preventive medicines in addition to patent medicines and other beliefs, such as 'putting a recently-killed animal on the patient's chest' (Phillips 1990a: 133–4). Canadian Aboriginal peoples utilised both their own and adopted healing systems, incorporating both Native and non-Native medicine. These included taking Western medicines and attending hospitals while indigenous treatments included the Heiltsuk people's use of devil's club, swamp gooseberry and water hemlock; the Gitsken people also used devil's club while the Tsilcotin people summoned a native healer. Okanagan people made a 'vile smelling, nauseating' tea from the mentholated sage brush in addition to sweat-bathing. There was also cross-fertilisation as non-Native products were used in Native ways and Native materials were used in Western ways; for example, the Tsilcotin elder Eagle Lake Henry 'used Lysol and rum to keep the flu away . . . rum was administered like a prescription, and the Lysol was added to water bath like Epsom salts'. This was done after cleaning the house with Lysol, daubing clothes in it and hanging them on the interior 'just as cedar might be hung in a house to purify it' (Kelm 1998). These were all responses to a disease that the medical or healing professions (of any tradition) were essentially incapable of dealing with. Not knowing what they were dealing with allowed for a great deal of conjecture and the promotion of all sorts of products and procedures for preventing and/or curing influenza and pneumonia. This was as true for the 'modern scientific' medicine of Britain as for anywhere, as in addition to his limited advice in the Memorandum, Newsholme recognised that influenza could not be 'stayed by organised measures. . . . I know of no public health measures which can resist the progress of pandemic influenza'. He also suggested that in light of this and the importance of 'mixed' or secondary infections that 'life under improved sanitary conditions was at present among the most hopeful lines of action' (Royal Society of Medicine 1918: 2–3). These comments reflect the sense of helplessness among medical professionals and recognise the lack of effective remedies and the hope held for preventive medicine.[14] One doctor recalled that 'We were helpless and felt silly and ignorant' (Henrikson 1959: 30). Newsholme argued that as they could not adequately combat the disease there was little point in warning about further waves of influenza (Royal Society of Medicine 1918: 12–13).

One of the more bizarre treatments employed in Britain was one that was administered by accident. After researching trench fever, William Hyam was brought back to a Hampstead hospital as the wards filled up with influenza patients, many of whom developed pneumonia and died exhibiting the purple–blue heliotrope cyanosis. The number of deaths rose and the 'mortuary became full of bodies piled one on another, up to the ceiling, because wood could not be obtained to make coffins for them'. Into this confusion arrived another influenza patient who developed the 'dreaded form of pneumonia'. Not only did he develop pneumonic complications with the cyanosis, but as they had 'not seen a case of "blue" pneumonia recover' and he was a heavy drinker they thought it particularly unlikely that he would survive. Hyam finally convinced the man's estranged wife to see the 'drunken sot'. As she had avoided him for some twenty years and had 'no intention of letting him get hold of her again', Hyam had to convince her that he was certain her husband would succumb to the influenza before she agreed to come to the hospital (Hyam 1963: 223–4).

When she did arrive she found an unconscious man with a weak pulse and a 'remarkable deep purple colour' who could neither swallow nor breathe properly. Hyam decided that to supply him with oxygen it was necessary to insert 'two huge hollow needles' under the skin of his chest and connect these to a large cylinder of oxygen (Hyam 1963: 224–5). The nurse on duty that evening, either from the fatigue brought on through overwork battling the pandemic or from the lingering effects of the gas that had been given to her by her dentist, fell asleep by the patient's bedside soon after checking on him. In her slumbers she must have slumped forward onto the valve regulating oxygen flow, opening the valve wide open, and when Hyam was called the large oxygen cylinder was completely empty. When the nurse had woken she had been horrified to find the patient

> closely resembled a fully-inflated balloon. His skin was tensely distended with oxygen; even his eyelids were inflated and so swollen that it

> was impossible to open them even with the finger. Pressure applied to any portion of the body produced a sensation of crackling such as might have been felt had the finger been pressing on a lemon sponge pudding. There was no concealing what had happened and in lachrymose mood nurse made her report to the Sister in charge of the floor.
>
> (Hyam 1963: 225)

Rather fortunately for almost everyone concerned this was not the terminal accident it first appeared it must be. Indeed, from that point the patient recovered and was able to leave hospital shortly after. The only person to take a dim view of this was his wife who accused Hyam of deceiving her. Hyam attributed the 'cure' to the delivery of oxygen under pressure that must have 'found its way into the blood stream' (Hyam 1963: 225).

While Hyam was a real doctor who unwittingly administered an unorthodox but successful treatment, not all those offering advice were recognised medical professionals. 'Professor J. Canarie', a self-confessed 'quack professor', published a little pamphlet in which he attributed influenza to the presence of lice! His preventive measures including 'a bath at least once a week' and a 'potion' concocted from ten packets of Epsom Salts, four packets of Cream of Tartar and hot water mixed with a jelly made from eucalyptus leaves (or oil) that was to be consumed each morning. His suggestions for those actually suffering from the flu included quinine thrice daily, 'as much medicine as you can get for a good sweating' and a mixture of rum and salt for gargling and 'douching the nostrils'. He also suggested that 'rum, whiskey and champagne are good' and serious cases should 'take strong drink, smoke to make you cough as much as you can, so as to bring up phlegm and expectorate as much as possible' (Canarie 1919).

In New Zealand, a Peter Macdonald claimed that a lack of hygiene of the tongue was the root of 'influenza and air-borne disease' as the 'rough posterior portion' of the tongue was 'the trapping place for all dust and germs' and that the pandemic is a 'deplorable vicious sequence' brought about by 'going to bed with a mouthful of germs in a world full of ignorance!' (Macdonald 1919: 7, 13). Consequently his advice was to keep the mouth clean, especially the tongue, and the best way to achieve this was to 'brush the back of your tongue or wipe it thoroughly with a wet rough cloth. Before ever swallowing, clean your mouth. . . . Cough, spit and expectorate as much as you like' (Macdonald 1919: 14). He believed that the universal adoption of such oral hygiene would make it 'easily possible to completely eliminate all these diseases from our midst, without masks, fumigation, vaccines, etc. by . . . the most attractive habit of perfect cleanliness of the mouth' (Macdonald 1919: 30). Macdonald perceived a world in which 'Just as we left empirical drugs and mystic charms for Vaccines, Surgery and Suggestion, so we must leave these for enlightened prevention and trophic control by physical culture' (Macdonald 1919: 28).

It was not only the pandemic period that saw the advocacy of various alternative therapies for influenza. During the 1920s there were a number of smaller epidemics of influenza and these maintained the stimulus for those devising unorthodox approaches. From the 'Edinburgh School of Natural Therapeutics', James Thomson claimed that homeopathic or naturopathic remedies were more effective than those of orthodox medicine and blamed the high mortality of the pandemic not on the disease itself but on those orthodox treatments (Thomson 1927). The following decade, Ethelbert Hoyle made similar claims for homeopathic treatments, suggesting that orthodox medicine had a 30 per cent case fatality rate in the pandemic, as opposed to 1 per cent for homeopathically treated cases (Hoyle 1935). However, Thomson's regimen was not restricted to homeopathy. Thomson considered disease as part of the body's attempt to cleanse itself: the disease should be allowed to run its full course, and the patient should assist by undergoing a two-day starvation, cold compresses and rest, followed by a fruit diet before resuming a normal diet.

Elements of the Thomson regimen were echoed in the post-Second World War advice of Clara Hofheinz who considered influenza to be a 'poisoning of your life stream by foreign influences' and that merely the fear of influenza could lead to 'influenza condition', to the extent that in epidemics as much as 75 per cent of cases were purely the result of 'fear of that illness'. She also claimed it was due to the concentration of 'toxins' in the 'Epigastrium' (region between the breast bone and the navel containing the stomach–liver–pancreas and the solar plexus). Her preference was not for cure, but prevention by 'leading a simple life'. Advocating a puritanical ethic, she considered disease the consequence of sin. For those who have 'sinned' and were suffering from influenza, she suggested the penitential practice of 'Felke' bathing treatments involving short cold baths and being wrapped in wet sheets for hours at a time, so as to draw out the 'poison' (Hofheinz 1948). As with Macdonald, Thomson and Hoyle, she railed against the use of drugs, vaccines and heat in treating influenza. While these may be regarded as 'anti-scientific' approaches, this is not the case with Frederick Alexander, who certainly would have considered himself to be 'scientific' and 'progressive' in advocating the use of electricity, particularly 'electro-therapeutical fluids' to prevent and cure infectious diseases, including influenza (Alexander 1929). Advice on countering flu did not cease to be proffered even once the influenza virus was isolated and identified in 1933.[15] One of the most remarkable pieces was the August 1936 letter written by a certain John Moss of Penzance, Cornwall:[16]

INFLUENZA

The temperature of the human body is maintained by an invisible combustion; consisting of a chemical combustion. The elements of the combination are carbon and oxygen.

The carbon is derived from the human body and the oxygen from the atmosphere.

The invisible combustion takes place on the surface of the body. In Influenza the carbon is forth-coming in abnormal quantities, and the combustion takes place too rapidly for the health.

In extreme cases the temperature rises until life is impossible. For this there is an automatic remedy. Requiring no services from an attendant.

It is an amazing discovery; solving a world-wide mystery.

Provide a good sized sheet for the top sheet of the bed.

Fold it down the middle; and place the patient in the fold.

The bed-clothes (blankets, etc.) that may be required can be placed over the top sheet as usual.

Two of the edges of the top sheet will come together on one side of the bed.

There the carbon from the patient will meet the oxygen from the atmosphere (between the edges).

And there the invisible combustion will take place. Instead of close to the body of the patient.

By this arrangement most of the oxygen from the atmosphere is prevented from free access to the body of the patient. So there is no combustion, and no influenza.

In an experiment the unaccountable disappearance of the pain seems like magic.

Moss' 'amazing discovery' is only hampered by a complete and utter lack of regard for reality. But such a lack does not seem to have hindered those who advertised the preventative and curative effects of all manner of products and treatments during the pandemic.

Advertising

In Britain, the advertising of flu remedies was delayed much as the domestic reporting of the pandemic had been. It is likely that the delay in reporting contributed to the delay in advertising, as did the restricted availability of newsprint through 1918.[17] As the reporting increased in the second and third waves, and with the easing of restrictions on newsprint, advertising became more common. The newspapers carried advertisements for a wide range of products, not all of which one necessarily associates with treating influenza. This advertising was most common after the peak of the second wave and was maintained in the third. Nor was advertising limited to the newspapers. One short book on the origin and prevention of influenza published in 1918 carried an advertisement for a brand of face masks on its inside front cover (Galli-Valerio 1918) while the Royal Society of Medicine's publication of its November 1918 'Discussion' on influenza carried an advertisement for Parke-Davis vaccines on the inside rear cover.

The widespread advertising of patent medicines and other products with claims of curing influenza was by no means restricted to Britain. In South Africa, the 'panicky atmosphere of the time' meant anything that

> promised protection or cure was tried. Newspapers were filled with advertisements for special flu remedies. ... In addition, a number of products not usually associated with combating flu or its after-effects were peddled as such. ... It is clear that many did not scruple to exploit a frightened and desperate public.

As a consequence many, including 'chemists – both registered and unregistered – had a field day' as those driven to desperation by the reporting, the advertising, the illness and, in some cases, the piles of bodies and coffins sought some defence (Phillips 1990a: 135). British pharmacists also gained much business during the pandemic. While advertising may have claimed that many products could aid in the fight against influenza, it was the pharmacist to whom many turned. Pharmacy registers show how business improved (Figure 6.1),[18] and this indicates that pharmacy sales only lagged slightly behind the mortality and rose shortly after the reporting (and

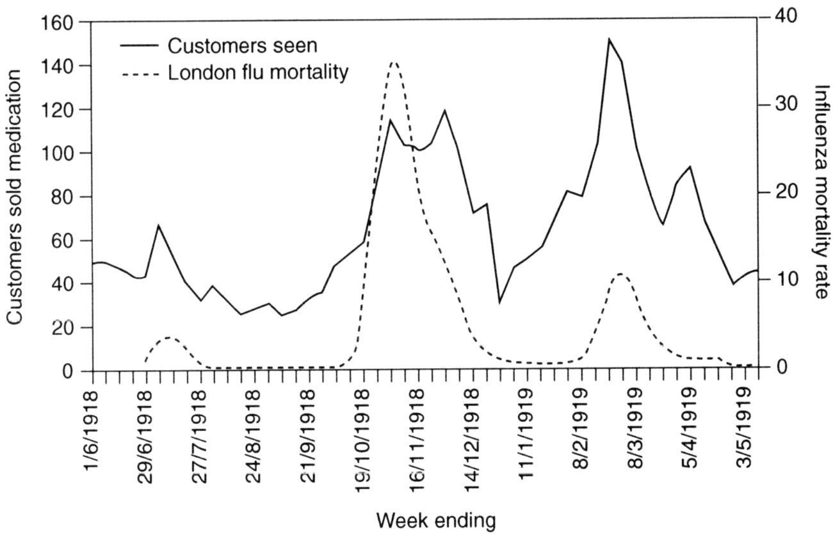

Figure 6.1 Pharmacy business and influenza mortality (source: CMAC GC/16 2 94 and GC/16 5 93 Savory and Moore).

advertising) increased. Once the influenza had entered the public consciousness, the pharmacies saw a surge in business. This is most clearly seen in the third wave where the sales reach their highest levels of all, despite mortality being much lower than in the previous wave. When the lower extent of the mortality became apparent, sales fell off dramatically.

It may have been this vast increase in business that saw a number of pharmacists incapable of coping. In one such example, the Pharmaceutical Service Sub-Committee of the Insurance Committee for the County of London's London Executive Council heard a complaint against the Torridon Road Drug Stores in Lewisham for failing to supply drugs. The pharmacist claimed it was only because of excessive overwork due to the influenza and

> conducting the business single-handed, and, as a result of the extreme pressure at which he had been working during the influenza epidemic in November, eye strain had developed to such an extent that he lost entirely the use of one eye and the partial use of the other. He was under treatment for this disability at a hospital for a period of three weeks from 11th November, and on certain occasions during that period and subsequently he felt that he was not in a fit condition to undertake the dispensing of medicines, as any work of this nature that he might attempt might be attended with serious risk to the patient.[19]

Recollections

Recent years have seen the preliminary examinations of the German collective and cultural memory of the Second World War, significantly prompted by the work of W.G. Sebald, whose stunning consideration of how Germany, and its writers, had avoided facing the massive devastation and loss of life that the Allied air bombing brought argued that one needed to consider the work of the writers 'whose task it was to keep the nation's collective memory alive' (2003: 98). However, he also noted that writings may be 'excluded from cultural memory because they threatened to break through the *cordon sanitaire* cast by society around the death zones' (2003: 97), a suggestion that may well have applied to any attempt to write of the flu. Furthermore, such avoidance of these issues may actually protect a society, and be a significant component of 'that active forgetting which Nietzsche, in the *Genealogie der Moral*, called the doorkeeper of mental peace and order' (Sebald 2003: 187). Certainly in popular culture and literature the First World War and its dreadful impacts overshadow the influenza pandemic to the point of virtual non-existence. In America only a handful of authors found a role for the pandemic in their works, despite more than 650,000 Americans dying of the flu. Works that had the pandemic as a major or notable feature include Thomas Wolfe's *Look Homeward, Angel: a story of the buried life*, published in 1929; Katherine Porter's 1964 work, *Pale Horse, Pale Rider: three short novels*; Sterling North and John Schoenherr's

1963 *Rascal, a memoir of a better era*; and, more recently, Ellen Voigt's 1995 *Kyrie: poems*. Ellen Voight's collection of sonnets, *Kyrie*, tells the story of a young schoolteacher, Mattie, in south-western Virginia, USA. They tell of her life, her family and her fiancé, Price. Price enlists in the US Army and is sent to France where he is struck by a shell, but actually succumbs to influenza. The influenza plays a major role in these vignettes of early twentieth-century rural American life. Indeed, the influenza is the major event in the lives of all those whose stories Voight tells.

William Maxwell found a place for the pandemic in a number of his short stories, including 'Period of Mourning' in his 1988 book, *So Long, See You Tomorrow* and in 'Billie Dyer' in the 1995 collection, *All The Days and Nights*. One of the few British works to showcase flu was a rather mediocre piece of crime fiction written by William Clunie Harvey, under the pseudonym of Sutherland Scott, and published in 1938 with the unimaginative title, *The Influenza Mystery*. A more recent work incorporating the pandemic into its storyline was Hari Kunzru's well-received debut novel *The Impressionist*, with the pandemic figuring early and continuing to influence the plot for a few years as the story unfolds (Kunzru 2002). The Canadian playwright Kevin Kerr wrote a play at much the same time, *Unity (1918)*, depicting the reactions of the people of the small town of Unity, Saskatchewan, as the pandemic arrives (Kerr 2002).

The pandemic was not to resonate long in the collective memory, and failed to have a substantial impact in the public spheres of society. Where it might be expected to have had a lasting impact was on the lives of individuals. However, this appears not to be the case either. Not only was the influenza overlooked for 'public' history, it seems to have little resonance in personal histories as it rarely appears in memoirs and biographies. This is a shame as it would be a tremendous way of understanding the world that the pandemic struck, how it struck, and how it was perceived and received. While Virginia Woolf may have recorded in her diary that 'we are, by the way, in the midst of a plague unmatched since the Black Death', she accorded it little more attention, other than to use it as a device to castigate another's writing: 'How I dislike writing directly after reading Mrs H. Ward! – she is as great a menace to the health of mind as influenza to the body' (Woolf 1979–85: 209, 211). However, Woolf did actually 'cast' the influenza in one of her works, *Mrs Dalloway* (Woolf 2000). Indeed, one literature/philosophy researcher has suggested that Woolf's major textual preoccupation with war can be understood not only as a literal critique, but also as a metaphorical/philosophical reflection upon the concept of boundaries. Invoking Derrida's notion of the *parergon*, which problematises the Western metaphysical binary opposition of the centre and margin (self and other) (Derrida and McLeod 1987), the same researcher argues that Mrs Dalloway's influenza (and post-influenzal malaise and debilitation) can be seen as the bridge/*parergon* that demonstrates the instability/futility of such borders: the war and the pandemic are conflated.[20] The significance of flu to

Woolf and her character(s) may well have been overlooked by readers of Woolf subsequently as they may not have perceived the disease in the way Woolf did when writing the work.

While there was something of a boom in the publishing of 'medical' memoirs following the Great War, these are marked for the absence of references to the pandemic. The few examples that do actually mention influenza tend to make only the most fleeting of references.[21] One of the few medics to record the pandemic's scale and impact was a London hospital supervisor, but his notes cover just a few modest pages in an unpublished notebook.[22] Recent work on the memoirs of British women, particularly of women on active service, found no mention of the pandemic in those writings either (Potter 1997, 2000). Yet again it is the absence that is so striking. We know from the few references we do have and from the newspapers that the pandemic caused massive disruption to life, made millions ill and killed hundreds of thousands in Britain, but in spite of this it barely rates a mention in the recollections of those who would have been attempting to treat and save its victims.

This is not to say the pandemic never appears in memoirs, just rather rarely. The few examples we have include brief mentions in Kathleen Clarke's autobiography (Clarke 1997: 165–6), in Virginia Carr's biography of John Dos Passos (Carr 1984), in Anthony Burgess' autobiography (Burgess 1987) (and in a recent biography: Lewis 2002), in the collection of Maxwell Anderson's letters, where it rated a mention in a 1956 interview (Anderson 1977). One of David Lloyd George's biographers has realised how close to killing him the flu came (Grigg 2002), while a biography of Groucho Marx has described how the flu affected the Marx Brothers (Kanfer 2000). The historian Robert McDowell discussed the influence of the pandemic on the course of his life but only in an afterword (McDowell 1997: 197–8), while Richard Schickel noted how the filmmaker D.W. Griffith had his productions severely disrupted. Griffith was forced to wear a mask on set and for his film *The Girl Who Stayed Home* was unable to cast his favourite actress, Lillian Gish, as she was so ill with flu. Budgets and schedules forced Griffith to make the film anyway. He noted that not only had the flu claimed his star, but that it also led many cinemas to shut during October 1918, and that there had also been a cessation of production on some Hollywood lots. He also insisted that the pandemic had hurt the earnings for one of his movies as it 'hit us just when we were starting to go strong' (Schickel 1984: 387–9).

When it does appear in biographies, and particularly autobiographies, the intensity of the pandemic does indeed become apparent, and this makes the forgetting all the more intriguing. One such powerful image (previously noted) of the influenza comes in Anthony Burgess' autobiography as his father returns to Manchester:

> In early 1919 my father, not yet demobilized, came on one of his regular, probably irregular, furloughs to Carisbrook Street to find both

> my mother and my sister dead. The Spanish influenza pandemic had struck Harpurhey. There was no doubt of the existence of a God: only the supreme being could contrive so brilliant an afterpiece to four years of unprecedented suffering and devastation. I, apparently, was chuckling in my cot while my mother and sister lay dead on a bed in the same room.
>
> (Burgess 2002: 17–18)

While, according to a recent biographer, Burgess took some artistic licence the basic facts are true – his mother and sister were taken by the flu (Lewis 2002: 59–62).

In the same city of Manchester just a few months earlier, September 1918, the Prime Minister David Lloyd George was all but killed by the flu. A recent biography has revealed what was certainly not in the newspapers in 1918: that he had been bed-ridden for nine days, that his valet had considered it 'touch and go' as to whether he would survive, and that when he travelled to Paris for the peace negotiations he was still very debilitated (Grigg 2002: 590–3).

The poet, playwright and author Robert Graves not only suffered familial loss but also suffered personally, and was one of the few to write anything of it. In his famous autobiography, *Goodbye To All That*, he recalled how when 'the first Spanish influenza epidemic began' it brought about the death of his mother-in-law on 13 July 1918. This is the first of a number of brief references to the influenza. He himself fell ill late in 1918 and this was then complicated by septic pneumonia in both lungs, 'but, having come through the war, I refused to die of influenza' (Graves 1998: 288, 297). However, the innovative French–Italian poet Guillaume Apollinaire, who also survived trench warfare (and military medicine, including trepanning, after being struck in the head by a shell fragment), did succumb to influenza, dying in Paris on 9 November 1918, aged 38 (Winter and Baggett 1996: 312–19). His fellow poet, Blaise Cendrars, encountered Apollinaire in Paris on 3 November when they 'spoke of the subject of the day, the epidemic of Spanish flu' (Winter and Baggett 1996: 317). Five days later, on learning that Apollinaire was ill, he went to visit. Greeted by Apollinaire's wife, Jacqueline, who was also ill, he found that Apollinaire was 'all black' (Winter and Baggett 1996: 317); the doctor Cendrars summoned could not prevent his death the next evening. A military guard of honour escorted the coffin from the church before burial in Père Lachaise two days after the Armistice. Cendrars said, 'Paris celebrating. Apollinaire lost. I was full of melancholy. It was absurd' (Winter and Baggett 1996: 319).

But the American humorist James Thurber was as determined as Graves, as he wrote to a friend on 15 October 1918:

> You mentioned Mary Flu in your letter, –(I refuse to call it John) Well, here's hoping Dover doesn't get in bed with it as badly and thoroly [*sic*]

> as Washington. All one sees here is nurses & hearses and all he hears is curses and worse. And such a heroic thing to pass out with,–Influenza! dying of influenza in these times of brave, poetical deaths. . . . I'd just as soon go with house-maid's knee. However, fear no fears for the J.G.T. I am in chipper condition with the correct psychological attitude of chestnuts and baseballs towards all flu. The influx of Enza will have to select a clever rapier and twist an adroit write to pink me, altho' I am in the pink of condition.
>
> (Bernstein 1975: 72)

And, at much the same time Graves was ill, the Irish political activist Kathleen Clarke was being held in Holloway Prison.[23] She later wrote of how, after Christmas 1918:

> we read of the terrible epidemic of flu raging all over England and Ireland. The newspapers were full of it. In a letter from home I got news that some members of the family were down with it, and for weeks after that there was no letter. I was sick with anxiety. What was wrong that I had no letters from home? Were they all dead? At the end of five weeks I got a big bunch of letters; they had been held up in the Censor's Office. I wondered if that Censor knew what suffering he had caused me, holding my letters up at such a time. However, the news was good. The family was neither dying nor dead, though some of them had had the 'flu.
>
> (Clarke 1997: 165–6)

Shortly after her release on 18 February 1919, she fell victim:

> Unfortunately, on my way home I contracted the 'flu, which was still raging, and by the time I reached Dublin I was utterly unable for the wonderful reception Dublin gave me. . . . Next morning I was removed to a nursing home, where I had to remain seven weeks, during which time death and myself had a big tussle.

The heart problems she suffered during her time in gaol made the influenza a life-threatening episode (Clarke 1997: 165–6).

Indeed, surviving the flu was itself no laughing matter. The American author John Steinbeck survived but only after his doctor operated on him in Steinbeck's parents' bedroom – wielding a scalpel to open up the teenage Steinbeck's chest, removing a rib and draining his purulent lung. Steinbeck was to say later that 'I went down and down, until the wingtips of angels brushed my eyes'. Steinbeck's lungs were to remain a problem and throughout his life he suffered for weeks at a time. One biographer has argued that the psychological damage 'inflicted by this illness of 1918, which had brought him close to death and required such intrusive surgery' was significant and that it gave Steinbeck a sense of living on the edge and of vulnerability (Parini 1994: 33–4).

Just as what is accepted and written as history, including the story of this pandemic, depends on 'the eye, angle and prevailing concerns' (Phillips 2004: 122), what forms the subject matter of any literary form may be as influenced by fashion, reaction and conceptualisations. Notwithstanding these few occurrences, the flu rarely appears in any literary form. Nor does it have much resonance in any other art form. Here was an event that tore through society on a global scale and yet our artists have given us precious little to remember it by: they seem to have had a selective recall, but that in itself may be an accurate reflection of wider society.

There is not even a decent song or even a nursery rhyme (remembering that the nursery rhyme *Ring-a-ring O' Roses* is a thirteenth-century plague song)! For the pandemic, few songs have been found – there are a couple of music hall songs (one includes sneezes in the score). Another song was one sung by schoolboys at St Andrews Preparatory School, Grahamstown, South Africa, while also in South Africa the Xhosa people had a song about the flu (Phillips 1990a: 237). Two songs published around the 1918–19 pandemic actually share the same title, the *Influenza Blues*. Both were published in the USA, one being a song from a musical, *A Lonely Romeo* (Franklin *et al.* 1919). It recounts the lonely Romeo's damp vigil, rendering him liable to come down with the flu. Klark and Brown's 1918 song, *The I-N-F-L-U-E-N-Z-A Blues*, was published in Oklahoma and is a lamentation of the singer's misfortunes – suicidal after the loss of his 'Honey', afflicted with the flu that came 'from the hun', and stuck 'without one drop of booze' and opining that 'if the blues don't kill me the Influenza must'. A few years later (in 1927), the composers Gallatly and Barber wrote *Love is Like the Influenza*. This is notable for being one of the very few instances in which influenza is used as a metaphor, the suggestion being that both conditions can strike quickly and once one does it is unstoppable, just as 'there's no pow'r in doctors' science 'gainst the deadly ill'. Just a few years after *Love is Like the Influenza* was published, 'Ace' Johnson was learning a song 'off a holiness boy in Amarillo, Texas'. This song from the 1929 epidemic in the USA tells of the influenza as 'God's almighty hand' slaying sinners as 'he was judgin' this old land'.[24]

One other theatrical example is not a mention of the flu but a theatrical failure that has been attributed to it. The Marx Brothers were trying to mount a new show, *The Street Cinderella*, and while the show had its shortcomings, 'the Brothers might have been able to save it except for a virus' according to biographer Stefan Kanfer. In America at the time theatres were restricted (more so than was the case in Britain) and 'members of the audience had to leave the seat on either side empty so that they would not breathe on one another. To further protect themselves many wore surgical masks, so that even when they laughed the sound was muffled'. Kanfer argues that *The Street Cinderella* can 'be chalked up as another victim of flu, succumbing in Michigan to bad reviews at empty houses' (Kanfer 2000: 56).

The Iconographic Collection at the Wellcome Library for the History and Understanding of Medicine in London is an extensive collection of illustrated books, prints, drawings, photographs, paintings and miscellaneous media relating to medicine. This collection is almost totally devoid of any material from this pandemic and the one work is a small pen and ink drawing described as: 'A large and grotesque monster symbolising an influenza virus hitting an old man over the head as he sits in his armchair. . . . by Ernest Noble, *c.* 1918' with the caption 'A-TICH-OO!! Good evening. I'm the new influenza' (Plate 7). The best-known artist to have depicted any aspect of the pandemic is Edvard Munch whose 1919 painting, *Selvportrett I Spanskeskyen*, shows the artist convalescing from an attack (Plate 8).

But Munch was a survivor; the expressionist painter Egon Schiele, later deemed 'degenerate' by the Nazis and (in)famous for the power and disquieting nature of much of his art, was not to survive. Indeed, Schiele, who died on 31 October 1918, All Saint's Day, aged just twenty-eight, is in many ways the perfect symbol, the 'poster boy', for this pandemic, dying, as he did, at the very peak of the pandemic and as a young man part of that group who suffered so disproportionately, the young adults. He is reported to have told his sister-in-law as he died that 'The war is over, and I must go. My paintings shall be shown in all the museums of the world' (Wilson 1980: 7). One of Schiele's very last works was a drawing of his wife, Edith, as she lay on her (flu) deathbed, her bout of flu made all the more serious by pregnancy and pneumonia. Egon realised the danger Edith was in, writing to his mother on 27 October 1918 that 'The illness is extremely serious and life-threatening. I am already preparing myself for the worst'. As Egon drew her that evening she managed to write him a last note: 'I love you eternally and love you more and more infinitely and immeasurably.' The next morning Egon wrote his own last note to his sister Gerti, informing her that 'Edith Schiele is no more' (Kallir 1998: 239).

The lack of collective cultural memory of the pandemic appears to be a particularly Western phenomena. Certainly, in parts of Asia and Africa there has been much greater retention of the pandemic in the collective consciousness. Anecdotal evidence suggests it is clearly in the public memory of Pacific island peoples (Boyd 1980; Herda 1998), Indians,[25] some African peoples (Echenberg 2003; Mueller 1998; Musambachime 1998; Phillips 1988, 1990a; Ranger 1988, 1992), and among some Canadian First Nations peoples (Kelm 1998: 21, 23–7). This is not so surprising when we recall that many of these areas endured massive mortality, including an estimated 18.5 million deaths in India (Mills 1986), while more than one-fifth of the total population of Western Samoa died (Tomkins 1992b). Could the lack of permanency in the Western public memory also be a reflection of our 'progressive' views? Could it be the fact that we had entered a time of scientific medicine when infectious disease was seen as something that killed our distant forebears but not us or generations close to us? Could it also be a consequence of how our societal structure and values have changed, changes that have meant reduced contact with older generations and whose experiences are progressively discounted?

Memory

It is ironic that the man who gave us one of our strongest symbols of remembrance was to die of something so lethal and yet almost forgotten or overlooked in history. The Canadian physician John McCrae served in the Canadian Field Artillery and, in May 1915, while he sat on the back of an ambulance looking out over thousands of crosses that marked the quickly dug graves of soldiers who died fighting on the battlefields of Flanders, Belgium, he wrote the poem *In Flanders Fields*, with its opening line of 'In Flanders fields the poppies blow'. This man, whose poem gave us the symbolism of the poppy as remembrance of the war dead, never lived to see his contribution to the remembrance and recognition of the lost generation as he died in 1918 at Wimereux near Boulogne, France, of influenza.[26]

The pandemic did not resonate long in the collective memory, and failed to have a substantial impact in the public spheres of society (McKenzie 2000). Nor does it feature strongly in personal memories, in memoirs or in biographies. Nor does it turn up too often in the archives or the official records of Britain and British institutions or the media.[27] The fact it has been forgotten is not a particularly recent realisation: writing in the 1930s, the British Major Greenwood observed that 'there is some psychological interest in the fact . . . that actually the emotional impression created was fainter than that produced by much less grave epidemiological happenings' (Greenwood 1935: 330). So why was it forgotten?

The first wave had been quite mild with low case-fatality rates. Perhaps that led to complacency, and then the mildness of the third wave revived this complacency – it was 'only' influenza. This was not an epidemic that struck a nation oblivious to its existence. Newspapers had certainly covered the 'story' of the influenza. This was not something that crept up on the British, either in the first wave or in the deadly second wave. The scale of the second wave was certainly known to Britons, especially the toll it had reaped in the Empire, particularly South Africa. Perhaps it is also an example of an unthinkingingly racist view – 'they' were struck by the pandemic because 'they' are backward, inherently weak and 'they' do not have the sophisticated and advanced medical care 'we' in Britain have.

The role of newspapers touches on the issue of collective memory of the pandemic. Was it forgotten or was it never known? Some tentative suggestions as to why there is little recollection of the pandemic have been put forward (Crosby 1989). These include the fact that case-fatality rates were generally no greater than for 'normal' influenza. Others suggest that the proximity of the Great War and desires to suppress, forget or 'leave behind' the hard times meant people actively denied it. Another possibility is that people failed to recognise the significance of the pandemic at the time. The latter is not supported in Britain as newspapers reported that the mortality was of the order of millions dead.

The influenza must have had a tremendous impact on life: the levels of morbidity, the lack of staff in businesses, the impairment of services, the sheer number of bodies could not have been ignored. However, it was an impact that seems to have been soon forgotten. The first wave seems to have had little noted impact. The second wave certainly had an impact with its massive mortality. The third wave attracted attention, as is evident from the increased coverage of influenza in both the newspapers and the medical journals, the increased advertising of flu remedies and increased pharmacy sales during this stage of the pandemic, but the mortality was far lower (particularly in London and the South). Perhaps it was the fact that the mortality did not reach the peaks of the second wave that contributed to the disappearance of influenza from the collective memory.

It is beyond doubt that, in Britain, the pandemic was overshadowed by war. The war also plays a rôle in the collective memory of the event (or lack thereof), particularly in nations highly involved in the conflict. The two events appear conflated; the flu has become a component of, or perhaps a bit player in, the larger story of the Great War. This was 'only' flu and, as such, may have been masked by the deep scars caused by the war and subsumed into the whole war experience. Such attitudes may have played a role in the downplaying of the scale of the pandemic and its failure to retain a prominent role in the collective memory that might otherwise be expected of a disease outbreak that brought so much illness and death.

Another aspect that may have contributed to the flu being overlooked was its duration. Did it not enter the collective memory because it came and went all too quickly? While this was a year of flu, with unprecedented and universal impact, in Britain the deaths were concentrated in about ten weeks across the year or so – three short bursts of flu killing a quarter of a million people.

It may well be that Camus identified the real reason for forgetting: scale. A disaster on a scale that cannot be imagined, cannot be personalised. Camus, in a quotation already cited, pondered:

> But what are a hundred million deaths? . . . since a dead man has no substance unless one has actually seen him dead, a hundred million corpses broadcast through history are no more than a puff of smoke in the imagination.
>
> (Camus 1947: 168)

The 100-million victims of flu are unimaginable, cannot be conceived of in human terms; we cannot put a face on so many and it becomes just a number.

7 Repercussions

Considering the massive scale of the pandemic, it is notable that its long-term impacts are not particularly obvious. The previous great plagues brought significant social, political and intellectual change in their wake. How could an outbreak of disease that may have killed as many as 100 million people lead to apparently such little change? What changes were wrought by the pandemic? Has the scope of the changes been understated or were there few or no long-term repercussions? And what were the connections between the flu and that other global conflagration, the World War?

Demographic impacts

An event of such a magnitude must have great demographic consequences and these must extend beyond the surge in mortality for the period. They may include changes in patterns of nuptiality and fertility, the effective loss of life years for a community or nation, increases in the number of orphans and changes in the age–sex structure of the population. Changes in nuptiality and fertility would almost certainly have occurred as the flu hit what are normally the most fertile and productive people in a population. Flu deaths would have increased the number of widows and widowers and would have brought a consequent reduction in marital fertility. However, there may be further dimensions to this reduction; there may have been reduction in fertility due to morbidity. There may have also been changes in nuptiality as weddings didn't occur due to the death of one of the intended or weddings that were delayed due to illness or death within the family. The level of mortality among pregnant women allied with abortions, miscarriages and stillbirths increased during the pandemic, and these deaths would also have influenced the fertility levels. However, quantifying these effects, particularly the portion due to influenza and that due to the war, is virtually impossible in most locations; some researchers have started to attempt to examine the dimensions of these impacts (Echeverri 2003; Mamelund 1998a, 1998b, 2003, 2004; Noymer and Garenne 1998; Phillips 1988, 1990a; Reid 2005; Rice 1988; Zylberman 2003). For Britain, it is unlikely that it will ever be possible to determine the true extent of many of these demographic impacts. It is extremely difficult, if not impossible, to separate out the demographic effects of the pandemic from those of the Great War. This is largely due to the fact that both events focused so heavily on the same segment of the population, the young adults. This population was the most heavily involved in the pandemic mortality – and that which suffered the most in the war – but would also otherwise have been the most fertile. Further, the disruption of the population by war rendered the basic population data unreliable and may have disrupted national and local registration processes. Eccheverri noted her fortune in that 'Precisely because of the fact that Spain was not a belligerent country, there is a wealth of medical and statistical data that neighbouring countries, implicated in the war, lack' (Echeverri 1998: 1), a situation also found in Norway (Mamelund 1998a, 1998b, 2003, 2004). Notwithstanding these difficulties, it is still possible to make some observations about the demographic outcomes of the pandemic.

In some cases it is difficult to find evidence of any impact. This is the case for the basic demographic measures such as crude death rate (CDR), crude birth rate (CBR) and infant mortality rate (IMR). Examining the CDR, CBR and IMR for England and Wales for the first thirty years of the twentieth century (Figure 7.1), it is readily apparent that, while the CDR jumped sharply in 1918, from 14.4 per 1,000 in 1917 to 17.3 per 1,000, before dropping to 13.7 in 1919, the CBR and IMR were less affected by the pandemic. The CBR had been in sharp decline throughout the war, stabilising in 1918 before a slight rise in 1919 that preceded a marked increase in 1920. Thus the natural increase of population was diminished markedly throughout the war, and the pandemic may have both added to this and ensured it continued for some time after the end of the war. Indeed, as was noted earlier, deaths exceeded births during this period and consequently a natural increase briefly became a 'natural' decrease. The pandemic diminished or delayed the later upturn in CBR in Britain to an extent. Neutral Norway saw a baby boom in 1920 for which it has been said 'the flu pandemic was indeed the main cause' (Mamelund 2004: 229). It seems natural that the end of the war and the improved world conditions would have been factors contributing to such a baby boom in neutral and belligerent countries alike, but its full extent and timing was affected by the influenza. Thus this was not purely a post-war baby boom, but a post-war *and* post-pandemic baby boom. Infant mortality had been tending downwards for some time and only saw a minor reversal of this trend during 1918. Again, this may be attributable in part to the influenza. Thus, the impact of the influenza is greatest on the CDR, with a lesser impact discernible in the CBR and IMR.

Accepting that IMR can be used as an indicator of prevailing health, then a comparison of IMR with the pandemic influenza mortality may give an indication of the role of existing health conditions in determining the level of mortality in the pandemic. If the prevailing state plays a role, then one

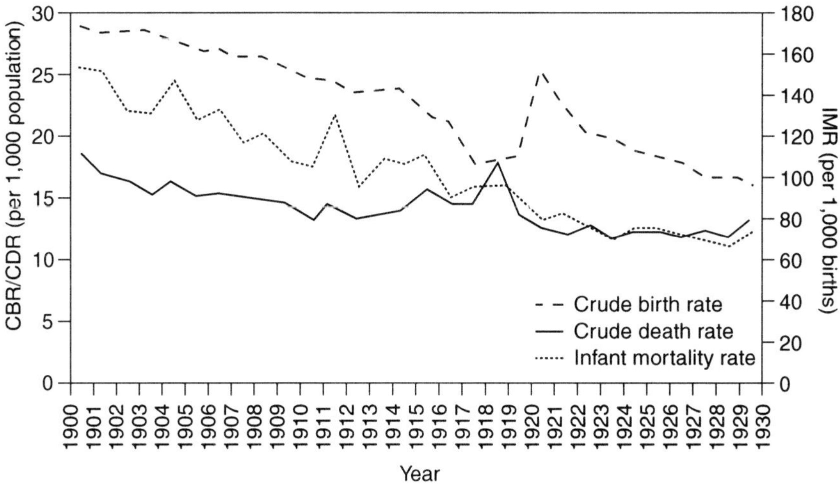

Figure 7.1 Vital statistics, England and Wales 1900–30 (sources: *ARRG*s 1900–30).

may expect a significant correlation between the IMR and the influenza mortality. Conversely, the lack of a significant relation between the two would indicate that the pandemic strikes irrespective of existing conditions, that it changes the situation so drastically that these existing conditions are immaterial in determining the excess mortality wrought by a pandemic. In this case the IMRs for 1911 and 1918 were correlated with the annualised influenza mortality for the entire pandemic period.

However, it is important to note that infant mortality in Britain had improved as 'the war years were the period of the most significant improvement in IMRs in the first thirty years' of the century (Winter 1982: 718). The improvement in British infant mortality and the narrowing of class mortality differentials have been claimed to be essentially a function of increasing quality of life/income and hence nutritional status as the war led to altered conditions to the extent that labour was made more valuable and was better paid, leading to claims such as that 'large sections of the working class were better fed during the war' than previously (Winter 1982: 727).[1] The primary factor was the 'rise in family incomes, especially among the poorest sections of the population, which reduced the economic distance between strata within the working class and between classes, and improved the life chances of the infant population of Britain during the First World War' (Winter 1982: 729).

The IMR for 1911 indicates conditions prior to the disruption of the war. The correlation coefficient with pandemic influenza mortality is 0.264, with a coefficient of determination of 0.069, suggesting a relatively insignificant association between the two; a slightly positive but by no means strong relationship. The Spearman's rank correlation coefficient (0.399, giving a *z*-score of 5.942 and an alpha-value percentage of <0.000001) confirms a degree of association between the two. The correlation between influenza mortality and the 1918 IMR values is slightly stronger at 0.346 (coefficient of determination is 0.120), but this is to be expected as the influenza mortality of infants would be a component of this IMR. The higher correlation value indicates a slightly stronger relationship between the influenza mortality and the 1918 IMR than that between flu mortality and the 1911 IMR. However, these are not strong relationships and indicate that influenza probably only had a small impact on infant mortality. It is this that is the unusual fact – that children, infants and the aged were not killed at markedly increased rates as the young adults were. Further, if one uses IMR as an indicator of the general health status, these results suggest that the existing conditions played a limited role in determining pandemic mortality.

While children were not taken at a substantially greater rate, it has been much discussed that young adults were. The illness and death of so many young adults must have had an effect on rates of nuptiality, family formation and fertility, with many potential marriages, conceptions and births either delayed or tragically prevented. The deaths of more than 2,500 pregnant women from flu were noted in the RG's reports in Scotland, England and Wales (Registrar-General 1920: 36; Registrar-General for Scotland 1919: 11), and these were only those deaths where the fact of pregnancy was recorded. Obviously, then, at least 2,500 births were foregone in Britain. It is impossible to quantify the additional deaths of pregnant women not recorded as such, but it is likely that they would not be insignificant. The RG believed that the unchanged mortality of premature infants and the only slightly lower than normal birth rate for 1918 indicated that a large number of births had not been lost as a result of the flu (Registrar-General 1920: 37). Additionally it is likely that with such high levels of morbidity, a reduction in conceptions would have occurred, although the effect of this may be reversed by the effect of returning troops.

However, it was those pregnancies terminated by abortion, miscarriage or death that were recorded, and even they are an understatement. This leaves another issue untouched. What about those pregnancies that never happened, the conceptions, pregnancies and births that may have otherwise been expected to occur? These would be the 'lost' or averted births due to the deaths of women who may have borne children. Using the concept of averted births, as invoked by Ó Gráda in claiming that 'there were 0.4 million missing births' in Ireland due to famine and emigration (Ó Gráda 1994: 179, citing Mokyr 1980, 1983), it may be possible to suggest the scale of the number of children who were not born due to the deaths of the potential mothers from influenza. Such a calculation is possible given fertility rates (Table 7.1) and the numbers of female deaths (Table 7.2).[2] The greatest limitation here is that these deaths are only those attributed to influenza in England and Wales for the pandemic period. Another consideration is that

Table 7.1 Fertility rates (births per 1,000 women in age group)

Year	*All ages*	*<20 (15–19)*	*20–24*	*25–29*	*30–34*	*35–39*	*40+ (40–44)*
1901	114	13	120	192	176	133	64
1911	98	11	106	170	150	104	45
1921	90	14	113	160	131	86	34

Source: Werner 1987: 8.

Table 7.2 Female influenza deaths by age group

Period	*Age group*						
	15–19	*20–24*	*25–29*	*30–34*	*35–39*	*40–44*	*Total*
Q2, 1918	30	35	48	30	27	37	207
Q3, 1918	447	520	647	514	389	330	2,847
Q4, 1918	3,732	5,549	7,724	6,251	3,643	2,450	29,349
Q1, 1919	901	1,451	2,290	1,919	1,184	885	8,630
Total	**5,110**	**7,555**	**10,709**	**8,714**	**5,243**	**3,702**	

Source: Registrar-General 1920: 9.

Table 7.3 Averted births, England and Wales

Fertility rate	*15–19*	*20–24*	*25–29*	*30–34*	*35–39*	*40–44*	*Total*
1901	66	907	2,056	1,534	697	237	5,497
1911	56	801	1,821	1,307	545	167	4,697
1921	72	854	1,713	1,142	451	126	4,357

of fertility rate and which rate is appropriate. Late 1918 and early 1919 were clearly a time of transition, a point of inflexion where fertility (and birth rate) reversed the war-time decline and led to a post-war baby boom. Given this constraint, all three fertility rates given have been used in calculating a range of values for averted births (Table 7.3).

In England and Wales, something in the vicinity of 5,000 births were averted due to the deaths of the potential mothers from influenza during the pandemic. This is in addition to the 2,500 deaths of pregnant women from influenza. Of course these numbers are based on the premise that there would have been enough males present to father all these potential children; given the mortality of the war, followed by that of the pandemic, this is not an insignificant consideration. It must be conceded that, in relation to the number of live births registered in England and Wales between 1 July 1918 and 30 June 1919 (some 623,740) and the RG's estimate of 750,000 pregnancies in the year (Registrar-General 1920: 36), this does not represent a major demographic impact. It is also plausible that these averted births were more than made up for in the surge in the birth rate in the next couple of years (Figure 7.1) as part of the post-war and post-pandemic baby boom.

Influenza and the war: causation, cessation and facilitation

There is much that links the influenza pandemic and the First World War beyond that of their coincidence, and various arguments have attempted to connect the two causally. These generally fall into three categories: those that claim the influenza was brought about or caused by the war; those that claim the influenza played a role in ending the war; and those that claim that the influenza pandemic was facilitated by the war.[3] No event concentrated the minds of the world's population in the early decades of the twentieth century as did the Great War. When an epidemic arose as that war was rumbling to its end, it is understandable that many thought they discerned a relationship between the two. For some, this was a direct causal relationship, others saw it as more of a coincidence, and some saw the disease as a cathartic or retributive measure brought about by a God or gods.

One of the more commonly claimed direct links between the war and the influenza revolved around the use of poison gas on the battlefields, particularly in France. On 10 October 1918, *The Times* reported a claim that the 'disease is directly traceable to the German use of poison gas, the after-effects of which have induced the growth of a new type of streptococcus', while others speculated that the disease may actually have been the product of German chemical warfare. This belief would have contributed to the blaming of Germany for the pandemic. Other explanations for the pandemic that gained some currency included the belief that the disease arose from the masses of decomposing unburied bodies on the battlefields.

In 1923, Rãjendra-Kumãra Sena, writing in India, also suggested that these unburied bodies were, in Rudyard Kipling's words, 'Senselessly tossed and retossed in stale mutilation/From crater to crater',[4] and could be the source of the affliction. They are but one of many causes Sena identified as being responsible. He attributed to a 'Hindu astrologer' the claim that the influenza 'emanated from the countless dead bodies' and that the emission of poisonous gases in the battlefields had 'vitiated the atmosphere and spread all over the world, affecting the human health' (Sena 1923: 13). Sena attributed a more general miasmic theory for disease to a Greek doctor, one M. Kouzas. Kouzas apparently argued that the majority of diseases were

> due to an invisible, unknown virus forming in our system, when mentally agitated. When we are sad or jealous, or harbour hatred we breathe

> out carbonic acid containing the virus, poisoning the atmosphere, and our blood during respiration, when the air is full of virus. This causes the out-break of epidemic such as influenza etc. The epidemics during the war were due to the general sadness and depression of the people.
> (Sena 1923: preface)

This combination of the centuries-old concepts of miasmas and the recently emerged concept of the virus form an arresting image. But beyond the miasmic explanations, there are other links people have attempted to make suggesting that the pandemic was caused by the war. For example, evolutionary biologists have contended that the conditions of war in France were the stimulus that gave rise to such a virulent strain of influenza (Ewald 1994). These explanations for the pandemic that have the war at their heart reflect the sense of horror at what was taking place on the Western Front. Howard Phillips has argued that, for many, the Western Front 'clearly was a place where terrible things were happening and could be expected to happen. When men so flagrantly broke the laws of humanity and nature every day, a deadly disease came as no surprise' (Phillips 1990a: 150). While this is undeniably the case, is it right to claim the war as a cause of the pandemic?

Reports to the Committee of the Office International d'Hygiène Publique in 1919 revealed how widespread the influenza had been. The British delegate reported that the 'contribution from Switzerland was particularly interesting as it showed the great intensity of the disease in 1918–19 on a neutral country which had escaped a great many of the war conditions to which the heavy incidence and mortality of the recent influenza epidemics have frequently been ascribed' (PRO MH 113 51 *Report 1*). This was a truly global influenza outbreak, encompassing almost every nation, whether they were at war or remained neutral. Whether the conditions in France provided some mechanism for enhancing the virulence of the virus or if that strain was inherently so virulent may well be impossible to determine. However, the latter appears the more likely as, once an entirely novel influenza virus had emerged, a pandemic was inevitable. Thus, the war did not per se cause the pandemic.

Accepting that the war did not directly cause the pandemic, is it possible that an effect actually worked the other way? Did the influenza have an impact on the prosecution of the war? Did it help hasten the end of the war? Certainly the influenza had a major impact on most, if not all, of the forces engaged in the war in France and elsewhere. Hundreds of thousands of military personnel suffered and certainly there are instances where particular actions or campaigns were delayed or cancelled due to illness. In a major work on the year 1918, Gregor Dallas recognised that such an impact was widespread and shared by all forces (Dallas 2000). He noted the tens of thousands of influenza cases among the many forces, the widespread misery caused by flu in the belligerent countries (but also that war was not a cause or a determinant of the pandemic), its affect on the amnesty celebrations in many locations, its influence on the Paris negotiations, and the illness striking important figures such as Woodrow Wilson. It is known that a number of the most senior political leaders suffered terribly from the flu, including the British Prime Minister David Lloyd George (bed-ridden for nine days in October 1918), the American President Woodrow Wilson and his senior adviser Edward House (who both came close to dying while in Paris), Prince Maximilian of Baden (who as German Chancellor in October 1918 spent much of that time ill in bed) and, in Moscow, Sverdlov (who had been the mediator between Stalin and Trotsky and 'the only brake on party centralization' (Dallas 2000: 403)) was killed by the flu, an event whose importance one can only guess at given the later history of the Soviet Union. Dallas also agreed that influenza mortality was several times greater than the combat-related mortality of the war and was greater than that caused by the Black Death in the 100 years following 1348.

The Royal Society of Medicine's 'Discussion' gave a number of military medics the opportunity to reveal how great the impact had been on their forces. For example, the British Colonel Soltau noted that

> Whole units were sometimes put out of action. One army brigade of artillery had at one time two-thirds of its strength laid up, and was unable to go into action, though badly needed, for three weeks. The German armies suffered heavily, and our Intelligence Branch had evidence that this was one of the factors which caused the postponement of a certain contemplated attack of very critical importance.
>
> (Royal Society of Medicine 1918: 27–8)

Influenza was made notifiable in the British Armies in France on 5 October 1918, and between then and the middle of March 1919 112,274 admissions and 5,483 deaths were recorded, and these were just those in the British forces located in France (MacPherson *et al.* 1920: 175). It was reported that, in just twenty-four weeks of 1918, the British forces in France and Flanders had 313,938 admissions at a rate of 157.81 'per 1,000 of ration strength', a rate which was nearly matched in Macedonia (154.27 from 19,862 admissions) (Butler 1943: 195). In Iran, the British and Bolshevik forces both suffered with the influenza, contributing to the Bolshevik surrender at Tashkent and to the British retreat in September 1918, 'leaving the Turks in control of Baku and the whole of western Azarbaijan' (Afkhami 2003: 374–5).

Harvey Cushing's journal of his time as a military surgeon reveals a number of instances where the influenza had a direct impact on military activity from the summer of 1918 through to November 1918. He also gives an insight into how military hospitals were faced with massive numbers of influenza cases in addition to their 'normal' workload of the war casualties. His diary entries reveal the impact on both the Allied and

German forces, including speculation that outbreaks of the flu, often known as 'three day fever', were hampering the German forces, and the scale of the problem in the autumn.

> *30 June, 1918*
> the epidemic of grippe which hit us rather hard in Flanders also hit the Boche worse, and this may have caused the delay . . .
>
> *7 July, 1918*
> Wonderful weather continues and yet no renewal of the Boche offensive. Many theories – shortage of men? internal troubles? an epidemic of the 3-day fever?
>
> *30 September, 1918*
> pneumonia in particular having become a real menace.
>
> *15 October, 1918*
> The weekly report of *Oct. 3rd* of the relation of patients to beds in the A.E.F. gave us a grand total:–

	Occupied	*Vacant*	*Normal*	*Emergency*
Base Hospitals	91,740	26,703	109,897	160,286
Camp Hospitals	15,138	2,850	16,264	17,798
Grand Total	106,878	29,553	126,161	178,084

> Thus 84.7 percent of the normal and 60 percent of the emergency beds were then filled and we were lacking personnel for 35 base hospitals. A few days ago it was reported that we had beds for only two days if wounded and sick continued to come in at the present rate, and the weekly report of *Oct. 10*, just come to-day, gives:–

	Occupied	*Vacant*	*Normal*	*Emergency*
Base Hospitals	119,739	12,906	110,994	162,068
Camp Hospitals	17,719	6,260	21,939	24,289
Grand Total	137,456	19,166	132,933	186,357

> In short, our base hospitals are 107.9 percent full, our camp hospitals 82.5 percent full, and 73.3 percent of our emergency beds are occupied.
> (Cushing 1936: 389, 396, 460, 472–3)

The poor conditions that medical personnel tending the military had to endure are well-known, as is their dreadful workload. Influenza ensured that even when the number of battle wounded dipped, there was still much to keep them busy, as in 'August and September [1918] the German retreat left some British units out of contact with the enemy. . . . At the same time came the Spanish 'flu epidemic and the advancing CCSs [Casualty Clearing Stations] and FAs [Field Ambulances] had to cope with an influx of sick men which more than made up for the decline in the number of wounded' (PRO MH 106 2387: 36). A doctor with one of those FAs, Ivo Geikie Cobb (who wrote his memoirs under the pseudonym Anthony Weymouth), later recalled that his efforts were rather wasted:

> One morning, not very long after I had joined the field-ambulance, a message came . . . that the influenza epidemic then raging in Europe had reached our part of the line. Would our C.O. please prepare to take in a large number of patients suffering from influenza? The C.O. groaned, then looked at me.
>
> 'Well, anyway, there is one real doctor amongst us. Now then, Weymouth, there are plenty of outbuildings here. Get 'em ready for patients.'
>
> As I left to carry out his orders, he called out, 'And for God's sake, don't get it yourself, or we *shall* be in the cart.'
>
> The next few days I was busily employed in lecturing to the orderlies on the avoidance of infection, and in converting stable-lofts into wards. On the morning of the fourth day I woke up with a splitting headache, and pains in my limbs. I took my temperature. It was nearly 104.
>
> 'Oh hell!' I thought, 'I'll be the first patient here after all.'
>
> Now, this was very awkward in view of the wise remarks I had uttered, when lecturing to the orderlies, on the prevention of infection.
>
> I shouted for my servant, and (mindful of my previous experiences with influenza and pneumonia) stayed in bed and sent a message to the C.O.
>
> (Weymouth 1936: 200–1)

By the time he had recovered from his bout of broncho-pneumonia and was discharged from hospital the war had ended. These examples demonstrate the scale of the flu among the military. It has been claimed that the Allied troops suffered but survived, whereas in

> Prince Rupprecht's Army . . . the percentage of those affected was higher, and owing to inadequate medical facilities and to general weakness caused by months of undernourishment, many of the sick did not recover . . . and as the epidemic was to roll in waves across Europe . . . it was to become a factor of increasing significance.
>
> (Pitt 1962: 166)

This account suggests that the influenza played a role in determining the outcome of the war and in bringing it to a close earlier than may otherwise have been the case. However, this view is a minority one and influenza is usually little more than a footnote in the histories of the First World War. Both of these are somewhat erroneous – the flu certainly had a major impact on all the forces, but it did not in itself directly determine the course of hostilities or even their cessation.

If the war had not caused the flu and the pandemic had not brought about the end of the war, what was the relationship, if any, between these two concurrent global events? Is it conceivable that they were not related at all and were merely coincident? No. The war played a significant role in facilitating the pandemic, largely through the mass movement of people that ensured the global reach of the disease. It was the (troop) ships that were to bring the disease to so many lands. For example, as the war ended in East Africa, thousands of porters were repatriated and brought the disease to places that had not yet encountered it. In many countries it was the returning forces that brought the flu from Europe and took it to their homes, working their way along the national and local transport networks to eventually spread the disease into every town and village. Such transport links and networks contributed to the spread of influenza to and within many countries, including Canada, Australia, New Zealand and South Africa.

The Times ran a story in October 1918 under the headline, 'The Summer Influenza' which shows how the importance of travel for spreading disease was appreciated:

> The epidemic was first reported in Spain. Generally speaking it moved northwards in Europe and eastwards in India. . . . In previous similar epidemics the progression has been westwards in Europe, the country of origin usually being Russia. The war has, however, fundamentally changed the general character of European traffic – that from east to west being suspended, while the north and south traffic has been greatly augmented; and in the absence of other definable factors it is reasonable to assume that the abnormal progression of the present epidemic has mainly been determined by the changed lines of inter-communication.
>
> (*The Times* 14 October 1918: 5)

Sir Arthur Newsholme at the LGB was in no doubt that 'the movements of the recent war have been responsible on a large scale for its increased virulence'. The mass movements of 'several hundred thousands persons' each month on a limited number of vessels took place at a time when influenza and pneumonia were present in a number of important military centres. Newsholme acknowledged that 'it would have been surprising had this marvellously rapid and successful transportation of troops been carried through without a heavy cost in communicable disease' (Royal Society of Medicine 1918: 16). War brings with it tremendous displacement and movement of people, often in appalling conditions.[5] This, in conjunction with the tremendous virulence of the newly emerged virus and the ease of transmission of influenza, set the scene for a calamitous pandemic and the disease was quickly dispersed to all parts of the globe. Thus it appears that the war in itself did not 'create' the pandemic, rather once the virus emerged it was destined to spread across the globe infecting peoples the world over and bringing hundreds of millions of deaths. But the war certainly played an important role in moving the disease, in facilitating its spread. For example, in South Africa it has been argued that the country's 'strategic maritime position had long laid it open to infection from visiting ships. World War I, with its expansion of this traffic and its shiploads of troops, multiplied this danger many times' (Phillips 1990a: 179)

Flu and the peace

September 1918 had seen the Prime Minister, David Lloyd George, in his native city of Manchester, with plans to receive the freedom of the city, make a number of speeches, including one that was to set the stage for a general election in the autumn, and to spend several days in the north of England. However, circumstances left these plans in tatters and kept Lloyd George in Manchester for much longer than he'd anticipated and incapacitated for some nine days. On 12 September 1918, the city of Manchester granted the freedom of the city to its most important native son. Lloyd George's acceptance speech at the Hippodrome lasted ninety minutes and was followed by a civic lunch at the Midland Hotel and a gathering of the local Welsh community. Lloyd George was meant to attend a dinner at the Reform Club but influenza drove him to his bed in the Town Hall and, as a recent biographer termed it, 'the Town Hall of Manchester was his hospital' for the next nine days. He was ill to such an extent that his valet, Newnham, considered it 'touch and go' as to whether he would survive. Naturally none of this was revealed to the press, and what bulletins that were issued 'were brief and made no suggestion that the Prime Minister was in any danger, no doubt because the truth would have been alarming to the British public and encouraging to the enemy' (Grigg 2002: 593–4).

When Lloyd George had recovered enough to return to London on 21 September, he did so still wearing a respirator. His post-influenzal malaise and weakness persisted and his public meetings were cancelled at least until the end of the month. His 4 October 1918 trip to Paris saw him accompanied by a specialist, Sir William Milligan, and Lloyd George wrote to his wife Margaret that 'I am off by the 8am train from Charing X. My temperature is still very low and my pulse too feeble'. His biographer is in little doubt that this bout of disease was 'one of the worst in his life' and that he was 'acutely, perhaps critically, ill at a time of mounting crisis in the world' (Grigg 2002: 594–5). Lloyd George later used the influenza as a rather odd metaphor in a heated discussion on 8 March 1919 on the issue of starvation and the blockade of Germany when he 'noted that the fruits of victory are notoriously perishable' and that one day the Allies might find the 'memories of starvation turned against them' and that it had been 'like stirring up an influenza puddle, just next door to one's self' (Vincent 1985: 117). Lloyd George was not alone among world leaders to suffer. As has been discussed, the King of Spain's tussle with the disease was one of the earliest reported cases and helped give rise to the name 'Spanish flu'. But of the warring nations, it was the German Chancellor, Prince Maximilian of Baden, who was also to face the wrath of influenza. Max was driven to his sickbed for a significant portion of his tenure as Chancellor. He was also well aware of how great a threat the disease posed to the German people, as he noted in his memoirs, on 15 October Berlin had seen 1,722 deaths from the disease (Maximilian 1928, II: 92, cited in Vincent 1985: 59).

By the time the Paris peace negotiations started, at least two of the senior figures had endured the agonies of flu – and many more of those in Paris were to share in that painful experience, many of them succumbing. The negotiations took place in a fug of flu and very large proportions of the British and American delegations were ill as the disease was extremely prevalent in Paris. Lloyd George had almost been killed by the flu not so long previously, and President Wilson and his aide Edward House were both taken very seriously ill (as with Lloyd George, their physicians had not been confident they would survive). The American delegation was struck heavily by the pandemic. It was also under great pressure from the other powers in the negotiations – pressure that eventually told. It has been suggested that Wilson's debilitation and post-influenzal malaise contributed to what is considered his failure to stand up for the Fourteen Points he had elucidated in his 8 January 1918 speech to a Joint Session of Congress[6] and his capitulation to the more extreme demands from other parties (on German reparations) (Crosby 1989: 171–96). Yet others have said that these demands for reparations contributed to the instability of the 1920s and 1930s and eventually culminated in the Second World War. Consequently a rather tenuous and over-extended chain of causation could be postulated to link influenza, the First World War, the Paris peace negotiations, the demands placed on Germany, the inter-war tensions and then the Second World War.

A tragic and ironic impact of war came in the form of those extra infections, further illness and death that stemmed from the celebration of the Armistice. There are many instances where celebrations became the foci of new or recrudescent outbreaks of influenza. People brought together in the exuberance of celebration and the relaxation of regulations governing meetings and the wearing of masks led to further influenza deaths. So even at the end of the fighting the war was still bringing death and many of those to die were those who had survived years of gruelling bloody warfare. Examples of such bittersweet suffering include the somewhat comic image of thousands of masked San Franciscans singing and dancing in the streets, deliriously happy celebrating the end of war, a scene repeated the world over (albeit not always including the face masks) (Crosby 1989). In Kenya, two major war-related social events have been identified as playing a major role in spreading the illness in Nairobi. The first was a military ceremony for the participants of the 1915 Turkana Expedition that brought many African soldiers and civilians together on 22 October. Many of the same worthies were doubtless present three days later when the city's European population celebrated the Red Cross Ball (Mueller 1995). Social events could be the focus for outbreaks, for example in Christchurch, New Zealand, the serious cases of the disease first appeared during Carnival Week and 'there was little doubt that [flu] was brought into the city by Carnival Week visitors, and quickly spread through the town and country districts' (Pearson 1919: 254). Elsewhere, *The Times* carried a report on 15 March 1919 that 'Carnival celebrations in Malta [were] blamed for . . . [a] fresh outbreak of influenza with many fatal cases'. In Spain, the St Isidro festival attracted many people to Madrid, many of whom returned to their homes across the country bearing influenza, and the subsequent autumn harvest festivals further 'served as potent diffusers of the virus'. The importance of such festivals could exert pressures of many types, including those seen in Valladolid where the chief health inspector, Dr Garcia Duran, agreed to delay the official declaration of an epidemic until late in September due to the economic and political interests and benefits of the week's activities (Echeverri 2003: 176–9).

Concerns about the possibility of further influenza cases contributed significantly to the British government's decision to inform the governments of a number of countries, including France, Belgium, Japan, Greece and China, that

> the influenza epidemic has rendered it unwise to receive contingents of Allied troops in London, and that the invitation for contingents to take part in the Lord Mayor's procession has therefore been regretfully withdrawn. It is pointed out that only troops of the United States, Portugal, Italy, and Serbia who are already in the United Kingdom will be able to take part.
>
> (PRO, CAB 24 149 Report for the week ending 7 November 1918)

This action may have helped reduce the number of influenza cases that were spread during the Procession slightly. It is notable that this is one of the very few mentions of the pandemic in the British Cabinet records. Indeed, there is relatively little on the influenza in the British records. The war obscures, if not obliterates, the influenza from the purview of the British government/establishment.

The war also plays a role in the collective memory of the event, particularly in those nations most involved in the conflict. The two events were quite frequently conflated with the flu becoming a component of the greater story of the war. Changes in society and attitudes are also attributed to the war. It marked a major time of change, not least in Britain. From the latter part of the nineteenth century, Britain had gone from being the dominant global power to one whose people now had to reconsider their place in the world. From the South African War and the carnage of the long years of the First World War, Britain's dominant position had been questioned. Changes in attitude brought about by war may well have contributed to how that society reacted to the pandemic. After years of sacrifice and having ideals of comradeship, of 'making do' and keeping a 'stiff upper lip' in the face of terrible war, surely these would influence the reaction to the minor inconvenience of flu? This was 'only' the flu and, as such, may have become masked by the deep scars caused by the war and subsumed into the whole war experience. Such attitudes may have contributed to the downplaying of the scale of the pandemic and its failure to retain a prominent role in the collective memory that might otherwise be expected of a disease outbreak that brought so much illness and death.

Political repercussions

Epidemics and the responses to them, particularly of public authorities and governments, can rapidly become politicised and potential sources of public disorder and change. It has already been noted that the 1918 influenza pandemic was largely free of such responses. One of the few threats to the governing elites recorded occurred in Brazil where it has been suggested that 'the fragility of the modernizing ideals of the Southern Brazilian bourgeoisie' were exposed and that the Rio Grande elite 'attempted to legitimate existing power relations and to prevent the erosion of established order' and denied the presence of an epidemic. It has been considered that 'it is surprising that this Southern Brazilian society survived this period of fear, desinformation [sic] and rupture' (Olinto 1993: 285).

Samoa also witnessed a political dimension to the pandemic as the influenza has been linked with the increase in the influence and motivation of the Samoan independence movement who regarded the extraordinarily high mortality there (22 per cent of the population) as indicative of New Zealand's failure to meet their responsibilities as the colonial power (Boyd 1980). Connections between the disease and relations between Canadian native peoples and the 'EuroCanadians' have also been suggested as the disease was 'incorporated into Aboriginal interpretations of the relationship between themselves, their non-Native neighbours and the government' (Kelm 1998: 21). These interpretations included attributing the disease to their contacts with whites, particularly confrontational contacts, while often using 'indigenous conceptions of disease causation' to explain the transmission of disease. First Nations' perspectives of the flu also often included a sense of betrayal: betrayal that the modernisation and medicine they had been encouraged to adopt failed to protect them, and also the failure to provide resources and assistance; it has been argued that this was tantamount to neglect (Kelm 1998: 23–7). Obviously such a perspective would give succour to political opposition and resistance.

Perhaps nowhere was the longer-term societal impact greater than in South Africa. This was to be a major event early in the development of the newly-founded Union of South Africa, an event that shaped much of South Africa in demographic, medical, social, racial and administrative terms. For example, it has been argued that the changes in South African legislation due to the flu actually laid the groundwork for the far more insidious apartheid laws that were to come later in the century. The new Public Health Act changed the Public Health Department from being the small advisory service that had been established in 1917 into a much more active and interventionist arm of the Union government (Phillips 1987, 1990a, 1990b). The pandemic permitted not only the creation of new health authorities with much-expanded powers, but also contributed to the 'hastened formulation and passing of some apartheid and health laws' (Mueller 1995). However, this view has been countered by the assertion that, while concerns about the spread of disease may have fuelled the fires of segregation, they were not in themselves a direct cause of the later laws, such as the Natives (Urban Areas) Act of 1923 (containing the main principles of residential segregation); rather, they may have acted as an enabling catalyst. This may have been particularly because the poor were seen as bringing the disease to the wealthier white population and so the 'epidemic added weight and urgency to demands for a comprehensive national policy to enforce residential segregation in South Africa's towns' (Phillips 1990a: 226–7).

National health systems

At the height of the pandemic, Harvey Cushing jotted in his diary that the 'pandemic of influenza may after all have served a worthy purpose. It takes a scourge . . . to rouse nations to constructive acts' (Cushing 1936: 492). One of the few long-term consequences of the pandemic that has been identified was the creation or alteration of national public health systems and administration (Afkhami 2003: 392 fn 101; Bryder 1982; Phillips 1990a; Rice 1988). For example, in South Africa and New Zealand the sudden and massive surge in deaths led to Commissions inquiring into the epidemic and the responses to it. These, along with public demand for change, led directly to major changes in the public health systems with major expansions in the remit, budget and personnel of those systems. In both these countries, these changes came about quite quickly. Indeed *The Times* reported on the introduction of the Public Health Bill in the South African parliament while the third wave of the pandemic was still striking Britain (*The Times* 7 February 1919: 7). The development of national public health systems and organisations in Canada, France, Australia, India, Iran and Russia can also be seen as a consequence of the pandemic. Exactly two months before reporting on the introduction of the South African legislation, *The Times* had reported that 'A public health bureau, associated with a national laboratory, is to be organized by the Canadian Government' (7 December 1918: 7). Calls for a national public health body in Canada had been made for some time, led by groups such as the Canadian Medical Association and the United Farm Women's Association, who argued for increased cooperation between the provinces on health, and for the establishment of a central health bureau. The pandemic gave this drive the extra momentum that saw its goals become reality and the 'bill to establish a federal department of health was given first reading in March 1919', and the department was operating later that year (Pettigrew 1983: 134–5).

However, the pandemic was by no means a universal opportunity for the spread of 'professional medicine' that it was in some countries (those countries where the profession was not perceived as having failed; rather it was thought to have been hindered by the lack of organisation, infrastructure, resources and support). The medical men and women were not blamed for the deaths; they were seen as having battled valiantly against an overwhelming foe. Instead it was the government, the lack of funding, the lack of public health systems and infrastructure that were seen as having contributed to the huge number of deaths. Criticism of the profession was generally rare. But this was not always the case, and there are a number of examples that reveal a different reaction. The experience of the pandemic in Puebla, Mexico, and Rio Grande, Brazil, for example, exposed greater tensions. In Puebla the pandemic led to a public health campaign, but this developed into a political conflict between apparently revolutionary groups and their opponents with the 'proprietary class' winning out both in political terms and in being able to impose their public health strategies (Gamboa Ojeda 1991). The southern Brazilian case 'demonstrated the fragility of the modernizing ideals of the Southern Brazilian bourgeoisie' and, in putting pressure on the health policies, it exposed 'the terrible health conditions of the majority of the population'. The medical profession, knowledge and policies 'could not respond to the needs of the bourgeoisie' and the loss of position and power seemed almost inevitable (Olinto 1993). The fact that the peaks of the pandemic were so brief, just weeks, prevented such tensions simmering long enough to actually boil over and precipitate major upheaval, and once the peak passed, most people were simply relieved to see it over and any political energy was dissipated.

In Australia, the pandemic played a significant role in the development of the Australian federal Department of Health and the Quarantine Service as Victor Heiser, the eminent American public health specialist who spent many years contributing to the international health work of the Rockefeller Foundation, recalled in his memoirs:

> in 1921, the idea of a Ministry of Health became a popular issue. The troops coming home from the War had threatened the introduction of malaria, typhoid, dysentery, and venereal disease. . . . The influenza epidemic, which spared no corner of the continent, brought to light the

> inefficiency and confusion of the states in dealing with a disease of such vital concern to all.
>
> (Heiser 1936: 351–2)

Australia had managed to delay the arrival of the flu by imposing a strict maritime quarantine (later followed by interstate quarantining). The Director of Quarantine in Australia, J.H.L. Cumpston, wrote a paper calling for the *Establishment of Department of Quarantine and Public Health*, and claimed that the quarantine service has been exemplary in keeping Australia free of the disease (though more than 12,000 Australians died of flu once it broke quarantine). However, he also warned of other epidemics and argued for a vigilant quarantine service, demanding more funding and staff (NAA A6006 1919/1/9. See also Cumpston 1919). The Australian Cabinet approved these requests and an increase in the Director's salary. The Australian federal Department of Health acknowledges that the 'panicked response to the 1919 influenza pandemic was a catalyst for founding the Commonwealth Department of Health in March 1921'.[7] Other factors influencing this decision included recommendations from the Premiers of the various Australian states, the British Medical Association of Australia (the forerunner of the modern Australian Medical Association) and a blunt appeal to the Prime Minister, Billy Hughes, by Victor Heiser, then of the Rockefeller Foundation's International Health Board. Heiser told Hughes that Australia would be considered backward until it had a national department of health. He also offered incentives of temporary expertise in industrial hygiene, public health engineering and administration, as well as training scholarships to encourage the government to agree. John Cumpston became the first Director-General of the new department established in 1921.

Richard Collier claimed that there was a similar outcome in Britain – that the pandemic led to the creation of the new Ministry of Health. However he overstates the case by explicitly linking the creation of the ministry with the pandemic. He suggests that the push to replace the Local Government Board (LGB) with a Ministry 'met at first with bitter reactionary opposition. But by 1919, backed by such powerful sponsors as Lady Rhondda, Lord Leverhulme and Major (later Lord) Astor, it had become reality' (Collier 1974: 289) and attributes the overcoming of such resistance to the pandemic. The end of the nineteenth century and the early decades of the twentieth century were a period of great change in British public health, from an ethos of laissez-faire small government towards the beginnings of a welfare state. Also there were changes in the conception of disease which occurred as medicine continued to establish itself as 'scientific' and 'professional', and changes in the government structures concerning health and disease as the Ministry of Health came to replace the LGB. Indeed, some did use the passivity of the LGB in the face of the pandemic to enhance their calls for a Ministry of Health. But whereas the pandemic did lead to the creation of new public health organisations in other countries, the British health ministry was already an idea whose time had come. Moves towards changes in British public health had already been underway for some time. Landmarks such as the Public Health Acts of 1875 and 1890, the 1906 Education (Provision of Meals) Act, and the 1911 National Health Insurance Act had all been passed and, as the medical historian Virginia Berridge has written, 'social reform in the health sphere has clear Victorian antecedents' (Berridge 1990: 217). However, *The Times*' medical correspondent was certainly keen on an active Ministry and argued the case on a number of occasions, as did a number of letter-writers, but only on occasion was the spectre of the pandemic invoked.[8] The war had delayed reform of the British medical and welfare policy as it 'distracted politicians and reformers alike' (Lees 1998: 328), so it may be that the pandemic aided in the revitalisation of this process.

While the LGB was criticised for its passivity and for the delay in its actions, it was not actually criticised for the nature of those actions. It acted wholly in keeping with the nature and beliefs of the medical establishment. It also justified its inactivity and failure to take more proactive measures, such as quarantine, by arguing that they would not work anyway and that in a country at war they were not possible or practicable. Sir Arthur Newsholme publicly admitted, when opening the Royal Society of Medicine's 'Discussion' on influenza, to having delayed the distribution of the LGB's first *Memorandum on Influenza* as he considered the nation's 'major duty is to "carry on" . . . the relentless needs of warfare justified incurring this risk of spreading infection and the associated creation of a more virulent type of disease or mixed diseases' (Royal Society of Medicine 1918: 13). So, in the national (military) interest it was 'business as usual' – an attitude encouraged by the press and the medical establishment. Any action and any treatment was then left to the local authorities as they had primary responsibility for public health, and this was discharged by the local MOHs. With no centralised or co-ordinating body, this led to a very mixed range of responses, with some MOHs effectively denying there was any such epidemic, whereas others provided as much assistance as they could.

Flu and the WHO

While the role of the pandemic in the creation or re-casting of national public health systems is recognised, there has been little recognition of the role the pandemic may have had in the development of international bodies such as the World Health Organisation (WHO). But there may indeed be links between the pandemic and such bodies. The root of this story may lie in South Africa, which was caught 'almost wholly unprepared', receiving 'no official notice that ships coming to the Union might be carrying the disease' (Phillips 1990a: 101). However, once infected, South Africa adopted a very proactive stance and information about the epidemic and warnings about the disease were quickly sent to many other nations, particularly other parts of the Empire and those nations that had major shipping connections with South Africa such as Australia, New Zealand, India, Mauritius, Madagascar and the Straits Settlements. South Africa also requested information from many nations as part of its Influenza Epidemic Commission's investigation.[9]

Much of this communication was not between Pretoria, the colonial periphery, and the imperial centre, London, but rather between members of the periphery, the colonies. It suggests that the members of the Empire were asserting a more independent role, a role emphasised by events such as the 1910 Union of South Africa and the 1900 Federation of Australia which were major staging posts on the route to each nation's statehood (rather than simply being colonial outposts). Communication between both Melbourne[10] and Pretoria and London were largely limited to copies of the LGB's *Memorandum on Influenza* and some other cursory communications, particularly regarding the payment of pensions.[11] However, the South Africans did also request that the King send a 'message of condolence', to which the British Secretary of State sent this message on 29 October 1918 (before the peaks of the second wave back in Britain but after them in South Africa) to the Governor-General:

> His Majesty the King has learnt with great concern of the ravages of influenza in the Union of South Africa and the South African Protectorates. Please convey His Majesty's sympathy to the sufferers and his condolences to those who have lost relatives through the epidemic.
>
> (NASA GG 1231 33/1026)

Both the South African and Australian governments had a similar level of correspondence with the USA[12] as they did with Britain, while the bulk of communication flowed between trading partners and fellow colonials. This information was certainly appreciated by at least some of the recipients.[13] The Australians regarded the situation as very serious and used it as justification for imposing the maritime quarantine that delayed the arrival of flu into Australia. New Zealand experienced a 'Black November' in 1918 (Rice 1988), but it was not until mid-1919 that Australia succumbed. The severity of the pandemic in New Zealand and its spread to a number of Pacific islands were of great concern and Australia was called upon by New Zealand to aid a number of these islands, including those that were New Zealand territories or protectorates as New Zealand itself was incapable. Australia continued to monitor outbreaks in many nations, particularly in the Pacific, for some years after the pandemic.

While Australia was grateful for the information and regarded it very seriously, the situation was very different in Britain. The scale of the epidemic in South Africa was no secret, being quite widely reported. In the colonial countries, central government viewed the epidemic very seriously indeed. In Australia they attempted to mobilise the states, to regulate interstate traffic when the disease was proclaimed, and gathered information from many sources. However, there is very little evidence of information flowing between London and Australia (and between London and South Africa). But while there is a real lack of information to and from London, there was a network operating across the southern hemisphere sending warnings, information on the disease, vaccines and so forth. Indeed, this network not only provided information but also organised for relief shipments of medical aid to stricken island nations.

Once the crisis was over and the flu had waned, South Africa wanted to formalise these networks and their flows. One of the recommendations of its Influenza Epidemic Commission was 'the establishment of an international organisation for the rapid dissemination of authoritative information regarding epidemics' (Union of South Africa 1919: 9). This wish was reported in Britain; for example, on 25 February 1919 *The Times* ran the headline, 'To Combat Influenza: An International Bureau Wanted' above their report of the Commission's report, and noting its call for both an international health organisation and a revised health administration in South Africa. The Union of South Africa offered to send out such information in return for information from other nations and 'over the next two years it expanded its epidemic notification network to neighbouring countries and other parts of the Empire' (Phillips 1990a: 207), and also joined the International Bureau of Public Health in Paris which issued monthly bulletins on outbreaks of disease and epidemics all over the world.[14]

Richard Collier suggested that, due to the pandemic, 'the medical frontiers stayed down' and that 'from January 1920 on the League of Nation's Health Organisation [now the World Health Organisation] ensured by a system of cables and weekly returns that flu fighters everywhere worked as an international team' (Collier 1974: 290), but this may be overstating the influence of influenza. It is recognised that the League of Nation's Health Committee owed its existence largely to concerns about disease among refugees, especially typhoid, in the years after the war, particularly in eastern and south-eastern Europe (Metzger 2001; Weindling 1995). However, the influenza pandemic may have played a role in the longer-term permanence of the international bodies and helped crystallise the need for some form of global public health organisation to combat large-scale health issues. Certainly the WHO Director General, Dr Gro Harlem Brundtland, reminded her audience in 2002 that 'the programme to confront influenza is WHO's oldest' (WHO 2002). When the fiftieth anniversary of the development of a cooperative network of influenza research and surveillance was marked by the WHO, a press release commemorating *50 Years of Influenza Surveillance* recognised that 'major strides have been made in combating influenza via surveillance of outbreaks in progress and preparation for upcoming influenza seasons', and announced the release of the WHO's influenza pandemic plan (WHO 1999d) that provided guidelines and information for combating future influenza pandemics. For the WHO, influenza remains a constant threat to be monitored, and by 1999 the WHO's Global Surveillance Programme for Influenza consisted of 110 national influenza centres in eighty-three countries, plus four Collaborating Centres for Virus Reference and Research in Australia, Japan, the UK and the USA. The Director-General of the WHO was quoted as acknowledging that 'We have to recognise that the unpredictability of an influenza pandemic, and the rapid and serious consequences which can occur when a pandemic strain does appear, gives us ample justification for constant vigilance and careful planning to improve preparedness' (WHO 1999e). The WHO's programme was established to set up and finance an international centre to collect and distribute information, co-ordinate laboratory work on influenza and train laboratory workers (WHO 1999b). Subsequently this has grown to include planning to mitigate future epidemics and pandemics, devising control methods to limit spread, severity and consequences of the disease, sharing information, viral isolates and laboratory diagnostic reagents among the national laboratories, including the development and standardisation of techniques and materials. More recently, in an effort to further improve influenza surveillance and promote the standardisation of reporting, the WHO, in collaboration with the Institut National de la Santé et de la Recherche Médicale in Paris, has created an Internet tool for linking the global network of flu research and surveillance centres (FluNet). This site allows each centre to enter data remotely and obtain access to real-time epidemiological and virological information. In addition, all information from the national laboratories is analysed and published by the WHO in the *Weekly Epidemiological Record*, and a summary of country reports is also available on the Internet.[15] The WHO convenes meetings twice a year to determine the composition of influenza vaccines, one in February for the northern hemisphere and then another in September for the southern. Influenza clearly has a significant role in the past, present and future of the WHO. The disease, and the pandemic particularly, may well have played a role in bringing about its predecessors, and thus the WHO may be claimed as one of the pandemic's lasting legacies, albeit somewhat indirectly.

8 Possible futures

The year 1918 saw both the end of the greatest war the world had seen to date, the First World War, and the greatest epidemic in modern history. Between them, these two global scourges probably claimed more than 100 million lives, with the flu claiming by far the greater proportion. The world in 1918 was a very different world to that prior to the war: empires had disappeared, maps were busily being drawn and re-drawn, nascent nations were trying to assert themselves, particularly due to the 'heady brew of self-determination', international and domestic power relations were altered irrevocably, and much of the world's financial and commercial structures had been swept away (Steiner 2005: 1). However, this was not simply an interregnum or a period of slowly and inexorably sliding into the next world war, as some have portrayed it; rather, there was a longing for peace, a sense of renewal and possibility, there was to be a time of potential and of reconstruction (Steiner 2005). But before any of this could be fully explored, the flu was to blight millions of lives.

The flu of 1918 was a pandemic in the truest sense, an epidemic that spread to reach almost every corner, afflicting neutral and belligerent countries alike, forming a melancholic coda or a dark epilogue to the war. It was the greatest outbreak of disease in centuries, and perhaps the greatest ever in terms of the number of people infected and the proportion of the world's population infected. Arriving as the First World War lurched toward its rather abrupt silence, the flu was known to be a danger but was still largely unregarded as it struck Britain. The British newspapers had reported on the vast numbers killed and sickened in many countries, yet the British authorities saw it as a lesser priority and that, with the war taking precedence over all else, it was essential to 'carry on'. Being 'only' flu meant it was much easier to argue the need to 'carry on', and also helped ensure the episode was not to lodge in the collective memory. Flu is too common, too banal and the crisis is brief with the waves of disease breaking quickly. It is something too familiar, too widespread and not really quite lethal enough. An 'exotic' disease with a high fatality rate, a bubonic plague or an Ebola, would be seared into the memory (even if the number of people taken were quite small), whereas an epidemic of the flu with its low mortality rate is far less conspicuous or terrifying, even if it is so pervasive that an unparalleled toll is exacted. But while largely unregarded and long unremembered, the pandemic was not without its impacts. These ranged from the delay in the postwar baby boom through to the political or societal changes, such as the creation and strengthening of public health as a prime concern of government. These changes could be seen as flowing through to bodies such as the League of Nations health programme and its successor, the World Health Organisation (WHO). In any coming pandemic it may be the WHO that plays a major role; indeed, it could be a vital factor in the prevention or diminution of a pandemic, thereby possibly condemning flu to further neglect.

Which raises the question of whether a pandemic is possible or even likely. Could humankind face the threat of a pandemic such as 1918 again? Further influenza epidemics and pandemics are highly likely; indeed, the introduction to an issue of a Royal Society journal reporting on a meeting devoted to influenza flatly stated that 'A devastating pandemic . . . is inevitable' (Laver and Webster 2001: 1813). The mechanisms of antigenic drift and antigenic shift mean that flu remains a threat, and potentially a very grave one. While influenza may not typically have a very high mortality rate, its ease of transmission and potential virulence means the bulk of the world's population could readily be infected once a novel strain emerges. Currently it is the possibility of a bird flu crossing the species barrier into humans and leading to a new avian–human strain that is focusing the attention of many in the healthcare professions.

Bird flu is not just a matter of a rapidly spreading disease that threatens the avian agriculture of a slew of Asian nations. Nor is it a threat solely because this bird disease could threaten the food industry, possibly globally. Indeed, this is not a food problem per se, and there is little reason to stop eating bird products from the afflicted region (but there is good reason not to transport live animals in and out of those countries). Rather, while it is a significant disease among birds, particularly commercially and economically important flocks, it is the potential of this disease to precipitate human illness on a scale that most of us cannot imagine that drives the WHO and influenza experts to urge such drastic action as the immediate culling of millions of birds across south-east and east Asia (and possibly elsewhere), and leads to headlines such as 'Mutated avian flu may kill millions' (*The Sun-Herald*, Sydney, 17 April 2005) and 'Killer flu: could the world cope?' (BBC 2005a).

The strains of bird flu that have killed people in these outbreaks have thus far shown little propensity for human-to-human transmission (whereas normal flu passes from one person to another so very freely) and it appears that almost all the human cases of bird flu have been contracted directly from birds, mostly from household birds rather than commercial flocks (WHO 2005b: 2). Of course the more widespread bird flu becomes, and the H5N1 strain has become endemic in parts of Asia, the greater the chances of such infections, but even so the numbers are likely to remain small. However, bird flu, when it does infect humans, has shown high virulence and a higher mortality rate than is usual for flu. Furthermore, it is apparent that the H5N1 strain has become both more pathogenic in birds and hardier, as well as also showing an increased range, with cases in various cat species and increased mortality in wild waterfowl (WHO 2005b: 2).

With the prevalence of bird flu increasing in spite of the extensive efforts of many public and animal health authorities, it appears increasingly possible that a pandemic strain may emerge, quite possibly an avian–human recombination first appearing in south-east or east Asia (Monto 2005; Stöhr 2005). While this development would naturally be most unwelcome, the possibility may itself generate an awareness and forewarning that may allow preventative and responsive measures to be taken, possibly including further study of the likely emergent strain(s), development of vaccines (perhaps using new techniques which may produce greater volumes of vaccine in shorter timeframes, and that are not dependent on the availability of chicken eggs), the preparation, development and dissemination of information campaigns for the medical professions, care-givers and the wider public, and other pandemic preparedness activities. However, much of this requires the will of public authorities, politicians and the medical community. Given how common and unregarded influenza is in many minds, this is by no means a given. An appreciation of how great a potential threat influenza may be is required.

A virulent and rapidly spreading epidemic of influenza in animals could be contained by slaughter and quarantine but, as Laver and Webster reassuringly note, 'this is not an option for people' (Laver and Webster 2001: 1813) should such a novel strain emerge in the human population. How successful influenza monitoring and surveillance is – and the rapidity with which such a strain could spread – may dictate whether or not there would be sufficient time to prepare, distribute and administer the millions, if not billions, of vaccines that would be required. With existing vaccines expected to be inefficacious, it may be that the modern anti-viral drugs become the frontline defence. It is for this reason that some nations, including the UK, Canada and Australia, have been stockpiling and/or securing contracts for the provision of these drugs.[1] Rapid, accurate diagnosis would aid in detecting an emerging epidemic or pandemic and in determining who should receive vaccines and/or other drugs. Such simple and accurate diagnostic tools are not currently widely available.

The real fear is that if we do not stop the bird flu quickly, it could undergo further changes within the bird population, or if a person (or bird) was infected by both a bird flu and a human influenza strain, this could lead to recombination of genetic materials from both strains, giving rise to a completely new strain, one easily transmissible between people and yet all but invisible to the immune systems of everyone in the world: a highly virulent and highly transmissible virus with no barriers. This happened in 1918 and the new virus surged through the world's population, exerting a massive strain on economies, on families, on medical personnel and facilities, and even on cemeteries and morgues. The funeral industry showed the strain as many towns ran out of coffins and coffin-makers, grave-diggers and others were put on extended hours, while cemeteries opened for longer hours. Reports in *The Times* recorded that:

> So many deaths have occurred [in Ilford] that local undertakers are finding it very difficult with their depleted staffs to cope. . . . All the schools in the town, which accommodate over 11,000 children, have been closed. Outside one doctor's surgery yesterday there was a queue of over 70 people.
>
> Enfield. . . . Undertakers are declining orders. One undertaker states that in Enfield and adjoining districts he has 97 funerals on his books for this week.
>
> Greenwich. . . . On account of the number of funerals permission has been given for interments in the borough cemeteries on Sundays.
>
> Mold. . . . There are queues of applicants for medicine outside the doctors' surgeries. Many bakers are ill and there is a shortage of bread.
>
> Stoke Newington. . . . The borough council have allowed a number of workmen to assist in digging graves at Abney Park Cemetery, as ordinary grave-diggers cannot do the extra work.
>
> Reading. . . . one third of the postmen and postwomen are suffering from influenza, and deliveries are much delayed. An insurance agent who visited 49 houses in the district found that in 46 the residents were affected.

What may happen if and when another pandemic does arise following the emergence of a completely novel influenza virus to which humanity has no immunity and which transmits from person to person as readily as 'normal' influenza does? If our worst fears were realised, would a new pandemic be as bad as 1918? What is the 'worst case' scenario? It would be 90 to 100 per cent infection with mass absenteeism, waves of illness striking quickly to cause great disruption to all aspects of life. Mortality in influenza epidemics and pandemics has rarely exceeded 3 per cent case fatality and is more typically around 1 per cent. But if half the world's population were infected, more than three billion people infected, this could translate into 300 million deaths globally, all in a very short space of time. With appropriate pandemic planning, the development and deployment of anti-virals and perhaps even new vaccines, and the availability of a degree of medical assistance and patient care, it should be possible to mitigate against such high mortality, at least in the developed world. Thus, this could be a influenza pandemic that does show a socio-economic bias – not necessarily in those it infects, but in those who succumb to it.

The monitoring of flu is the WHO's oldest single programme and its 1999 and 2005 Influenza Pandemic Plans and 2002 Global Agenda on Influenza Surveillance, Prevention and Control provide a 'strategic roadmap' for reducing morbidity and mortality from both the annual influenza outbreaks and 'to prepare for the next influenza pandemic' (Stöhr 2002: 517). They have also been encouraging individual countries to develop their own contingency plans for if and when we face such a scourge. This awareness and preparedness (if countries realise the potential danger and prepare and act appropriately), in conjunction with vaccines (if they can be developed in time), anti-virals (where available) and antibiotics (to stem the bacterial complications that claimed so many in 1918) may ameliorate the impact of a new pandemic strain, particularly in the developed world and has 'led to the belief that it might be possible to . . . perhaps even prevent a pandemic' (Monto 2005: 324). However, given that the global population is far larger than it was in 1918, and is so much more inter-connected and inter-dependent, it is perfectly plausible that billions of us could be ill and then, even if the fatality rate remains as low as normal, the numbers of deaths could be in the tens, even hundreds, of millions. Expert estimates for the possible mortality of the next pandemic ranged from '2 million to over 50 million' (WHO 2004b). The actual nature of the virus itself will also be a major determinant of the severity of the pandemic. The 1918 virus had a penchant for young adults – unusual for flu – and so how pathogenic a novel virus might be, and which age groups are affected, could greatly alter its impact.

Beyond factors of the virus, the response and level of preparedness of governments and healthcare systems would also influence the final death toll. Even moderate pandemics inflict a considerable burden on the unprepared and disadvantaged, thus planning of healthcare responses will be crucial. Good healthcare could substantially ameliorate the impact of a pandemic, yet the pandemic itself may disrupt the provision of essential medicines and healthcare workers themselves could be hard-hit, especially if anti-virals and vaccines have limited efficacy against the new strain of flu. Consequently, pandemic response plans need to be both strong and flexible to cope with a wide range of possibilities. We are better placed to face a pandemic now than they were in 1918, but not so well-placed as to be confident, let alone complacent. It would still be a very major stress on the public health systems of every nation – a major test of the wealthier nations and an overwhelming one in many other countries.

In 2001, more than 250 million doses of influenza vaccine were used for a global population of more than six billion, with those considered at the greatest risk of dying (those aged over sixty-five) already numbering more than 380 million (Stöhr 2002: 517). The bulk of these vulnerable people live in developing countries where there has been little access to or provision of vaccines or anti-virals. Consequently many millions would face the prospect of no medical assistance, even in the burgeoning economies of those most populous states, India and China. The WHO believes that in a future pandemic the 'greatest impact [will be] on developing countries where there is no vaccine or antiviral production' (Stöhr 2002: 517). Consequently their Global Agenda on Influenza has the themes of strengthening influenza surveillance both within nations and internationally, increasing knowledge on the burden of influenza to societies, increasing vaccine usage and accelerating national and international action on preparing for pandemics (Stöhr 2002). However, if surveillance and co-operation are not forthcoming, or a strain emerges to which the anti-virals have no efficacy or for which we cannot rapidly develop vaccines, then the mortality could indeed be great. Any failure to distribute medication and assistance to all affected populations could lead to great political and social pressures within and between nations. The economic costs, even if mortality is low, would be enormous. Failure to assist countries and/or communities and any perceived failing of governments to protect their peoples could lead to rancour and unrest.

The WHO's global influenza preparedness plan is designed to guide states and those responsible for public health, medical and emergency preparedness in planning and responding to the possibility and occurrences of pandemic influenza. The 2005 version revised the existing plan, which had focused on the role of the WHO and national governments in the event of a pandemic, and specifically considered the possible presence of an influenza virus of pandemic potential, such as the bird flu subtypes seen in poultry flocks in Asia. The revised plan covered the possibility of simultaneous pandemic viruses with different levels of threat, as was the case in 2004 with outbreaks in poultry of H7N3 in Canada and H5N1 strains in Asia. The phases of increasing public health risk associated with the emergence of a new influenza virus subtype that may pose a pandemic threat were re-examined, recommendations for actions by national authorities at the various stages of a possible pandemic were given and the measures to be taken by the WHO during each phase outlined. This planning should result in greater surety of the measures to be taken by the various actors involved, including the WHO, during the different phases of a pandemic, and should improve international co-ordination and transparency in recommended national measures. The plan also provided guidance for national authorities in developing their own pandemic plans in line with the pandemic phases. National governments must allocate appropriate resources to both the planning and execution stages of their pandemic response. The plans must co-ordinate the activities of many agencies and tiers of government. They must also take into account the national and local conditions. These are not simple tasks but the effort thus far has been lamentable as there has been slow progress as many countries seem to have failed to appreciate the potential danger from influenza. Few national pandemic plans have been devised, fewer put into operation and even fewer given significant legislative backing or real powers in the event of a pandemic (the Canadian plan being the most notable exception).[2]

Existing vaccines are manufactured using influenza virus grown in fertile chicken eggs that are then inactivated by either formaldehyde or β-propiolactone. These vaccines can consist of whole virus, split-product or purified haemagglutinin and neuraminidase. The whole-virus vaccines are not widely used as adverse reactions in young children can occur. The split-product or purified haemagglutinin and neuraminidase vaccines have been shown to be effective, well-tolerated and very safe (Nicholson *et al.* 2003: 1737). The production of these vaccines is a time-consuming process and is heavily dependent on a steady supply of eggs. Even during inter-pandemic periods, at least six months is required to organise sufficient fertile chicken eggs for annual vaccine manufacture, thus making it untenable in the event of a pandemic unless we are so fortunate as to have long advance warning. Furthermore, two of the influenza strains of greatest concern, those of the highly pathogenic H5 and H7 subtypes, cannot be successfully grown in eggs (Webby and Webster 2003: 1520–1). Advance warning in itself may lead to false alarms and see much time and effort spent on producing a vaccine whose disease threat never materialises.

Currently, anti-virals and inactivated vaccines offer the only immediate means of mass prophylaxis, but the supply of these is hampered by limited production capacity of vaccines and limited stocks of anti-virals. Tissue-culture-based and live attenuated vaccines are licensed in some countries and these could augment the supply of inactivated vaccine supplies. Recent years have seen research attention focus on vaccines and vaccine production, including cell-culture vaccines (which could 'offer the potential of being able to respond quickly . . . and avoid the risk of contaminated eggs . . . Moreover, influenza viruses grown in mammalian cells more closely resemble those present in clinical samples . . . hence offering the potential for more effective vaccine'), live vaccines (which may offer 'the advantage of mimicking natural infection . . . [thereby] providing a broader immunological response and more durable protection'), parenteral adjuvants, mucosal adjuvants, recombinant vaccines, reverse genetics and nucleic acid vaccines (Nicholson *et al.* 2003: 1737–9). One research direction that is considered among the more promising is the use of plasmid-based reverse genetic systems to construct influenza virions and vaccines. These systems also offer a successful alternative means of producing H5 and H7 vaccine seed strains (Webby and Webster 2003: 1521).

Collaboration and co-operation between governments, industry, and academia are necessary to overcome the various hurdles and to ensure rapid production of any candidate vaccines. The severe acute respiratory syndrome (SARS) outbreak demonstrated that international collaboration in the face of a global medical threat is possible. There may actually be benefits to be gained from the outbreaks of SARS and bird flu, in terms of better disease surveillance, better co-operation between states and different tiers of government, improved resourcing and greater awareness of the potential dangers of a fast-spreading respiratory disease. These benefits may be short-lived and there is also the danger of 'crying wolf', but the lessons of SARS (and bird flu) must be learned. The fact that SARS was initially denied and that an earlier admission of its existence and prompter action may have saved lives are important lessons. International monitoring and co-operation are vital as such outbreaks are no respecter of borders or political systems.

There are also concerns about potential vaccines with regard to their safety as well as their efficacy. The 1976 swine flu scare in the USA saw how such safety issues can stymie an otherwise well-intentioned campaign. Would any modern government be willing to allow an essentially untested vaccine to be widely used? Would a population accept such a vaccine, except under the most severe of circumstances (when many lives had already been lost)?

That children can play a major role in the propagation of influenza and the possibility of the vaccinating of children in reducing or preventing influenza outbreaks has already been identified (Glezen 1980; Glezen *et al.* 1980; Kendal 1987; Kendal and Glezen 1998; Schoenbaum 2003: 246–248, 251). There is an argument that school-age children should be a prime concern in vaccination, not simply for their own protection but also for that of the greater community. Currently many countries with influenza vaccination policies tend to focus on those at greatest risk of death, that is, young children, the elderly, those with underlying or chronic respiratory conditions, women who may be pregnant during the flu season, residents of nursing homes, health-care workers and so on (for example, CDC 2004). It may well be that an effective approach would be a vaccination programme in which school-age children are vaccinated, thus slowing down the transmission of the disease and possibly even inducing a degree of herd immunity. Mass vaccination of children could be implemented where there is a limited quantity of vaccine and by giving the vaccine to the group most likely to spread the disease rather than the groups at highest risk from the disease itself as this could delay or lessen the intensity of an epidemic; such a delay would gain time for the further production, distribution and administration of vaccine to other people. However, as Schoenbaum noted, health policy-makers have tended to favour vaccination of high-risk groups and 'essential' personnel and, before they could switch to a policy of giving a vaccine of which there are limited stocks to healthy children, proof of the efficacy of such a policy would be required (Schoenbaum 2003: 249–50).

Several measures have been suggested to ensure communities can face a new pandemic with some degree of confidence. These have included: the stockpiling of a sufficient supply of anti-virals and other drugs to reduce the severity and spread of infection; developing vaccines matching the subtypes of an emerging influenza strain, testing these in clinical trials and having manufacturers prepared to 'ramp up' production if and when necessary; the preparation, testing and provision of a reverse genetics-derived vaccine;[3] and an improvement in influenza vaccine manufacturing capacity around the world, particularly in the developing world.

If and when a new flu strain arrives, we will face a grave threat. This threat could emerge in the coming days or months or it may not happen for decades, but as the virologists Richard Webby and Robert Webster warned in *Science*, 'nature's ongoing experiments with H5N1 influenza in Asia and H7N7 in Europe may be the greatest bioterror threat of all. The time for talking is truly over. We must be prepared' (Webby and Webster 2003: 1522). It has been claimed that the emergence of these bird flu strains 'may resemble that leading to the 1918 pandemic' (WHO 2005b: 3) as the gradual adaptation of an avian to a human-like virus, the severity of the disease, the concentration among young and healthy people, and the occurrence of primary viral pneumonia in addition to secondary bacterial pneumonia are all considered to parallel the circumstances prior to the 1918 pandemic. While it is probable that any avian influenza virus would have reduced pathogenicity if it acquired the enhanced transmissibility needed to develop into a pandemic form, it is apposite to remember that no H5 virus has circulated among humans and therefore the vulnerability to an H5N1-like pandemic virus would be total and universal (WHO 2005b). For the foreseeable future flu is going to remain with us, regularly bringing illness to many and death to a relative few, with the threat of a massive pandemic always present. For this reason we must continue the monitoring and the research.

Notes

2 The history of influenza: a long history of affliction

1 Phillips (2004) argued that it had gone through an initial 'epidemiology as history' phase before being followed by a 'high drama as history' phase prompted by the 1957 'Asian' flu. This was followed by a 'social science and ecology as history' stage as social and environmental histories presaged the social history of medicine movement. These were followed by a more recent 'scientific saga as history' which coincided with the SARS and bird flu outbreaks in east and south-east Asia. He also noted that the influenza pandemic is still largely overlooked in historical surveys or overviews of the twentieth century.

2 Crookshank later wrote a rather vitriolic attack on 'mongols' and degenerates titled *The Mongol in our Midst* (1931).

3 Charles Creighton was long considered to be one of Britain's most learned medical historians, but his views on Jennerian vaccination and the germ theory of infectious disease saw him ostracised by much of the medical profession.

4 As Chief Medical Officer of the Local Government Board (hereafter LGB), Newsholme was effectively the individual primarily responsible for public health (policy) in England and Wales. The LGB's health functions were assumed by the Ministry of Health on its creation in 1919.

5 Smith has discussed how during the 'Russian' flu of the 1890s the bacteriological view so readily merged with the 'centuries-old contexts of airs, waters and places' (1995: 62).

6 Examples of works recording wide assortments of micro-organisms include Carnwath 1919; Crookshank 1922; Cummins 1919; Donaldson 1922; Frost 1919; King 1922; Léon 1921; Levinthal *et al.* 1921; Lister and Taylor 1919; McIntosh 1922; Ministry of Health 1920c; Opie *et al.* 1921; Royal Society of Medicine 1918.

7 Van Helvoort discusses at some length the prevailing bacteriological paradigm, including Koch's postulates, and how this affected research into influenza (1993). Many of the issues surrounding the discovery (and earlier failure) are also discussed by Crosby in Chapter 13, 'Research, frustration and the isolation of the virus' (Crosby 1989: 264–94).

8 Some of Pfeiffer's more notable achievements were in bacteriology and immunology as he revealed the lifecycle of cocci, developed methods for immunising against typhus and cholera, and discovered endotoxins. He also discovered specific bacteria-dissolving immune bodies in cholera and typhus. In 1894 he found that live cholera vibrios could be injected without ill-effect into guinea pigs previously immunised against cholera, and that plasma from these animals added to live vibrio caused them to become motionless and to lyse, and that this could be inhibited by previously heating the serum. He termed this

process 'bacteriolysis' and it later became known as the Pfeiffer Phenomenon, or Isayev–Pfeiffer phenomenon. Pfeiffer also invented a universal staining for histological preparations.

9 Not all of these examples were quite so obsequious as Galli-Valerio's 1918 book, *L'Étiologie et la Prophylaxie de la Grippe ou Influenza*, with its dedication 'A Richard Pfeiffer dans le 60me anniversaire de sa naissance, 36me de la découverte du Bacterium influenzae', recognising Pfeiffer's sixtieth birthday and the thirty-sixth anniversary of his discovery of the bacillus.

10 Indeed, of the printed summary of this meeting, many of the pages recount these discussions. The discussants mentioning bacteriology and possible causative agents include Sir Arthur Newsholme (Chief Medical Officer to the LGB), General W.S. Thayer (MC, USA), Sir Kenneth Goadby, Dr Harold E. Whittingham, Major T.R. Little (CAMC), Captain Hallows (RAMC), Surgeon-Lieutenant G. Roche Lynch (RN), Major T.A. Malloch (CAMC), Captain J.G. Hopkins (MC, USA) and Professor John Eyre (Royal Society of Medicine 1918: 2, 31–2, 32–4, 34–6, 36–41, 41–3, 44, 45–50, 50–4 and 93–7 respectively).

11 Reports in *The Times* include 19 October 1918: 3; 28 October 1918: 7; 29 October 1918: 10; 31 October 1918: 7; 1 November 1918: 7; 2 November 1918: 7; 4 November 1918: 7; 12 November 1918: 5; 18 December 1918: 5; 7 February1919: 5; 14 February 1919: 5; 14 March 1919: 7; 11 April 1919: 10; 21 October 1919: 11 and 2 February 1921: 7. Similar stories can be found in the medical and general press all over the world. For example, the *Medical Journal of Australia*, having lauded the Australian Quarantine Service for 'the greatest triumph of its kind in the history of epidemiology' (30 November 1918: 455), in apparently stopping the passage of influenza into Australia, then spent much of the following year documenting the pandemic and its impact on Australia, including discussions of the causative agent, leading to the possibility of a 'filter-passing agent'. For example, 25 January 1919 was an 'Influenza Number' that was 'devoted almost entirely to the subject of the pandemic known as pneumonic influenza' where the editor also noted that 'the causal organism of the disease is in doubt' (p. 73). A 17 January 1920 'Retrospect' (pp. 59–63) noted the problems of causation, including that '[t]he frequency of the association of Bacillus influenzæ of Pfeiffer and the disease called influenza is said to have varied between 5% and 93% of the cases investigated' and that '[i]t is [now] generally recognised that the virus of the disease is still unknown' though some were claiming 'the discovery of a filter-passing virus in connexion with influenza' (p. 59).

12 Considered one of Australia's greatest scientists, Burnet's work as a virologist and physician led to many awards and honours, including the Nobel Prize in Physiology or Medicine in 1960 and a knighthood.

13 For example, personal correspondence with Professor John Oxford, Head of Academic Virology Department, St Bartholomew's and the Royal London School of Medicine and Dentistry, 13 October 1998.

14 There was, however, another 'side-effect' of the discovery of the influenza virus (and particularly that Pfeiffer's bacillus was *not* the cause). Pfeiffer's bacillus (later renamed *Haemophilus influenzae*), now better known as 'Hib', can cause various forms of infection, but is most feared for its role as an agent of meningitis. Once the influenza virus was isolated, attention swung away from Pfeiffer's bacillus and onto the newly-identified influenza virus. While this proper identification was a boon to influenza researchers, it also meant that 'Hib' was then little researched, being 'relegated to the footnotes of medical textbooks and dismissed as the microbe that did *not* cause flu' (Dixon 1994: 101). Consequently it was not until 1987 that a Hib vaccine was first introduced following somewhat belated research.

A more positive offshoot of influenza research was Alexander Fleming's vital discovery of penicillin as a direct, if accidental, consequence of his work on influenza. In attempting to find something to inhibit the growth of cocci, so as to allow the growth of pure cultures of Pfeiffer's bacillus, Fleming inadvertently left a number of culture plates containing staphylococci out, exposing them to open air and contamination. Shortly after he noticed the staphylococci around an 'uninvited colony of penicillium' mould had died. This mould was then found to kill all cocci while not affecting Pfeiffer's bacillus. Fleming's discovery led to his 'quiet little article . . . and the discovery of the most miraculous of all antibiotics' (quotes come from Crosby's account of Fleming's work (Crosby 1989: 273). Fleming's 'quiet little article' (Fleming 1929) was a follow-up to his 1919 article (Fleming 1919).

15 Much of this is based on personal conversations with Professor John Oxford, Head of Academic Virology Department, St Bartholomew's and the Royal London School of Medicine and Dentistry who was a leading member of the Spitzbergen expedition. A detailed account of the expedition has appeared more recently as one of the prime instigators and leaders of the expedition gave an unvarnished account of her experiences (Duncan 2003).

16 Papers presented at 'Influenza – Past, Present and Future: Genetics of Virulence and Pathogenicity' conference, London, 15–16 November 1999, in addition to Goto and Kawaoka 1998; Guan *et al.* 1997; Scholtissk *et al.* 1978.

17 Guillain–Barré Syndrome, also known as Guillain–Barré–Strohl syndrome, acute inflammatory demyelinating polyneuropathy, acute idiopathic polyradiculoneuritis, acute idiopathic polyneuritis and Landry's ascending paralysis, is a form of acquired neuropathy affecting both sexes, most frequently affecting young adults and believed to be a form of autoimmune disease with a delayed hypersensitivity reaction.

18 Professor Edwin Kilbourne in discussions at 'The Spanish 'Flu 1918–1998: Reflections on the Influenza Pandemic of 1918 after 80 Years' conference, University of Cape Town, September 1998.

19 One of the authors of the 1999 Plan discussed it and the role of the 1918–19 pandemic in shaping it in his presentation at the Cape Town conference in 1998 (Snacken *et al.* 1998). This Plan has subsequently been revised (WHO 2005c).

20 There has also been evidence found of direct transmission of avian H9 strains to humans (Guan *et al.* 1997; Peiris *et al.* 1999).

21 Winner of the 1958 Nobel Prize in Physiology or Medicine for his work in genetic structure and function in micro-organisms.

3 Pandemic geographies

1 And also in the history and literature of many other nations, including those colonies that sent so many of their people to fight for the 'mother country' or 'fatherland' on distant battlefields.

2 For example, *The Times*, 1 October 1918: 7; 3 October 1918: 7.

3 One of the earliest representations of the 'Spanish lady' was a cartoon in the German magazine *Simplicissimus* on 23 July 1918 (No 17: 205) where 'she' is pictured stalking past a weary-looking *Friedensengel* (angel of peace)

4 *Sherbrooke Daily Record*, 5 October 1918: 6, quoted in Rioux (1983).

5 However, lack of evidence is no evidence of absence of illness, especially with something as apparently commonplace as influenza, and this claim is regarded with pronounced scepticism.

6 Indeed, when the Ministry of Health came to update their *Memorandum on Influenza* in the late 1920s (Ministry of Health 1927), Sir George Buchanan wrote on a minute sheet attached to the various draft revisions that 'It is well to

remember the evidence that the 1918/19 epidemic came to us from the West' (PRO MH 55 57). This revision of the Memorandum, first issued in 1918 (Local Government Board 1918, 1919b), was driven by an epidemic in America and the fear that the disease could be brought from the West to England, as it was thought to have done so in 1918.

7 It was the specimens taken from Vaughan that allowed Jeffrey Taubenberger's team to first sequence the DNA of the virus (Taubenberger 1998; Taubenberger *et al.* 1997, 2000, 2001).

8 Also providing genetic samples for DNA sequencing by Taubenberger's team (Basler *et al.* 2001; Fanning *et al.* 2002; Larson 1998; Reid *et al.* 1999, 2000, 2001; Reid and Taubenberger 1999, 2003; Taubenberger 1998).

9 From whom samples were recovered for further sequencing work (Davis *et al.* 2000; Duncan 2003; Gladwell 1997).

10 Also reported in MacPherson *et al.* (1920).

11 Personal communications with Professor John Oxford, Head of Academic Virology, St Bartholomew's and Royal London School of Medicine and Dentistry. Also refer to Kobasa *et al.* 2004; Reid *et al.* 1999; Reid and Taubenberger 2003, Taubenberger *et al.* 2001.

12 Cushing is considered to be possibly the greatest neurosurgeon of the twentieth century and served as a war surgeon. These entries come from Cushing's published war-time journal. This quite long journal is notable for its lack of references to the influenza, despite it being recognised as having a major impact on the forces. However, unlike a number of other such journals, it does actually make some reference to the influenza.

13 The Norwegian data on the pandemic are unusually good as a comprehensive registration system had existed since 1801 and there was no disruption of the Norwegian demographic data collection (or the population) as a consequence of the war due to Norway's neutrality.

14 This pattern can be masked where the data plotted are monthly or quarterly due to the short duration of the waves of influenza. It is most clearly seen where daily or weekly data is plotted.

15 For further discussion of the application of models to influenza see Elveback *et al.* 1976; Fine 1982; Fortman 1976; Riordan 1986; Sattenspiel and Herring 1998; 2000; 2003; Selby 1982; Spicer and Lawrence 1984.

16 The New Zealand and consequent South Pacific events are investigated in Bryder 1982; Edwards 1986; Herda 1998; Rice 1988; Tomkins 1992b. The impact of the influenza in New Zealand and its 'responsibility' for its spread in the South Pacific led to the Australian government being asked to assist throughout the South Pacific (NAA files A1/15 1919/287; A2 1919/452; A2 1919/701; A2 1919/998; A457/1 501/5; CP78/22 1918/254; CP78/22 1919/224; CP78/22 1919/957; CP78/22 1921/53; CP103/11 432). This concern over influenza also led the Australians to monitor influenza activity in the South Pacific for some years after (NAA files A1/15 1925/6310; A2 1919/219; A2 1920/1006; A457/1 501/17; A457/1 501/40; A457/1 501/42; A457/1 I501/3).

17 'A Brief Report on Pandemic Influenza in Korea With Special Reference to its Etiology', by Frank W. Schofield and H.C. Cynn, of Union Medical College, Seoul, contained in PRO FD 1 F33 Medical Research Committee, Influenza General Research in UK.

18 The suggestion was made in a 19 February 1919 letter to the Australian Prime Minister from the Premier of Victoria. The Commonwealth authorities declined to implement such a system (NAA A2 1919/1328).

19 Burnet and Clark considered that the introduction of influenza into England was by way of troops returning from France. However, they suggested it may

have occurred in June 1918 (Burnet and Clark 1942: 70, citing Carnwath 1919).

20 These claims were supported by Carnwath (1919: 142–3).

21 For example, Canada (Johnson 1993) and South Africa (Phillips 1990a).

22 The 1911 Census notes the changes to the boundaries of a number of cities, including Manchester, Birmingham, Liverpool, Bath, Bury, Reading, Sheffield, Southport and Cambridge (1911 Census of England and Wales, Vol. I, Administrative Areas: xx).

23 Something Kearns (1988) suggested was generally no longer the case.

4 The human cost

1 William Sidney Thayer (1864–1932), awarded the Bright Medal in 1927, had research interests including the study of the circulatory system and blood in malaria, leukaemia and typhoid fever, and was Professor of Clinical Medicine at Johns Hopkins University, Baltimore.

2 This association of the influenza with black death was reflected in some of the names given to the pandemic. Furthermore, the nineteenth-century cholera epidemics had been noted for leaving victims blue, leading to the phrase 'a blue funk' and an understandable horror of diseases that could alter the colour of sufferers (Bourdelais and Raulot 1987).

3 The proportion of the total population that was under arms was 10.3 per cent in 1917 and 10.7 per cent in 1918 (source: *ARRG* 1917, 1918).

4 Data prior to 1911 is not easily comparable as 1911 saw changes in reporting areas and the disease definitions used.

5 For further detail, see Johnson 2004b; 2001: 235–45.

6 PRO MH 10 83, LGB letter (Item 227~18) accompanying the *Public Health (Acute Encephalitis Lethargica and Acute Polio-Encephalitis) Regulations, 1918* and *Report of an Enquiry into an Obscure Disease, Encephalitis Lethargica.*

7 PRO MH 113 51. It was noted in *Reports by the Delegate of Great Britain on the Sessions of the Committee of the Office International d'Hygiène Publique, Paris and of the Health Committee of the League of Nations* for May 1922, August 1922, February 1924 and May 1924. In 1922 there are separate discussions of influenza and encephalitis lethargica, whereas in 1924 they were discussed together in a single section of the report.

8 A connection between the two conditions was also made in Benussi *et al.* 1983.

9 Work by Professor John Oxford (Head of Academic Virology, St Bartholomew's and the Royal London Hospitals) and others attracted media interest, leading to a documentary on the encephalitis lethargica and its links to the influenza pandemic (BBC 1998).

10 *ARRG* 1920–1930. At other times it was included in omnibus categories of various forms.

11 Spink gave a figure of 21,642,283, which rather suggests an implausible degree of precision. Spink's tally recorded deaths in England and Wales as being only 112,239, whereas eighty years previously the Registrar-General had estimated mortality at 200,000 (Spink 1979: 215–16).

12 Particularly around the September 1998, *The Spanish 'Flu 1918–1998: Reflections on the Influenza Pandemic of 1918 after 80 Years* conference held at the University of Cape Town.

13 For further details on estimating global mortality, see Johnson and Mueller (2002).

14 Estimates for Second World War mortality can range from twenty to sixty million. The *Grolier Encyclopaedia* (online edition at http://gi.grolier.com/wwii/wwii_16.html. Accessed 6 March 2005) notes that total mortality has been

stated as twenty million. However, a figure of approximately sixty million can be tallied from the work of historians such as Lord Bullock (1993: 987), John Keegan (1989: 204–5) and Richard Overy (1998: 288).

15 As did those of many nations, including many colonial nations.

16 An argument put forward by Kendal and Glezen (1998), and reiterated by Kendal in personal and group discussions at *The Spanish 'Flu 1918–1998: Reflections on the Influenza Pandemic of 1918 after 80 Years* conference (Cape Town, 1998). That children can play a major role in the propagation of influenza and the possibility of vaccination in children in reducing or preventing influenza outbreaks has also been raised (Schoenbaum 2003: 246–8, 251).

17 Western Samoa lost more than 20 per cent of its population. Tomkins suggested that in all the Pacific islands struck, the mortality was at least 5 per cent of the total population (Tomkins 1992b: 181). A history of the London Missionary Society recounted how the 'violent epidemic' had 'swept away' so much of the Western Samoan native population, including many 'Christian pastors and leaders'. Of the 220 pastors the Society had or knew of, 103 had died and the Native Advisory Council, the leading body of the Samoan Church, had only one survivor from its thirty members. One of the missionaries wrote: 'Everything is chaotic. . . . I do not need to speak of our organisation, we have none. We have to begin all over again' (James 1923: 35). In New Zealand the Maori population endured an influenza death rate of 42.4 per 1,000 population while the pakeha (white) rate was 5.8 per 1,000 (Rice 1989).

18 The Inuit in Alaska and other parts of North America suffered terribly; whole villages were wiped out and others lost their entire adult population. Across the USA there was a terrible toll as 'American Indians suffered hideously in the pandemic . . . 24 per cent of reservation Indians caught flu . . . and the case mortality rate was 9 per cent, about four times as high as that in the nation's big cities. Two per cent of all American aborigines died' (Crosby 1989: 228). To the north the situation was at least as bad, as the disease 'hit the First Nations hard with nearly universal morbidity and shocking mortality rates especially as compared to non-Natives', with examples cited including a First Nations death rate in British Columbia of 46 per 1,000 population as opposed to a rate of 6.21 per 1,000 in the non-Native population, with some reserves reporting 100 per cent morbidity (Kelm 1998: 2). Elevated levels of mortality were found among many First Nations and Inuit peoples throughout Canada (Herring 1994; Herring and Sattenspiel 2003; Kelm 1998; Pettigrew 1983).

19 In England and Wales there were 2,285 deaths (Registrar-General 1920: 36) and 266 in Scotland (Registrar-General for Scotland 1919: 11).

20 The MOH reports cited are those for Leicester, South Shields, Warrington and Newcastle-on-Tyne (Ministry of Health 1920c: 445–55, 529–38, 539–55 and 556–63).

21 This is one of the few clear links between the influenza and the nascent Ministry of Health, nearly all of which built upon the sanitary argument.

22 For Newsholme's views, see Eyler (1992, 1997) and Hammer (1995). Hammer's work reveals the contrasts and tensions between Newsholme and George Newman who was to succeed him as the leading public official on public health.

23 Further analysis appears in Johnson 2001: 281–4, including scatterplots of epidemic mortality and each factor.

24 Residuals examined by residuals versus fit, residuals normal quantile–quantile and Cook's distance plots from linear regression of each variable against the annualised influenza mortality.

25 In this report only influenza mortality in the period 1921–23 was considered.

26 For example, Phillips found miners died in Kimberley, South Africa, at alarming rates. In the De Beers compounds there were high morbidity and mortality

rates and the 'mortality was far higher among underground workers (both Black and White) than among men who worked on the surface, indicating a greater susceptibility on their part or a more congenial environment for man-to-man infection underground' (Phillips 1990a: 52).

27 He gave his report this rather long-winded title: *A few notes on the epidemiology of the recent epidemic of 'influenza' among the workers in gas works, in a cordite factory, and in a tin mine – together with – A preliminary investigation into the germicidal power of gaseous fumes in those works of micro-organisms, and on the post-nasal flora of the workers and others.*

28 PRO FD 1 537, quotation is from Fletcher's 29 January 1919 letter to the Heads of various schools.

29 Including Repton School, Derby, King's School, Canterbury, Loreto, Musselbourgh, Trinity College, Perth, Lancing College, Worthing and the Leys School, Cambridge.

30 PRO FD 1 537, 31 January 1919 letter from Dr A.H. Penistan.

31 PRO FD 1 537, 6 February 1919 letter from Dr J. Tremlett Wills.

32 PRO FD 1 537, 26 January 1919 letter from Dr C. Perry.

33 PRO FD 1 537, report received by the MRC on 5 February 1919.

34 PRO FD 1 537, 2 February 1919 letter from H.G. Armstrong.

35 PRO FD 1 537, 30 January 1919 letter from Dr W.H. Bown, Medical Officer, Leys School, Cambridge.

36 S. Monckton Copeman, 'Report on Incidence of Influenza in the University and Borough of Cambridge, and in the Friends' School, Saffron Walden' (Ministry of Health 1920c: 388–440). This is a report by the Cambridge MOH published in the Ministry of Health's 1920 report on the pandemic. Discussion of King's College School appears on pages 400–1.

37 S. Monckton Copeman, 'Report on Incidence of Influenza in the University and Borough of Cambridge, and in the Friends' School, Saffron Walden' (Ministry of Health 1920c: 388–440). These school figures appear on pages 398 and 439–40.

38 S. Monckton Copeman, 'Report on Incidence of Influenza in the University and Borough of Cambridge, and in the Friends' School, Saffron Walden' (Ministry of Health 1920c: 388–440). Discussion of the epidemic in the university and colleges appears on pages 388–94 and 414–39. This also includes discussion of the epidemic among the military contingents that were occupying some of the colleges.

39 Nor was this a new phenomenon. Creighton had discussed the tragic history of influenza outbreaks onboard ships. These tales illustrate how contagious the disease is and how much it depends on human-to-human transmission, as do the story of St Kilda and most of the section 'The Influenzas of Remote Islands' (Creighton 1965: 425–31).

40 Examples of shipping being identified as importing the disease include India (Gill 1928), western Africa (Mueller 1995), South Africa (Phillips 1990a), Argentina (*The Times* 1 November 1918: 7), Canada (Johnson 1993; Pettigrew 1983) Australia, New Zealand and other parts of Oceania (McQueen 1976; Rice 1988; Thomas 1998 and National Archives of Australia files A457/1 501/17; A457/1 501/19; A1/15 1919/287; A6006 1919/1/9, 1919/2/3; A2 1919/452, A2 1919/482 Part 2, A2 1919 701, A2 1919 742, A2 1919 887 Part 2, and A2 1919/952. In other instances, for example Portugal, the railways have been cited (Echeverri 2003). Many of these works also illustrate the role of national transport networks in dispersing influenza across the country.

41 Examples of individual cases of influenza and pneumonia in the services include the following PRO files: PIN 26 7921; PIN 26 15039; PIN 26 22103; PIN 26 20251. The records of the 85th General Hospital (PRO MH 106 2384) also contain many cases, often fatal.

42 Other similar recollections include Bourne 1963; Bryson 1966; Cushing 1936; Hagmeier 1981; Henrikson 1956; Hyam 1963; Millard 1936; Morton 1973; Wauchope 1963; Weymouth 1936.

5 Impacts and responses

1 It was also proclaimed as a notifiable disease in South Africa (NASA files URU 378 2468, URU 378 2468A, URU 378 2469 and URU 393 479) and in various states of Australia (NAA files A2 1919/482; A2 1919/742; A2 1919/953 Part 2; A2 1919/993; A2 1919/1319; A2 1919/1664; A2 1919/2959).

2 The Ministry's Circular 1499 described the change in thinking which had 'recently been revised in the light of present-day knowledge'. The accompanying memorandum (*Memorandum on Pneumonia*, Memo 189, 1935) placed emphasis on pneumonia, with influenza reverting to a lower level of consideration (PRO files MH 10 83, MH 10 84 and Wellcome CMAC file SA/BMA Box 210 F.75).

3 In comparing the experiences of Japan and New Zealand, Rice claimed that 'just over one third of the total population' of Japan were infected and in New Zealand there was an 'estimated 40 per cent morbidity'. However, Rice notes that this estimate 'was only a guess and masked considerable variation' across New Zealand with some towns reporting estimates as low as 10 per cent, while the North Island towns of Inglewood and Taumarunui reported 60 and 80 per cent infected, and Southland reporting 90 per cent (Rice 1998: 15). Mueller reported similar variation in Kenya, 30–90 per cent (Mueller 1995: 10), and Kelm claims up to 100 per cent of some First Nations communities in Canada were infected (Kelm 1998: 2). In another Canadian community with very few (if any) natives, overall morbidity was estimated in excess of 53 per cent, while some businesses in that city reported 95 per cent absenteeism (Johnson 1993: 127). Similar ranges, generally from 25 per cent and up to entire populations, can be found in much of the pandemic literature.

4 Reports of all these events can be found in most newspapers of the period, for example *The Times* 21 October 1918: 5; 22 October 1918: 3; 23 October 1918: 3; 24 October 1918: 3; 25 October 1918: 3; 28 October 1918: 3; 31 October 1918: 7; 1 November 1918: 7; 7 November 1918: 3; 27 November 1918: 5; 29 November 1918: 3; 4 December 1918: 3. Wilshere described the disruption experienced in Leicester (Wilshere 1986).

5 CMAC SA/HVA Box 78 F.1/7 Chelsea Health Society and School for Mothers, *Eighth Annual Report for the year ended March 31st, 1919*.

6 Dyhouse discussed Wauchope's experiences as one of the first women who gained a medical education in Britain (Dyhouse 1998).

7 Westminster was one of the last of the London boroughs to show an increase in influenza mortality.

8 Examples of these debates can be found in much of the literature on the pandemic in the USA, Canada, Australia and South Africa.

9 For example, the Manchester MOH, James Niven, promoted their use, as did a number of commentators in the press (van Hartesveldt 1992). *The Times* repeatedly advised the wearing of masks: 1 November 1918: 5; 11 December 1918: 5; 19 December 1918: 5; 30 January 1919: 5; 31 January 1919: 5; 22 February 1919: 10; 1 March 1919: 7.

10 Durey's discussion of the 1832 cholera epidemic examined the 'cholera riots' that had included attacks on doctors and hospitals. Durey relates the unrest to the prevailing social and political contexts. While disavowing the belief that the cholera riots were closely linked to the passing of the Reform Bill, he suggests

that they had much to do with a perception that doctors were using the cholera as a cover under which to kill the poor, particularly for medical purposes. He argued that while there is 'no clear evidence for class antagonism . . . most eruptions were narrowly focused on antagonism towards the medical profession.' This is understandable in a context were the poor feared the medical profession for practices such as 'Burking' (from Burke and Hare's procuring of bodies for medical examination and education). The 1918–19 influenza pandemic occurred in a greatly altered context, one in which the medical profession was far better regarded and far more secure (Durey 1979, particularly chapters 7 and 8. Quotation taken from page 3).

11 The Pacific Islands spared included the Solomon Islands, Papua New Guinea, Norfolk Island, Gilbert and Ellice Islands (now Kiribati and Tuvalu respectively) and New Caledonia (Burnet and Clark 1942: 74; Collier 1974: 174–5; Graves 1969: 160).

12 The French and British Resident Commissioners for the New Hebrides (now Vanuatu), Nielly and King, did promulgate quarantine (Condominium of the New Hebrides 1919).

13 For documentation on Australia's concerns and actions with regard to influenza, quarantine and other Pacific islands see NAA files A1/15 1919/287; A1/15 1925/6310; A2 1918/3705; A2 1919/219; A2 1919/224; A2 1919/452; A2 1919/701; A2 1919/957; A2 1919/998; A457/1 501/5; A457/1 501/17; A457/1 G501/6; A457/1 I501/3; A457/1 501/40; A457/1 501/42; A8510/1 68/24A; CP78/22 1918/254; CP78/22 1919/224; CP78/22 1919/957; CP78/22 1921/53; CP103/11 432.

14 For primary documentation on Australian quarantine and the spread of the disease, refer to NAA files A1/15 1919/2364; A2 1919/482 Part 2; A2 1919/742; A2 1919/887 Part 2; A2 1919/953 Part 1; A2 1919/953 Part 2; A2 1919/964; A2 1919/965; A2 1919/967; A2 1919/971; A2 1919/993; A2 1919/1182; A2 1919/1302; A2 1919/1311; A2 1919/1319; A2 1919/1657; A2 1919/1658; A2 1919/1659; A2 1919/1661; A2 1919/1664; A2 1919/1922; A2 1919/2959; A199 FCL1919/238; A361 DSG19/1582; A361 DSG20/82; A361 DSG21/52; A457/1 501/20; A457/1 501/53; A457/1 C501/3; A2487 1919/2104; A6006 1919/1/9; A6006 1919/2/3; A6006 1919/12/31; CP103/11 404; CP103/11 407; CP103/11 411; CP103/11 413; CP103/11 424; CP103/11 430. Also see NAA files held at the PROV MP472/1 19/19/3740; MP367/1 527/21/493; MP367/1 612/32/332; MP367/1 556/16/84. See SRNSWs file 4/6247 Premier's Department – influenza epidemic; 8/2035.8 Quarantine – influenza; 5/5348.1 Health – Pneumonic influenza; 6/4461 Health – Minutes 1917–1921 and SLV manuscript MSB422 for further documents and images of quarantine camps. Quarantine, especially interstate quarantine, became a widely debated subject, frequently mentioned in the various Parliaments around Australia (also see Hyslop 1994, 1998a, 1998b).

15 *Full Text Citations For Award of The Navy Cross For World War 1 – Era Actions*, Available from: www.homeofheroes.com/verify/1_Citations/nc_03era_miscelaneous.html (Accessed 1 April 2005).

16 *Report by the Delegate of Great Britain on the Autumn Session of the Committee of the Office International d'Hygiène Publique, Paris 1919*: 7 (Epidemic Influenza – Inquiry as to the Epidemics of 1918–19 and Replies to the Questionnaire which has been sent out by the Office International).

17 Gill's argument is rather undermined by the fact that so many other southern-hemisphere countries, including New Zealand, South Africa and Argentina, often with similar climates, did endure the pandemic in 1918–19 and did not show the climatically determined timing he suggests. Furthermore, his selection of Adelaide as his major example is unfortunate as Adelaide exhibited the same

pattern as the rest of the country, although the city's climate is recognised as being of a 'Mediterranean' type and quite different from elsewhere in the country, except for the far south-western corner of Western Australia.

18 See PRO MH 55 57 for the creation of this Memorandum. Quarantine was also considered in the re-framing of the powers of the Port Sanitary Authorities in 1919–20. An issue that arose there was the use of the phrase 'any endemic, epidemic or infectious disease'. This was specifically questioned as, while the intention was the 'prevention of the importation of dangerous diseases such as smallpox, typhus, &c.' such wording would allow for the removal 'to hospital any person on a ship . . . suffering from influenza'. The implicit assumption was that influenza was not an important disease yet these words were written less than a year after the peak of the third wave of the pandemic in Britain (PRO MH 58 418. Quotations from 3 February 1920 minute from Mr Maclachlan to Mr Gwyer). A year earlier, another Ministry of Health officer had noted newspaper advocacy of 'the application of quarantine to all ships arriving with cases of influenza' but suggested that quarantine was 'impracticable' and that it was 'desirable to retain the power of dealing with influenza on board ship', thus absolving the on-shore authorities of responsibility (PRO MH 58 418. 9 February 1919 minute from Mr Reece to Mr MacLachlan). The published Regulations eventually carried a definition referring to 'any epidemic or acute infectious disease' (*The Port Sanitary Authorities (Infectious Diseases) Regulations, 1920*).

19 City of Kitchener, Board of Health minutes, 7 October 1918.

20 Living in the New South Wales town of Queanbeyan, the mail coach driver met the Sydney trains and conveyed passengers and mail across the state-territory border from Queanbeyan to Canberra (NAA A192 FCL1921/295).

21 There are many NAA files documenting the scale of the concern (and debates) around national and interstate quarantine, including A2 1919/452; A2 1919/482 Part 1; A2 1919/482 Part 2; A2 1919/742; A2 1919/887 Part 2; A2 1919/953 Part 1; A2 1919/953 Part 2; A2 1919/971; A2 1919/993; A2 1919/1182; A2 1919/1302; A2 1919/1311; A2 1919/1319; A2 1919/1601/4; A2 1919/1657; A2 1919/1658; A2 1919/1659; A2 1919/1661; A2 1919/1922; A2 1919/2959; A457/1 C501/3; A457/1 501/20; A6006 1919/2/3; A6006 1919/12/31. The dispute was also continued in the report on the pandemic to the New South Wales Parliament (New South Wales 1920: 161–2). Quarantine was also often raised in the *Medical Journal of Australia* throughout the pandemic period.

22 The roles and actions of the various levels of government are discussed in Tomkins (1989, 1992a) and Tanner (2002). For examples of the debate in the press, see *The Times* 1 November 1918: 7; 11 December 1918: 5; 19 December 1918: 5; 30 January 1919: 5; 31 January 1919: 5; 22 February 1919: 10; and 1 March 1919: 7.

23 In 1922, Crookshank contributed chapters to and edited *Influenza: Essays by Several Authors* (Crookshank 1922).

24 For example, see reports in *The Times* 25 October 1918: 3; 26 October 1918: 7; 28 October 1918: 3; 31 October 1918: 7; 1 November 1918: 7.

25 20 November 1918 letter to local authorities accompanying copies of the *Public Health (Influenza) Regulations, 1918*. Reported in *The Times*, 21 November 1918: 3.

26 22 November 1918 letter to local authorities accompanying copies of the *Public Health (Influenza) Regulations (No. 2), 1918*. Reported in *The Times*, 27 November 1918: 5.

27 Examples from *The Times* include 8 November 1918: 3 and 3 February 1919: 5.

28 By the 1927 revision of the *Memorandum on Influenza*, these restrictions were being considered rather ambiguously. That version of the Memorandum, while

specifically drawing attention to 'public places of entertainment' and their role as 'important foci for the spread of disease', noted that the 1918 'emergency regulations' were 'admittedly incomplete' (PRO MH 55 57; Ministry of Health 1927: 12).

29 Member of the House of Representatives, the lower house of the Australian Parliament. Kelly represented the Sydney seat of Wentworth from 16 December 1903 until his retirement on 3 November 1919.

30 Reports of school closures came in all three waves of the pandemic. For example, *The Times* carried reports of school closures as early as 26 June 1918 and throughout July, and from mid-October to early 1919 there was at least one report on school closures every week.

31 In Vancouver, for example, the schools were initially kept open as the city's medical health officer, Dr F.T. Underhill, believed that closing the schools

> would be positively harmful to the health of children who, with schools closed, would be removed from the close surveillance of teachers and school medical staff on guard for influenza symptoms, and would instead be free to roam the streets, exposing themselves to various sources of infection and neglecting early signs of the disease.
>
> (Andrews 1977: 30)

The Cape Education Department in South Africa also believed that the closure of schools was 'highly objectionable from the public health point of view, as it tends to prevent the supervision of school-going children' and made little sense unless other places of assembly were also closed and children kept in the home. They also suggested that it was a waste of money and educational resources, disrupted life unduly and would cause panic and worry (Phillips 1990a: 213, 246).

32 Hamer's views, and those of the Board of Education and the LGB, were echoed in the Ministry of Health's 1927 revision of the *Memorandum on Influenza* in which the issue of school closures was again discussed. The opinion expressed then was that it is a measure that 'may sometimes be employed with advantage', especially outside urban areas where the 'excluded children have few opportunities of coming in contact with each other outside' school. The Memorandum also notes that where 'day schools' are closed, then the same should apply to Sunday schools. Other elements of the 1918 advice that were repeated were the exclusion of sick children, but here it was also suggested that children so excluded should not be re-admitted before 'a careful medical examination of the heart and lungs has been made to eliminate possible latent complications and sequelæ' (PRO MH 55 57; Ministry of Health 1927: 12).

33 This is a feature common to many of the local and national histories written on the pandemic. Works that touch on the volunteer efforts and the published local and national histories include Adamo 1992; Arrington 1990; Baird 1976; Belyk and Belyk 1988; Borza 2001; Brito 1997; Bryder 1982; Buelow 1992; Cavina 1959; Clark 1991; Crosby 1977, 2003; Daniel and Gerstner 1991; de Gooyer 1968; Decker 1996; Doherty 1977; English 1986; Ensley 1983; Fanning 1995; Fatovic Ferencic and Sain 1991; Fee *et al.* 2001; Figura 1998; Fritz 1992; Garner 1921; Gavrilovic 1995; Gear 1983; Gernhart 1999; Guillaume 1978; Hamilton 1992; Hildreth 1992; Hoehling 1961; Irwin 1981; Johnson 1993, 2003; Kass 1993; Katz 1974, 1977; Katzenellenbogen 1988; King 1992; Kirkpatrick 1986; Knibbs 1920; Koblenz 1998; Langford and Storey 1992; Lautaret 1971; Linnanmäki 2000; Luckingham 1984a, 1984b; McConnell 2000; McCreery 1992; McFadden *et al.* 2001; McGinnis 1976, 1977; McPherson 1990; McShane 1968; Melzer 1982; Mullen and Nelson 1987; Müller 1996; Niven 1923; Noll 1989; Noyes 1968; Olm 1998; Palmer and Rice 1992; Pankhurst 1989; Peterson 1992; Pettigrew 1983; Phillips 1990a; Porras Gallo

1994a, 1994b, 1996, 1997; Puklin 1992; Quincy 2002; Ramanna 1998; Reddi 1998; Rice 1979, 1983, 1985, 1988; Rockafeller 1986; Rodies 1998; Sanford 1983; Schoch Spana 2001; Scott 1988; Smallman-Raynor *et al.* 2002; Spears 1979; Thalman 1968; Tomkins 1989; van Hartesveldt 1992; Vasold 1996, 1998; Wakimura 1998; Weiler 1988; White 1985; Wilshere 1986.

34 Sir Auckland Geddes (1879–1954) trained as a surgeon but spent much of his career in public service. After active service in South Africa, he was Assistant Professor of Anatomy, Edinburgh University (1906–09), Professor of Anatomy, Royal College of Surgeons in Ireland (1909–13), and Professor of Anatomy, McGill University, Canada. Geddes was a Major in the 17th Northumberland Fusiliers (1914–15) and then Director of Recruiting at the War Office (1916–17) before serving as MP for Basingstoke (1917–20), as well as Director General and Minister for National Service (1917–19). During 1918–19, he was President of the Local Government Board before being Minister of Reconstruction (1919), President of the Board of Trade (1919–20) and the British Delegate in Washington to the Conference on Limitation of Armaments (1917–20) before his appointment as Ambassador Extraordinaire and Minister Plenipotentiary to the USA (1920–24). He was also Chairman of the Rio Tinto Company (1924–47) and the Rhokana Corporation.

35 The Victorian notice lists draconian penalties for not notifying authorities of cases whereas such compunction was not present in the UK (or even considered).

36 Also see NAA files (held at the PROV) MP367/1 612/32/332; MP367/1 527/21/1272; and MP367/1 556/49/714.

37 Documentation, including volumes of completed 'Influenza Epidemic Distress Relief' forms along with receipt books, etc. can be found in the PROV files 8291/P/0001 INFLUENZA; 3183/P/0000 (boxes 000050, 000051 and 000052).

38 New South Wales Parliamentary Debates, Session 1919, 10 George V, Second Series, Vol. 75: 89–90.

39 Reports come from PRO MAF 60 307; MH 79 7; NATS 1 797 and NATS 1 849 and *The Times* 23 October 1918: 3; 25 October 1918: 3; 29 October 1918: 10; 30 October 1918: 7, 8; 10 December 1918: 5; 17 December 1918: 5.

40 Chief Medical Officer of the Ministry of Health from its outset (1919) until 1935.

41 Such enquiries were established in South Africa (Union of South Africa 1919), New Zealand (1919) and New South Wales (1920).

42 For example, Löwy has argued that before action, particularly public action, could be deployed to combat yellow fever in Brazil, the visualisation of the disease/problem was essential (Löwy 1998).

43 Newsholme's career took in the New Poor Laws, the changing medical functions of the LGB and ceased as his role was taken over by George Newman shortly before the LGB was supplanted by the Ministry of Health, where Newman assumed the same role.

44 For example, *The Times* 24 February 1919: 10.

45 The entries on October 29 and 30 about meetings with Newsholme and then the President of the LGB about influenza are the only references to influenza in Newman's diaries for 1918 and 1919. However, it seems possible he himself may have suffered as he wrote 'Sept. 26. Bad cold –29' which may suggest he had a case of 'three-day fever' (the term British troops used for the influenza).

46 Cabinet committee endorsed the principle of a Ministry in June 1917, and it was discussed by Cabinet in January 1918, but the Bill was not passed until June 1919 and the Ministry established in July 1919 (Hammer 1995: Chapter 6; Honigsbaum 1970). However, the early years of the Ministry under Newman did not live up to his or the country's expectations (Hammer 1995: Chapter 7).

47 Honigsbaum also considers Newsholme to have failed in his handling of the pandemic (Honigsbaum 1970: 51).

48 Descriptions of the activities undertaken by MOHs can be found in Tomkins (1989, 1992a) and van Hartesveldt (1992).

49 For discussion of the bacteriological paradigm and its impact on the discovery of the virus, see Hildreth (1991), van Helvoort (1993), and Witte (1998).

50 This seems to be the suggestion in South Africa, where the authorities had not enacted a quarantine as they felt it was not practicable, they did not have the powers to do so, and also because the first cases had apparently come from Sierra Leone – they

> believed that Sierra Leoneans were particularly vulnerable to diseases such as influenza as they were 'physically the worst type of native, very subjected to Malaria and Pneumonia'. Surely the 'flu which had come from there would remain as mild as the first cases which had appeared in South Africa?
>
> (Phillips 1990a: 103)

51 Quotation is from 2 December 1918 letter from Fletcher to Major Gibson. Further documentation on influenza research activity is contained in PRO files FD 1 530, FD 1 532; FD 1 534; FD 1 535; FD 1 536; FD 1 545; FD 1 553; and FD 1 554.

52 Quotation is from 17 February 1919 letter from Fletcher to S.L. Cummins. Gibson co-authored parts of Cummins (1919), including *The Etiology of Influenza. A Filtrable Virus as the Cause, with some Notes on the Culture of the Virus by the Method of Noguchi and The Bacteriological Flora of the Respiratory Tract in Cases of Influenza.*

53 Mill Hill has also housed the specimens recovered from the Spitzbergen exhumations (BBC 1999b; Davis *et al.* 2000; Duncan 2003; Gladwell 1997; Oxford *et al.* 1999)

54 Quotation is from 6 December 1918 letter from Fletcher to Cummins.

55 The Royal Society of Medicine 'Discussion' (1918) heard varying views on vaccines from Newsholme (12), Dr W.E. Carnegie Dickson (78–83), Surgeon Captain P.W. Bassett-Smith (83–4), Sir Humphrey Rolleson, the RSM President (84) and Mr E.B. Turner (87–90). Equally divergent reports were carried in *The Times*, including 22 October 1918: 3; 31 October 1918: 7; 4 November 1918: 5 (reporting the LGB vaccine); 5 November 1918: 6; 9 November 1918: 3; 12 November 1918: 5; 24 December 1918: 5; 20 February 1919: 5; 22 February 1919: 10; 1 March 1919: 7; and 14 March 1919: 7. Newspaper reports on vaccine seem to correspond to peaks in mortality (November 1918 and February 1919). Newman encouraged vaccines in his Ministry of Health publications (Ministry of Health 1919a, 1920a). Also see PRO FD 1 529; FD 1 535.

56 Reports and correspondence on the supply and return of medical personnel come from PRO MH 49 7; MH 65 51; MH 65 60; MH 79 7; NATS 1 797 and NATS 1 849; *The Times* 23 October 1918: 3; 25 October 1918: 3; 29 October 1918: 10; 30 October 1918: 7, 8; 10 December 1918: 5; 17 December 1918: 5; the *Western Morning News* 30 October 1918; *Glasgow Herald* 30 October 1918.

57 For example, the records of Prime Ministers, Governors-General and the Cabinets of South Africa and Australia include many references to the pandemic.

58 Cases where doctors failed to attend include M. 18/73, M. 18/75, M. 19/12, M. 19/17, M. 19/18, M. 19/19, M. 19/22, M. 19/37 and M. 19/40. Cases of misdiagnosis: M. 19/2, M. 19/3, M. 19/5, M. 19/26 and M. 19/47. Cases where pharmacists would not dispense the required material: P. 19/2, P. 19/4. Such cases appear throughout the volume as they were heard throughout 1919.

59 As Galishoff noted in the USA where the 'pattern was the same in nearly every major city: one or two weeks of rapid spread followed by two or three weeks of

high morbidity and mortality, whereafter the epidemic rapidly subsided' (Galishoff 1969: 249).

60 Similar reactions can be found in Musambachimc (1998), Phillips (1988, 1990a) and Ranger (1988, 1992). Watts also noted that the pandemic was an 'example of a disease crisis which in most polities elicited little novel medical or political response . . . However in recently British-colonized Yoruba land in the Nigeria regions, the death of 250,000 people from influenza led to the establishment of locally managed Aladura faith-healing churches' (Watts 1997: 282 fn 10).

6 Cultural dimensions

1 For example, regarding China as the source of bubonic plague, as in Sydney, Australia, where the Chinese community was held responsible (Curson and McCracken 1989).

2 For example, over the centuries the French and English adopted names for sexually transmitted diseases that implicated and blamed the other.

3 The Tuskegee Syphilis Study was started as a study into the effectiveness of treatments considered harmful and ineffective and to show that non-treatment was less harmful. During the study, penicillin had been recognised as an effective and safe treatment but the Tuskegee patients, mostly poor, illiterate African-Americans, were allowed to sicken and die for many years, with some prevented from accessing effective treatments. This 'experiment' is considered one of the greatest failures of American medical ethics, and was the subject of a presidential apology to the survivors and their relatives decades after the fact.

4 One of the '4 Hs' risk categories (heroin-users, homosexual, haemophiliac and Haitian).

5 Rather than Haiti being the source of HIV/AIDS, it was North Americans or Haitians returning from North America that in all likelihood brought the condition to Haiti. Contaminated blood and sexual transmission account for the great proportion of early cases in Haiti.

6 Personal communications. See also Echeverri (2003).

7 Article by 'Craftman' 'Occasion'd by an Article of News from Rome of a contagious Distemper raging there, call'd the Influenza', *The London Magazine: and Monthly Chronologer*, 26 March, No. 874: 145. A copy is held by the University of Cambridge university library.

8 Wellcome Library for the History and Understanding of Medicine, CMAC, GC/21 Hood, Volume 1.

9 This downplaying of the disease was found in many places. Belyk and Belyk found it in the Vancouver press where the emphasis was on reporting the disease only as experienced elsewhere, a similar approach to that of *The Times* in London. In Vancouver, as the situation grew more serious the newspapers

> appeared more concerned with preventing public panic, than keeping their readers informed. No matter how terrible the situation, no matter how many residents had fallen with the flu or died from pneumonia, local newspapers seemed able to find some spot where the situation was worse. And when it was difficult to convince their readership it was worse elsewhere, newspapers refrained from telling the entire story.

The most extreme example Belyk and Belyk cite is of the *Free Press* in Nanaimo, British Columbia, that, once mortality started to 'spiral upward', simply stopped printing any figures (Belyk and Belyk 1988).

10 Reports from Tangiers that included extensive discussion of the pandemic appeared over several weeks. These included *The Times* 8 October 1918: 7; 12

October 1918: 5; 14 October 1918: 7; 15 October 1918: 7; 22 October 1918: 5; 23 October 1918: 7; 29 October 1918: 5; 1 November 1918: 5.

11 Just such an effect was seen in parts of Africa in 1919 and 1920 when 'a recrudescence of the Spanish Influenza appeared in some regions, a panic reaction was recorded in some areas that had been hard hit by the second wave' (Mueller 1995: 2).

12 In Senegal indigenous peoples were given rum or wine while the French were prescribed champagne (Echenberg 2003: 234).

13 PRO FD 1 537 Medical Research Committee – Influenza – Schools reports on cases and treatments of, 17 November 1918 letter. Repeated by Fletcher in a 13 February 1919 letter when he noted that 'This powder can hardly be germicidal' (PRO FD 1 531).

14 Many medical professionals reported feeling helpless in dealing with the influenza as the pandemic brought the 'medical profession face to face with the limitations of its own skills and knowledge' (Phillips 1990a: 133. See also 118–19). Other works on the powerlessness of the medical professions include Bristow 1998; Gribble 1997; Hagmeier 1981; Millard 1936; Sage 1995, 1998.

15 Examples include the two anonymous authors who produced *Colds, Catarrh and Influenza (By A Civil Service Doctor)* in 1934 and *How to Escape Colds and Influenza* in 1937.

16 Held in the British Library, neither the letter nor the British Library catalogue indicate to whom this was sent.

17 Certainly in October and November 1918 *The Times* regularly published a notice reading, 'Owing to the continued shortage of paper The Times cannot insert advertisements in large type, or with large illustrations, which would encroach upon the daily quantity of space devoted to public intelligence.' Examples include 31 October 1918: 7; 1 November 1918: 7.

18 The data comes from the pharmacy registers from Savory & Moore, Dispensing Chemists, Chapel Street, Belgravia SW1. These registers are held at the Wellcome Library for the History and Understanding of Medicine: CMAC GC/16 2 94 and GC/16 5 93 Savory & Moore.

19 PRO MH 65 3 Ministry Health, National Health: Insurance Committee for the County of London, London Executive Council, Agenda, April report: 9. Identification of the pharmacy comes from PRO MH 65 91 Ministry Health, National Health: Insurance Committee for the County of London, Pharmaceutical Service Sub-Committee, Minutes.

20 Emma Simone, personal communications, March–April 2005.

21 Examples include Anonymous, *A Doctor's Diary* 1925; Bourne 1963; Bryson 1966; Cushing 1936; Fletcher 1957; Heiser 1936; Henrikson 1956, 1959; Hyam 1963; Mackie 1949; Millard 1936; Schofield 1928; Wauchope 1963; Weymouth 1936.

22 Wellcome Library for the History and Understanding of Medicine, CMAC, GC/21 Hood, Volume 1.

23 Kathleen Clarke was married to Tom Clarke, who was the first signatory of the Easter 1916 Proclamation. Tom Clarke and Ned Daly, Kathleen's brother, were both executed after the Easter Uprising.

24 Ace Johnson, *Influenza* (Washington, DC: Library of Congress, 1939). Recording made by John and Ruby Lomax at Clemens State Farm, Brazoria, Brazoria County, Texas, for the Library of Congress.

25 Personal communication with Dr Stuart Corbridge, University of Cambridge, 1997.

26 Veterans Affairs Canada, *John McCrae*, www.vac-acc.gc.ca/general/sub.cfm?source=history/firstwar/mccrae (accessed 8 April 2005).

27 A fact made all the more stark when compared with the situation in the official records of other countries, for example, Australia and South Africa.

7 Repercussions

1 The point has been contested, for example Harris (1993).
2 The calculation is simply multiplying the number of women who died in each age group (divided by 1,000) by the fertility rate (per 1,000) for that age group and then adding all the age groups to give total averted births. This has been done using the three different sets of fertility rates, thus giving three possible averted births figures (Table 7.3).
3 However, it has been noted that the 'absence of any systematic investigation of the connection between the influenza pandemic of 1918–19 and World War I' is one of the more unexpected aspects of recent historiography that has otherwise seen the pandemic come back into the purview of academic historians (Phillips 2004: 131).
4 From his poem, 'The Children'.
5 The mass movements of people after the war, particularly the refugee movements in eastern Europe, and concerns about disease played a significant role in the development of the League of Nations' health activities (Metzger 2001; Steiner 2005; Weindling 1995).
6 Wilson announced to the US Congress what he considered the basic premises for a just and lasting peace. The Fourteen Points included basic principles such as freedom of the seas and open covenants, a variety of geographic arrangements carrying out the principle of self-determination, and a League of Nations that would enforce the peace (Link 1984: xlv, 534–9).
7 Commonwealth of Australia, Department of Health and Ageing, *1920–1929 The Early Years*. Available at: www.health.gov.au/pdf/fact2.pdf (accessed 15 April 2005).
8 For example, *The Times* 15 July 1918: 3; 28 October 1918: 7; 29 October 19: 7; 30 October 1918: 7; 2 November 1918: 7; 4 November 1918: 7, 11; 7 November 1918: 3; 19 December 1918: 5; 24 December 1918: 3; 19 February 1919: 8; 25 February 1919: 7.
9 This flow of information is evident in various archives, including the National Archive of South Africa (NASA files GG 1232 33/1014; GG 1232 33/1036; GG 1232 33/1051; GG 1232 33/1064; GG 1232 33/1068; GG 1232 33/1079; and GG 1232 33/1082A) and the National Archives of Australia (NAA files A2 1919/452; A2 1919/482 Part 2; A2 1919/952; A6006 1919/12/31; and CP78/22 1921/53).
10 The seat of the Australian federal government at the time.
11 NASA files GG 232 33/1073A; VWN 3637 PG291; VWN 3637 PG292; VWN 3700 PG384.
12 For example, Australia not only contacted the UK for information on the pandemic (receiving the LGB memoranda) (NAA A2 1919/966), but they also instructed their representatives in the USA to investigate New York's responses and American vaccines (NAA A2 1919/1663). For Australia, moving away from a British influence to fall under that of the USA was to be a continuing trend, possibly peaking in Australia's participation in the Vietnam war (a conflict that the British and other Commonwealth nations largely remained apart from) and then the Gulf wars, including active participation in Afghanistan and Iraq.
13 This flow of information around the Pacific may have been facilitated by a personal network among the various Governors. For example, the New South Wales Governor informed the Australian Governor-General that the reason the

Governor of Fiji had communicated to him in both public and personal channels was due to previous personal contact in South Africa (NAA file CP78/22 1918/254).

14 These monthly mailings could be regarded as the predecessors of the WHO's *WER* (*Weekly Epidemiological Record*) that are available via email or from the World Wide Web at www.who.int/wer.

15 The FluNet website is www.who.int.

8 Possible futures

1 The British pandemic plan includes plans to stockpile sufficient anti-virals to treat 14.6 million people (Meikle 2005). The same report suggested that at least 50,000 Britons would die, with 80,000 requiring hospitalisation and that the UK might also impose travel restrictions, voluntary quarantine, school closures and the postponing of many hospital procedures in the event of a pandemic. In April 2005 the Australian Minister for Health claimed Australia was the nation with largest stockpile of anti-viral drugs on a per capita basis (*Sun-Herald*, Sydney, 15 April 2005) but Canada has also been buying anti-virals to cover a quarter of the population, as has the UK (BBC 2005b). Similarly, the USA, Germany, Japan and the Netherlands have been purchasing anti-virals, while Italy and France were placing orders for millions of doses of vaccine, as had the USA (BBC 2005a, 2005b).

2 Some of the national pandemic plans (and their precursors) are available from the WHO website at: www.who.int/csr/disease/influenza/nationalpandemic/en/index.html.

3 It has been argued that the scientific knowledge technology exists to achieve this goal, but that 'manufacturing, intellectual property, and liability issues remain unresolved' and that in the event of a pandemic, 'reverse genetics would be the most rapid means by which to produce an antigenically matched vaccine'. However, in order 'to be truly prepared, such a vaccine needs to be produced and tested now to identify and resolve the issues, rather than doing so in direct response to an emergency' (Webby and Webster 2003: 1522).

Bibliography

Unpublished official records

PRO

CAB 23 Cabinet minutes to 1939.

CAB 24 Cabinet Memoranda to 1939 GT series.

CAB 26 1 Home Affairs Committee, *Minutes – 1918–19.*

CAB 26 2 Home Affairs Committee, *Minutes.*

ED 50 34 Education, *School Medical Service.*

ED 50 56 Education, *School Medical Service – Nurses.*

ED 50 71 Education, *School Medical Service.*

FD 1 529 Medical Research Committee, *Influenza – Research by Colonel Cumming with British Forces in France.*

FD 1 530 Medical Research Committee, *Influenza – Research by Dr Fildes.*

FD 1 531 Medical Research Committee, *Influenza – Report by Captain A Gregor on tin mines in Cornwall.*

FD 1 532 Medical Research Committee, *Influenza – Research by Dr Twort.*

FD 1 533 Medical Research Committee, *Influenza – General research in UK.*

FD 1 534 Medical Research Committee, *Influenza – General research in UK.*

FD 1 535 Medical Research Committee, *Influenza Committee: Correspondence with LGB and War Office.*

FD 1 536 Medical Research Committee, *Influenza – Conference on Influenza.*

FD 1 537 Medical Research Committee, *Influenza – Schools Reports on Cases and Treatments of.*

FD 1 545 Medical Research Committee, *Influenza – 1920 Epidemic: Informal Conference of Research Workers.*

FD 1 546 Medical Research Committee, *Influenza – 1922 Epidemic Reports and Correspondence.*

FD 1 553 Medical Research Committee, *Pneumonia: Grant to Prof. E.E. Glynn; Observations on Bacteriological Diagnosis of Acute Pneumonia.*

FD 1 554 Medical Research Committee, *Pneumonia: Grant to Prof. E.E. Glynn; Observations on Bacteriological Diagnosis of Acute Pneumonia.*

MAF 60 307 Ministry of Food and Board of Trade, *Diary of Sir W.H. Beveridge, K.C.B. 1918.*

MH 10 83 Ministry of Health, *Circulars, Local Government Board 1918.*

MH 10 84 Ministry of Health, *Circulars, Local Government Board 1919.*

MH 10 85 Ministry of Health, *Circulars, Local Government Board 1919.*

MH 49 7 Ministry of Health, *Welsh Insurance Commission – Minutes of Meetings of Commissioners, 1918.*

MH 55 57 Ministry of Health, *Influenza and Common Colds.*

MH 58 418 Ministry of Health, *General Health – Infectious Diseases – Powers of Port Sanitary Authorities.*

MH 58 419 Ministry of Health, *General Health – Encephalitis Lethargica.*

MH 65 2 Ministry of Health, *National Health: Insurance Committee for the County of London – London Executive Council – Agenda.*

MH 65 3 Ministry of Health, *National Health: Insurance Committee for the County of London – London Executive Council – Agenda.*

MH 65 51 Ministry of Health, *National Health: Insurance Committee for the County of London – General Purposes Sub-Committee – Minutes.*

MH 65 60 Ministry of Health, *National Health: Insurance Committee for the County of London – Medical Benefit Sub-Committee – Minutes.*

MH 65 91 Ministry of Health, *National Health: Insurance Committee for the County of London – Pharmaceutical Service Sub-Committee – Minutes.*

MH 79 5 Ministry of Health, *Epidemic Disease Circulars.*

MH 79 7 Ministry of Heath, *War Office Demand for Medical Practitioners.*

MH 96 738 Ministry of Health, *Welsh Health Services – Extension of Infectious Diseases Act.*

MH 106 Ministry of Health, *Representative WWI medical records.*

MH 106 2384 Ministry of Health, *Medical Sheets – 85th General Hospital – 1917–1920.*

MH 106 2387 Ministry of Health, *Papers Based on the 1914 War Medical Records Section – Compilation and Usage.*

MH 113 51 Ministry of Health, *Reports by the Delegate of Great Britain on the Sessions of the Committee of the Office International d'Hygiène Publique, Paris and of the Health Committee of the League of Nations (Reports 1–12).*

MH 139 3 Ministry of Health, *Newman Diaries (1916–1920).*

NATS 1 797 National Service Department, *Influenza Epidemic.*

NATS 1 849 National Service Department, *Influenza Epidemic.*

PIN 2 4 National Health Insurance Joint Committee, *Minutes 1918.*

PIN 26 7921 War pension file, *John Jones Jenkins.*

PIN 26 15039 War pension file, *Sydney Thomas Varney.*

PIN 26 20251 War pension file, *Nelly Stevenson.*

PIN 26 21568 War pension file, *Harold T. Eking.*

PIN 26 22103 War pension file, *Alan John Mawson.*

RECO 1 847 Ministry of Reconstruction, *War Cabinet.*

RG 26 38 Registrar-General, *Influenza Deaths 1919–1922; Weekly Return Proof.*

Wellcome CMAC

GC/16 *Savory and Moore, Dispensing Chemists, Chapel Street, Belgravia SW1.* Particularly 16 4 92 and 16 5 93 (Registers).

GC/21 *Hood, Dr Basil.* Volume 1 – notebook, 1918.

SA/BMA *British Medical Association.* Particularly SA/BMA Box 197 F.16; Box 197 F.9; Box 198 F.17; Box 202 F.44; Box 204 F.50; Box 206 F.58; Box 206 F.59; Box 207 F.60; Box 208 F.66; Box 208 F.67; Box 210 F.75.

SA/CMO *Association of County Medical Officers* Box 1 A.2 (Minutes).
SA/HVA *Health Visitor's Association* Box 1 A.1/12 (Annual Reports); Box 1 A.1/13; Box 78 F.1/7; Box 82 G.2/1; Box 82 G.2/2; Box 82 G.2/3.

National Archives of Australia

A1/15 1919/287 Home and Territories Department, *New Zealand – Restriction on Issue of Passports or Permits a/c Influenza Epidemic.*
A1/15 1919/2364 Home and Territories Department, *Pneumonic Influenza. Application to be Made Notifiable Disease ACT.*
A1/15 1919/3646 Home and Territories Department, *Mr. C. Lett. Use Canberra Hospital as Isolation Ward for Influenza Patients.*
A1/15 1925/6310 Home and Territories Department, *Medical. Influenza at Sabai Island Papua.*
A2 1918/3627 Prime Minister's Department, *Admission of Clergymen to Sydney Quarantine Station During Influenza Epidemic of 1918.*
A2 1918/3705 Prime Minister's Department, *Spanish Influenza. S.S. 'Makura'.*
A2 1919/219 Prime Minister's Department, *Spanish Influenza. Gilbert, Ellice, Ocean Island.*
A2 1919/224 Prime Minister's Department, *Spanish Influenza. Outbreak at Fiji.*
A2 1919/452 Prime Minister's Department, *Spanish Influenza.*
A2 1919/472 Prime Minister's Department, *Spanish Influenza: Solomon Islands.*
A2 1919/482 Part 1 Prime Minister's Department, *Influenza Epidemic. Border Regulations.*
A2 1919/482 Part 2 Prime Minister's Department, *Spanish Influenza. Conference at Melbourne. Precautionary Measures.*
A2 1919/701 Prime Minister's Department, *Influenza Epidemic. Samoa.*
A2 1919/742 Prime Minister's Department, *Influenza: Victoria Declaration of Infected Area.*
A2 1919/887 Part 2 Prime Minister's Department, *Influenza Epidemic Misc. Papers unregistered. Relation of Influenza to Quarantine of Ships.*
A2 1919/952 Prime Minister's Department, *Spanish Influenza. Information Required by Influenza Commission – South Africa.*
A2 1919/953 Part 1 Prime Minister's Department, *Influenza Epidemic Broken Hill.*
A2 1919/953 Part 2 Prime Minister's Department, *Influenza – New South Wales.*
A2 1919/957 Prime Minister's Department, *Spanish Influenza. New Zealand.*
A2 1919/964 Prime Minister's Department, *Pneumonic Influenza – Compulsory Inoculation.*
A2 1919/965 Prime Minister's Department, *Pneumonic Influenza Inoculation of Commonwealth Public Servants.*
A2 1919/966 Prime Minister's Department, *Influenza. United Kingdom.*
A2 1919/967 Prime Minister's Department, *Pneumonic Influenza. Serum.*
A2 1919/971 Prime Minister's Department, *Pneumonic Influenza Mails.*
A2 1919/993 Prime Minister's Department, *Influenza. South Australia Proclamation as Infected Area.*
A2 1919/998 Prime Minister's Department, *Influenza Epidemic. Australia. Information for Nauru.*
A2 1919/1182 Prime Minister's Department, *Transports. Use of for Coastal Work during Influenza Outbreak.*
A2 1919/1302 Prime Minister's Department, *Influenza Epidemic. Commonwealth Regulations.*

A2 1919/1311 Prime Minister's Department, *Spanish Influenza. Miscellaneous. Transcontinental Railway. (Correspondence with West Australian Government.)*

A2 1919/1319 Prime Minister's Department, *Influenza. New South Wales. Proclamations Issued by New South Wales Government.*

A2 1919/1328 Prime Minister's Department, *Influenza Epidemic. Commonwealth Departments. Hours of Service.*

A2 1919/1601/4 Prime Minister's Department, *Influenza Epidemic. Claim for Compensation.*

A2 1919/1657 Prime Minister's Department, *Influenza. Tasmania. Troops.*

A2 1919/1658 Prime Minister's Department, *Influenza Epidemic. Interstate Traffic. South Australia.*

A2 1919/1659 Prime Minister's Department, *Influenza Epidemic. Interstate Traffic. Victoria.*

A2 1919/1661 Prime Minister's Department, *Influenza Epidemic. Interstate Traffic (NSW).*

A2 1919/1663 Prime Minister's Department, *Influenza. America.*

A2 1919/1664 Prime Minister's Department, *Pneumonic Influenza Queensland. Proclamation as Infected Area.*

A2 1919/1922 Prime Minister's Department, *Shipping. Effect of Influenza Epidemic on Interstate Shipping.*

A2 1919/2930 Prime Minister's Department, *Influenza Epidemic. Theatres.*

A2 1919/2959 Prime Minister's Department, *Influenza Epidemic. Tasmania. Declaration as Infected Area.*

A2 1920/1006 Prime Minister's Department, *Spanish Influenza. Miscellaneous.*

A192 FCL1919/146 Home and Territories Department, *Inoculation against Pneumonic Influenza at Jervis Bay.*

A192 FCL1921/295 Home and Territories Department, *Influenza Inoculations Federal Territory.*

A199 FC1919/238 Home and Territories Department, *Influenza at Canberra.*

A361 DSG19/1582 Home and Territories Department, *Influenza Outbreak.*

A361 DSG20/82 Home and Territories Department, *Advertising of Inoculation Depots in Connection with Pneumonic Influenza Epidemic.*

A361 DSG21/52 Home and Territories Department, *Inoculation against Pneumonic Influenza.*

A457/1 C501/3 Prime Minister's Department, *Medical. Influenza. Claims by Commonwealth Railways against W.A.*

A457/1 G501/6 Prime Minister's Department, *Medical – Reports, etc. – Influenza Epidemic in Savannah.*

A457/1 I501/3 Prime Minister's Department, *Medical. Influenza Outbreak at Solomon Islands.*

A457/1 501/5 Prime Minister's Department, *Medical. Influenza. (Spanish) in Samoa and Fiji.*

A457/1 501/17 Prime Minister's Department, *Medical. Influenza at Thursday Island.*

A457/1 501/19 Prime Minister's Department, *Medical. Influenza on the S.S. 'Kursk'.*

A457/1 501/20 Prime Minister's Department, *Medical. Influenza. South Australia.*

A457/1 501/36 Prime Minister's Department, *Medical. Influenza. Tasmania. Claims by Staff Nurses.*

A457/1 501/40 Prime Minister's Department, *Medical. Influenza. Epidemic. New Caledonia.*

A457/1 501/42 Prime Minister's Department, *Medical. Outbreak of Influenza at Tonga.*
A457/1 501/51 Prime Minister's Department, *Medical. Influenza. Miscellaneous.*
A457/1 501/53 Prime Minister's Department, *Medical. Influenza. Victoria. Use of Base Hospital by State Departments.*
A458 M368/1 Prime Minister's Department, *Medical – Influenza – Pneumonic Epidemic 1919.*
A2487 1919/1494 Department of Reparation, *Vocational Training: Effect of Influenza Epidemic on.*
A2487 1919/2104 Department of Reparation, *Sustenance to Returned Men Suffering from Epidemic Influenza.*
A2487 1919/2211 Department of Reparation, *Ambulance for Bendigo – Pneumonic Influenza.*
A2487 1919/3034 Department of Reparation, *Pneumonic Influenza: Loan of Adelaide Street Drill Shed Premises for Free Public Inoculation, Brisbane.*
A2487 1919/4575 Department of Reparation, *Tents Appropriated by Dept. of Labour and Industry for Emergency Accommodation at Wagga – Influenza Epidemic.*
A2487 1919/5445 Department of Reparation, *Brisbane Office, Clerical Arrangements Due to Staff Shortage Resulting from Influenza Epidemic.*
A6006 1919/1/9 Cabinet Records, *4th Hughes Ministry Jan. 1919 to June 1921 – 9 January 1919.*
A6006 1919/2/3 Cabinet Records, *4th Hughes Ministry Jan. 1919 to June 1921. 3 February 1919.*
A6006 1919/12/31 Cabinet Records, *4th Hughes Ministry Jan. 1919 to June 1921. 31 December 1919.*
A8510/1 68/24A Advisory Council of Science and Industry, *Executive Committee. Influenza.*
CP78/22 1918/254 Governor-General's Office, *Influenza.*
CP78/22 1919/224 Governor-General's Office, *Influenza.*
CP78/22 1919/957 Governor-General's Office, *Influenza.*
CP78/22 1921/53 Governor-General's Office, *Influenza.*
CP103/11 404 Prime Minister's Department, *Influenza Epidemic. Miscellaneous Papers Unregistered.*
CP103/11 406 Prime Minister's Department, *Quarantine – Tasmania – Shipping.*
CP103/11 407 Prime Minister's Department, *Influenza Epidemic. Sydney Chamber of Commerce Resolutions.*
CP103/11 411 Prime Minister's Department, *Influenza Epidemic. King Island. Port of Entry.*
CP103/11 413 Prime Minister's Department, *Influenza Epidemic. Cabinet Decision re Sub-committee.*
CP103/11 416 Prime Minister's Department, *Tasmania – Permits to Leave, Ports of Entry.*
CP103/11 420 Prime Minister's Department, *Quarantine – Cockburn.*
CP103/11 421 Prime Minister's Department, *WA – Declaration of Infected Area.*
CP103/11 422 Prime Minister's Department, *Qld. – Tas. Shipping – Quarantine.*
CP103/11 424 Prime Minister's Department, *Pneumonic Influenza. Press Notices.*
CP103/11 425 Prime Minister's Department, *Qld. – NSW Control of Traffic.*
CP103/11 427 Prime Minister's Department, *Qld. – Passage Across Border.*
CP103/11 428 Prime Minister's Department, *Interstate Passenger Restrictions.*

CP103/11 430 Prime Minister's Department, *Influenza. {Miscellaneous correspondence re incidents occurring during train travel.}*

CP103/11 432 Prime Minister's Department, *Influenza. Miscellaneous Correspondence.*

NAA files held at PROV

MP367/1 527/21/1272 Department of Defence – Influenza Expenditures.

MP367/1 527/21/493 Department of Defence – Pneumonic Influenza.

MP367/1 556/16/84 Department of Defence – Influenza Pay.

MP367/1 556/49/714 Department of Defence – Influenza Expenditure – Claims – Public Health Department.

MP367/1 612/32/332 Department of Defence – Materials Provided to Quarantine Service.

MP367/1567/7/4467 Department of Defence – Liverpool Concentration Camp – Arrangements for Influenza Outbreak.

MP472/1 19/19/3740 Department of Defence – Special Influenza Leave – Civilian Officers.

MT487/1 MEDLEY W Department of Defence – Corporal William Medley.

National Archives of South Africa

CES 188 ES70/4647/14 Commissioner for Enemy Subjects, *Influenza Outbreak.*

GG 1231 33/1014 Office of the Governor-General of South Africa, *Health: General. Spanish Influenza: Outbreak of in Union.*

GG 1231 33/1015 Office of the Governor-General of South Africa, *Health: General. Outbreak of Spanish Influenza in Basutoland.*

GG 1231 33/1018 Office of the Governor-General of South Africa, *Health: General. Spanish Influenza: Outbreaks of in the Bechuanaland Protectorate.*

GG 1231 33/1019 Office of the Governor-General of South Africa, *Health: General. Spanish Influenza at Uitenhage: Proposed Supply of Medicine for Needy Doses at Government Expense.*

GG 1231 33/1024 Office of the Governor-General of South Africa, *Health: General. Suspension of Recruitment of Native Labour in Basutoland on Account of Outbreak of Spanish Influenza.*

GG 1231 33/1026 Office of the Governor-General of South Africa, *Health: General. Outbreak of Spanish Influenza in the Union: Suggests that Message of Condolence and Sympathy be Sent from His Majesty.*

GG 1232 33/1029 Office of the Governor-General of South Africa, *Health: General. Spanish Influenza: Outbreak of at Kimberley: Report on by Colonel Orenstein.*

GG 1232 33/1031 Office of the Governor-General of South Africa, *Health: General. Spanish Influenza: Outbreak of in Northern Rhodesia.*

GG 1232 33/1032 Office of the Governor-General of South Africa, *Health: General. Spanish Influenza: Outbreak of in East Africa.*

GG 1232 33/1034 Office of the Governor-General of South Africa, *Health: General. Spanish Influenza: Suggests Appointing a Day for Humiliation and Prayer in View of.*

GG 1232 33/1035 Office of the Governor-General of South Africa, *Health: General. Outbreak of Spanish Influenza in Union: Expresses Sympathy with the People who has Suffered from the Epidemic.*

GG 1232 33/1036 Office of the Governor-General of South Africa, *Health: General.*

Outbreak of Spanish Influenza in the Union: Requests Information re Vaccine Used in Connection with Prevention of Pneumonia.

GG 1232 33/1040 Office of the Governor-General of South Africa, *Health: General. Report Regarding Outbreak of Spanish Influenza in South West Africa.*

GG 1232 33/1042 Office of the Governor-General of South Africa, *Congo. Spanish Influenza Epidemic: Regulations Regarding Admission to the Katanga.*

GG 1232 33/1051 Office of the Governor-General of South Africa, *Health: General. Spanish Influenza in Union: Requests Certain Information Regarding Vaccines for Treatment of.*

GG 1232 33/1052 Office of the Governor-General of South Africa, *Health: General. Spanish Influenza in Bechuanaland: Transmits Further Information Regarding.*

GG 1232 33/1053 Office of the Governor-General of South Africa, *Commissions: Appointment of Commission to Enquire into the Influenza Epidemic in the Union.*

GG 1232 33/1061 and 33/1066 Office of the Governor-General of South Africa, *Health: General. Influenza Epidemic: Offers Her Services.*

GG 1232 33/1064 Office of the Governor-General of South Africa, *Health: General. Influenza Epidemic: Certain Information Required From the Surgeon-General, United States Army, Regarding.*

GG 1232 33/1068 Office of the Governor-General of South Africa, *Health: General. Influenza Epidemic: Request Certain Information Regarding from the Government of Australia.*

GG 1232 33/1073A Office of the Governor-General of South Africa, *Health: General. Transmits Copies of a Memorandum on Epidemic Catarrhs and Influenza Which has been Issued by the Local Government Board.*

GG 1232 33/1079 Office of the Governor-General of South Africa, *Health: General. Influenza Epidemic: Transmit Telegram to be Forwarded to the Governor-General of Australia Regarding the Outbreak of in Australia.*

GG 1232 33/1082A Office of the Governor-General of South Africa, *Health: General. Reports on Influenza Epidemic.*

GG 1233 33/1089 Office of the Governor-General of South Africa, *Report of the Influenza Epidemic Commission.*

GG 1236 33/1333 Office of the Governor-General of South Africa, *Health: General. Notifies Increase of Influenza Epidemic in Great Britain UK.*

GG 1236 33/1341 Office of the Governor-General of South Africa, *Health: General. Influenza Epidemic in England: Transmit Further Copy of a Telegram from Secretary of State London Notifying Decrease of Epidemic.*

GG 1308 36/135 Office of the Governor-General of South Africa *Immigration. Nyasaland: Prohibition of Immigration of Europeans or Natives into on Account of Spread of Spanish Influenza.*

GG 1308 36/136 Office of the Governor-General of South Africa, *Immigration. Nyasaland: Cancellation of Restrictions re Immigration on Account of Spanish Influenza.*

GG 1417 45/82 Office of the Governor-General of South Africa, *Governor-General: Tours, Inspections, Treks, Et Cetera of His Excellency. Potchefstroom: Proposed Visit Abandoned on Account of Outbreak of Spanish Influenza.*

GG 1548 50/746 Office of the Governor-General of South Africa, *Natives: Labour on Mines. Suspension of Repatriation of Natives from Transvaal to Mozambique Owing Development of Spanish Influenza in Mozambique.*

GG 1689 51/4922 Office of the Governor-General of South Africa, *Sentences: Abdulla Jamat and Others. Remission of Sentences in Respect of Special Duties Performed During the Prevalence of Spanish Influenza in Cape Town.*

GNLB 300 370/18 Native Affairs, *Part file No. 370/18/203 Spanish Influenza. Witwatersrand General.*

GNLB 301 370/18 Native Affairs, *Influenza Among Natives.*

JUS 467 and 468 1/249/18 Justice Department, *Spanish Influenza Epidemic.*

MNW 438 MM2826/18 Mines & Industries, *'Spanish Influenza': Organisation of Relief Committees at London, Kameelfontein and Bleshok Diggings.*

MNW 438 MM2838/18 Mines & Industries, *Spanish Influenza: Closing of Miners Phthisis Medical Bureau Owing to Epidemic. Release of Medical Officers of Bureau to Assist in Connection with.*

SAS 718 G119/5 Transport/Immigration, *Traffic Restrictions Owing to Outbreaks of Smallpox and Influenza.*

TES 9334 F131/3/3 Treasury, *Social Welfare. Children's Protection Act (No. 25 of 1913): Expenditure in Connexion with Influenza Epidemic 1918.*

URU 378 2464 Prime Minister's Office, *Outgoing Correspondence.*

URU 378 2468 and 2468A Prime Minister's Office, *Proclamation – Natal.*

URU 378 2469 Prime Minister's Office, *Issue of a Proclamation Proclaiming Epidemic Influenza to be a Disease with the Meaning of Section 58 of Ordinance 58 of 1902. Transvaal.*

URU 378 2470 Prime Minister's Office, *Issue of a Proclamation Proclaiming the Disease Epidemic Influenza to be a Contagious or Infectious Disease Within the Meaning of the Cape Health Acts.*

URU 384 2934 Prime Minister's Office, *Appointment of a Commission to Enquire into Matters Concerning the Influenza Epidemic in the Union.*

URU 393 479 Prime Minister's Office, *Proclamation Declaring Epidemic Influenza to be a Contagious or Infectious Disease Within the Meaning of the 27th and 48th Section of the Public Health Amendment Act, No. 23 of 1897 (Cape).*

URU 397 788, 790 and 792 Prime Minister's Office, *Influenza Correspondence.*

URU 400 959 Prime Minister's Office, *Influenza Correspondence.*

URU 401 1070 Prime Minister's Office, *Medal Using Red Cross.*

VWN 3637 PG291 Treasury (Pensions), *Spanish Influenza. Compensation to Dependants of Discharged Soldiers who here Died from.*

VWN 3637 PG292 Treasury (Pensions), *Spanish Influenza. Question of Relief to Dependants of Victims who were Pensionable Officers but where Relative Pension Laws Contain no Provision for Awards to Dependants.*

VWN 3700 PG384 Treasury (Pensions), *Spanish Influenza.*

Public Record Office, Victoria

3183/P/0000 Boxes 000051, 000051 and 000052 Charity Welfare Health – Influenza Epidemic 1919.

8291/P/0001 Influenza File labelled 'Pneumonic Spanish Influenza'.

State Library of Victoria

MSB422 Chandler, Horace Arthur. *Diary and Papers 1915–1919.*

State Records of New South Wales

4/6247 Premier's Department – Influenza Epidemic.

4/7776 Minutes Book, Hospitals Advisory Board.

5/5348.1 Department of Health – Pneumonic Influenza.

6/4461 Department of Health – Minutes 1917–1921.
8/2035.8 Quarantine – Influenza.

City of Kitchener, Ontario

City of Kitchener. 'Board of Health Minutes.' Kitchener, Ontario: City Clerk's Office, 1918.

Published sources

Abler, R., Adams, J.S. and Gould, P. (1971) *Spatial Organization: The Geographer's View of the World*, Englewood Cliffs: Prentice-Hall.

Abrahams, A., Hollows, N.F., Eyre, J.W.H. and French, H. (1917) 'Purulent bronchitis: its influenza and pneumococcal bacteriology', *The Lancet*, ii: 377–80.

Abrahams, A., Hollows, N. and French, H. (1919) 'A further investigation into influenzo-pneumococcal and influenzo-streptococcal septicaemia: epidemic influenzal "pneumonia" of highly fatal type and its relation to "purulent bronchitis"', *The Lancet*, January 4: 1–11.

Adamo, S. (1992) 'Rio de Janeiro', in F.R. van Hartesveldt (ed.) *1918–1919 Pandemic of Influenza: the Urban Impact in the Western World*, London: Edwin Mellen Press.

Afkhami, A. (2003) 'Compromised constitutions: the Iranian experience with the 1918 influenza pandemic', *Bulletin of the History of Medicine*, 77(2): 367–92.

Aiach, P. and Curtis, S. (1990) 'Social inequalities in self-reported morbidity: interpretation and comparison of data from Britain and France', *Social Science & Medicine*, 31(3): 267–74.

AIHW (Australian Institute of Health and Welfare) (2004) *Australia's Health 2004*, Canberra: AIHW.

Albert, Edward (1986) 'Illness and deviance: the response of the press to AIDS', in D. Feldman and T. Johnson (eds) *The Social Dimensions of AIDS: Method and Theory*, New York: Praeger.

Alexander, Frederick William (1929) *Electro-Therapeutical Fluids: Prevention and Abolition of Influenza and Epidemic Infectious diseases*, London.

Åman, Margareta (1990) 'Spanska sjukan: den svenska epidemin 1918–1920 och dess internationella bakgrund (Spanish influenza: the Swedish epidemic, 1918–1920, and its international background).' PhD thesis, Uppsala University.

Anderson, M. (1977) *Dramatist in America: Letters of Maxwell Anderson, 1912–1958*, Chapel Hill, NC: University of North Carolina Press.

Andrews, Margaret A. (1977) 'Epidemic and public health: influenza in Vancouver, 1918–1919', *BC Studies*, 32 (Summer): 21–44.

Anonymous (1925) *A Doctor's Diary*, London: Hutchinson & Co.

Anonymous (1934) *Colds, Catarrh and Influenza (By A Civil Service Doctor)*, A.D. Baker (ed.), London: Cassell and Company.

Anonymous (1937) *How to Escape Colds and Influenza*, London: Leonard Hill Limited.

Arrington, Leonard (1990) 'The influenza pandemic of 1918–19 in Utah', *Utah Historical Quarterly*, 58(2): 164–82.

Australia (annual) *Official Yearbook of the Commonwealth of Australia*. Canberra: Commonwealth Bureau of Census and Statistics.

Baird, N.D. (1976) 'The "Spanish Lady" in Kentucky 1918–1919', *The Filson Club History Quarterly*, 50: 290–301.

Baldwin, Peter (1999) *Contagion and the State in Europe 1830–1930*. Cambridge: Cambridge University Press.

Barnett, D. (2001) 'Clinical effectiveness and cost effectiveness of zanamivir (Relenza): translating the evidence into clinical practice, a National Institute for Clinical Evidence view', *Philosophical Transactions: Biological Sciences*, 356 (1416): 1899–1903.

Barry, J.M. (2004) *The Great Influenza: the Epic Story of the Deadliest Plague in History*, New York: Viking.

Basler, C.F., Reid, A.H., *et al*. (2001) 'Sequence of the 1918 pandemic influenza virus nonstructural gene (NS) segment and characterization of recombinant viruses bearing the 1918 NS genes', *Proceedings of the National Academy of Sciences of the United States of America*, 98(5): 2746–51.

Baxter, J. and Eyles, J. (1999) 'Prescription for research practice? Grounded theory in qualitative evaluation', *Area*, 31(2): 179–81.

BBC (1998) *QED: Prisoners of the Forgotten Pandemic*, TV programme.

BBC (1999a) *Cost Warning on Flu Drug*. Available from: news.bbc.co.uk/hi/english/health/newsid_435000/435874.stm.

BBC (1999b) *Doctors Fear Over Flu Drug*. Available from: news.bbc.co.uk/hi/english/health/newsid_383000/383992.stm.

BBC (1999c) *Flu Hospital Uses Lorry as Mortuary*. Available from: news.bbc.co.uk/1/hi/health/249038.stm.

BBC (1999d) *Flu Kills Thousands*. Available from: news.bbc.co.uk/hi/english/health/newsid_255000/255244.stm.

BBC (1999e) *Horizon – Pandemic*. TV programme.

BBC (1999f) *Race to Find Key to Killer Flu*. Available from: news.bbc.co.uk/hi/english/health/newsid_272000/272081.stm.

BBC (1999g) *Watchdog stories – Relenza Watchdog Healthcheck*. Available from: news.bbc.co.uk/watchdog/stories/hcrelen.shtml.

BBC (2005a) *Killer Flu: Could the World Cope?* Available from: news.bbc.co.uk/1/hi/health/3497355.stm.

BBC (2005b) *Britain Reveals Flu Pandemic Plan*. Available from: news.bbc.co.uk/1/hi/health/4305813.stm.

Belyk, Robert C. and Belyk, Diane M. (1988) 'The Spanish influenza 1918–1919: no armistice with death', *Beaver*, 68(5): 43–9.

Benison, Saul (ed.) (1967) *Tom Rivers, Reflections on a Life in Medicine and Science*, Cambridge, MA: MIT Press.

Benussi, G., Barbone, F., Monai, L. and Gasparini, V. (1983) 'Sequele Neurologiche Dall'Influenza: Pandemia del 1918–19 ed. Encefalite Letargica a Trieste', *Acta Medicae Historiae Patavina*, 30: 11–19.

Bernstein, B. (1975) *Thurber: a Biography*, New York: Dodd, Mead.

Berridge, Virginia (1990) 'Health and medicine', in F.M.L. Thomson (ed.) *The Cambridge Social History of Britain 1750 1950*, Cambridge: Cambridge University Press.

Beveridge, W.I.B. (1977) *Influenza: the Last Great Plague*, London: Heinemann.

Beveridge, W.I.B. (1991) 'The chronicle of influenza epidemics', *History and Philosophy of the Life Sciences*, 13: 223–34.

Blücher Von Wahlstatt, E.M. (1920) *An English Wife in Berlin. a Private Memoir of Events, Politics, and Daily Life in Germany Throughout the War and the Social Revolution of 1918*, London: Constable & Co.

Borza, T. (2001) 'Spanish flu in Norway 1918–19', *Tidsskrift for den Norske laegeforening*, 121(30): 3551–4.

Boseley, S. (2000) 'Something in the air: the virulence of the 1918 outbreak is the biggest unsolved mystery', *Guardian*, 11 January 2000.

Bourdelais, Patrice and Raulot, Jean-Yves (1987) *Une peur bleue: Histoire du choléra en France, 1832–1854*, *Médecine et sociétés*, Paris: Payot.

Bourne, Aleck W. (1922) 'Influenza: pregnancy, labour, the puerperium and diseases of women', in F.G. Crookshank (ed.) *Influenza: Essays by Several Authors*, London: William Heinemann (Medical Books) Ltd.

Bourne, Geoffrey (1963) *We Met at Bart's*, London: Frederick Muller Limited.

Boyd, Mary (1980) 'Coping with Samoan resistance after the 1918 influenza epidemic: Colonel Tate's problems and perplexities', *Journal of Pacific History*, 15(3): 155–74.

Brainerd, E. and Siegler, Mark V. (2003) 'The economic effects of the 1918 influenza epidemic', London: Centre for Economic Policy Research, Discussion Paper Series (No. 3791).

Braithwaite, Max (1953) 'The year of the killer flu', *MacLean's Magazine*, 1 February: 10–11, 43–4.

Bristow, Nancy (1998) '"You can't do anything for influenza": doctors, nurses and the influenza epidemic in the USA,' paper presented at The Spanish 'Flu 1918–1998: Reflections on the Influenza Pandemic of 1918 after 80 Years, Cape Town, 12–15 September.

Brito, Nara Azevdeo de (1997) 'La dansarina: a gripe espanhola e o cotidiano na cidade do Rio de Janeiro (La dansarina: the influenza epidemic and the quotidian report of the Rio de Janeiro city', *História Ciências Saúde – Manguinhos*, 4(1): 11–30.

Brockbank, E.M. (1934) 'Pneumonia', in W.R. Bett (ed.) *A Short History of Some Common Diseases*, Oxford: Oxford University Press.

Brown, Colin (1987) 'The influenza pandemic of 1918 in Indonesia', in Norman G. Owen (ed.) *Death and Disease in Southeast Asia: Explorations in Social, Medical and Demographic History*, Oxford: Oxford University Press.

Brown, D. (2003) 'Killer virus', *Washington Post*, 4 June: CO1.

Brownlee, G.G. and Fodor, E. (2001) 'The predicted antigenicity of the haemagglutinin of the 1918 Spanish influenza pandemic suggests an avian origin', *Philosophical Transactions of the Royal Society of London. Series B: Biological Sciences*, 356(1416): 1871–6.

Bryder, Linda (1982) '"Lessons" of the 1918 influenza epidemic in Auckland', *New Zealand Journal of History*, 16(2): 97–121.

Bryson, Elizabeth (1966) *Look Back in Wonder*, Dundee: David Winter & Son.

Buelow, Paul (1992) 'Chicago', in F.R. van Hartesveldt (ed.) *1918–1919 Pandemic of Influenza: the Urban Impact in the Western World*, London: Edwin Mellen Press.

Bullock, Alan (1993) *Hitler and Stalin: Parallel Lives*, London: Fontana Press.

Burgess, Anthony (1987) *Little Wilson and Big God: Being the First Part of the Confessions of Anthony Burgess*, London: Heinemann.

Burgess, Anthony (2002) *Little Wilson and Big God: Being the First Part of the Confessions of Anthony Burgess*, London: Vintage.

Burnet, F. MacFarlane (1945) *Virus as Organism: Evolutionary and Ecological Aspects of Some Human Virus Diseases, E.K. Dunham Lectures 1944*, Cambridge, MA: Harvard University Press.

Burnet, F. MacFarlane and Clark, Ellen (1942) *Influenza: a Survey of the Last 50 Years In the Light of Modern Work on the Virus of Epidemic Influenza*, Monographs from the Walter and Eliza Hall Institute of Research in Pathology and Medicine, Melbourne – Number Four. London: Macmillan.

Butler, A.G. (1943) *The Official History of the Australian Army Medical Services, 1914–18*, Canberra: Australian War Memorial.

Calfee, D.P. and Hayden, F.G. (1998) 'New approaches to influenza chemotherapy. neuraminidase inhibitors', *Drugs*, 56(4): 537–53.

Camus, Albert (1948) *The Plague {La Peste}*, trans. S. Gilbert, London: Hamish Hamilton.

Canaris, J. (1919) *A Remedy for the 'Flu'*, London.

Caplan, A.L., Engelhardt H.T., Jr. and McCartney, J.J. (eds) (1981) *Concepts of Health and Disease: Interdisciplinary Perspectives*, Reading, MA: Addison-Wesley Publishing Company.

Carnwath, T. (1919) 'Lessons of the Influenza Epidemic 1918', *Journal of State Medicine*, 27(5): 142–57.

Carr, V.S. (1984) *Dos Passos: a Life*, New York: Doubleday & Co.

Cartwright, Frederick F. (in collaboration with Michael D. Biddiss) (1972) *Disease and History*, London: Hart-Davis, MacGibbon.

Cartwright, Frederick F. (1983) 'Pandemics past and future', in Gerald D. Hart (ed.) *Disease in Ancient Man: an International Symposium*, Toronto: Clarke Irwin.

Cate, Thomas (1987) 'Clinical manifestations and consequences of influenza', *American Journal of Medicine*, 82(Suppl. 6A): 15–19.

Cavina, Giovanni (1959) *L'Influenza Epidemica Attraverso I Secoli*, Rome: Edizioni Pozzi.

CDC (2004) *Key Facts About the Flu and Flu Vaccine.* Available from: www.cdc.gov/flu/keyfacts.htm.

Chan, Chi-Ho and Liu, W.T. (1998) 'The evolution of influenza A/H1N1 in Taiwan', paper presented at The Spanish 'Flu 1918–1998: Reflections on the Influenza Pandemic of 1918 after 80 Years, Cape Town, 12–15 September.

Channel 4 and Granada Media (2003) *Secrets of the Dead.* TV programme.

Channel 4/WGBH (1998) *Secret Histories: Killer 'Flu.* TV programme.

Clark, Sean Hannon (1991) 'The impact of the 1918–1919 influenza pandemic on Fresno, California', unpublished MA thesis, California State University, Fresno.

Clarke, Kathleen (1997) *Revolutionary Woman: My Fight for Ireland's Freedom*, Helen Litton (ed.), Dublin: The O'Brien Press.

Cliff, A.D., Haggett, P., Ord, J.K. and Versey, C.R. (1981) *Spatial Diffusion: an Historical Geography of Epidemics in an Island Community*, Cambridge: Cambridge University Press.

Cliff, A.D., Haggett, P. and Ord, J.K. (1986) *Spatial Aspects of Influenza Epidemics*, London: Pion.

Cole, Festus (1994) 'Sierra Leone and World War I', unpublished PhD thesis, University of London.

Colinvaux, Paul (1983) *The Fates of Nations: a Biological Theory of History*, Harmondsworth: Penguin.

Collier, Richard Hugheson (1974) *The Plague of the Spanish Lady: the Influenza Pandemic of 1918–1919*, London: Macmillan.

Collins, S.D. (1932) 'Excess mortality from causes other than influenza and pneumonia during influenza epidemics', *Public Health Report*, 47: 215–19.

Collins, S.D. and Lehmann, J. (1953) *Excess Deaths from Influenza and Pneumonia and from Important Chronic Diseases During Epidemic Periods, 1918–1951*, Public Health Monograph No. 10; Public Health Service Publication No. 213, Washington, DC: US Government Printing Office.

Condominium of the New Hebrides (1919) *Quarantine Regulation (Amendment Regulation) 1919*, Vila.

'Craftman' (1743) 'Occasion'd by an Article of News from Rome of a contagious Distemper raging there, call'd the Influenza', *The London Magazine: and Monthly Chronologer*, March, 2nd edn: 145.

Creighton, Charles (1965) *History of Epidemics in Britain*, 2nd edn, London: Frank Cass & Co.

Crookshank, F.G. (ed.) (1922) *Influenza: Essays by Several Authors*, London: William Heinemann (Medical Books) Ltd.

Crookshank, F.G. (1931) *The Mongol in our midst*, 3rd edn, London: Kegan Paul, Trench, Trubner & Co.

Crosby, Alfred W. (1976) *Epidemic and Peace, 1918*, Westport, CT: Greenwood Press.

Crosby, Alfred W. (1977) 'The pandemic of 1918', in June E. Osborn (ed.) *Influenza in America 1918–1976*, New York: Prodist.

Crosby, Alfred W. (1989) *America's Forgotten Pandemic: the Influenza of 1918*, Cambridge: Cambridge University Press.

Crosby, Alfred W. (1993) 'Influenza', in Kenneth F. Kiple (ed.) *The Cambridge World History of Human Disease*, Cambridge: Cambridge University Press.

Crosby, Alfred W. (1997) 'Influenza: in the grip of the grippe', in Kenneth F. Kiple (ed.) *Plague, Pox and Pestilence: Disease in History*, London: Weidenfeld & Nicolson.

Crosby, Alfred W. (2003) *America's Forgotten Pandemic: the Influenza of 1918*, 2nd edn, Cambridge: Cambridge University Press.

Cummins, S.L. (1919) 'Studies of influenza in hospitals of the British Armies in France', Special Report Series No. 36. London: Medical Research Committee.

Cumpston, J.H.L. (1919) *Influenza and Maritime Quarantine in Australia*, Melbourne: Albert J. Mullett, Government Printer.

Curby, P. (1998) *Memories of the 1918 Influenza Pandemic*, Ryde: Ryde City Council.

Curson, P.H., and McCracken, K. (1989) *Plague in Sydney: the Anatomy of an Epidemic*, Kensington, NSW: New South Wales University Press.

Cushing, H. (1936) *From A Surgeon's Journal*, Boston: Little, Brown, and Company.

Dallas, G. (2000) *1918: War and Peace*, London: John Murray.

Daniel, Thomas M. and Gerstner, Patsy A. (1991) 'The 1918–1919 influenza pandemic', *Journal of Laboratory and Clinical Medicine*, 117(3): 259–60.

Davis, J.L., Heginbottom, J.A., Annan, A.P., *et al.* (2000) 'Ground penetrating radar surveys to locate 1918 Spanish Flu victims in permafrost', *Journal of Forensic Science*, 45(1): 68–76.

de Gooyer, A.C. (1968) *De Spaanse griep van '18*, Amsterdam: Philips-Duphar Nederland n.v.

Decker, N. (1996) 'Spanish 'Flu in Leipzig 1918–1920', *Archiwum historii i filozofii medycyny/Polskii Towarzystwo Historii Medycyny i Farmacji* 59(1): 67–72.

Denmark (annual) *Statistik Aarborg*, Copenhagen.

Derrida, Jacques and McLeod, T.I. (1987) *The Truth in Painting*, Chicago: University of Chicago Press.

Dillner, Luisa (1995) 'A pig of a problem', *Guardian*, 14 October: 12.

Dixon, Bernard (1994) *Power Unseen: How Microbes Rule the World*, New York: W.H. Freeman.

Doherty, W.T. (1977) 'A West Virginia county's experiences with the 1918 influenza epidemic', *West Virginia History*, 38: 136–40.

Donaldson, R. (1922) 'The bacteriology of influenza – with special reference to Pfeiffer's Bacillus', in F.G. Crookshank (ed.) *Influenza: Essays by Several Authors*, London: William Heinemann (Medical Books) Ltd.

Dowdle, Walter and LaPatra, Jack (1983) *Informed Consent: Influenza Facts and Myths*, Chicago: Nelson Hall.

Duncan, K. (2003) *Hunting the 1918 Flu: One Scientist's Search for a Killer Virus*, Toronto: University of Toronto Press.

Durey, Michael (1979) *The Return of the Plague: British Society and the Cholera 1831–2*, London: Gill and Macmillan.

Dutton, Diana B. (1988) *Worse than the Disease: Pitfalls of Medical Progress*, Cambridge: Cambridge University Press.

Dyhouse, C. (1998) 'Driving ambitions: women in pursuit of a medical education, 1890–1939', *Women's History Review*, 3: 321–43.

Echenberg, Myron (1993) 'L'histoire et l'oubli collectif: L'épidemie de grippe de 1918 au Sénégal', in Dennis D. Cordell (ed.) *Population, reproduction, sociétés: perspectives et enjeux de démographie sociale: mélanges en l'honneur de Joel W. Gregory*, Montréal: Presses de l'Université de Montréal.

Echenberg, Myron (1998) 'The dog that did not bark: evidence for the 1918 influenza pandemic in Senegal', paper presented at The Spanish 'Flu 1918–1998: Reflections on the Influenza Pandemic of 1918 after 80 Years, Cape Town, 12–15 September.

Echenberg, Myron (2003) 'The dog that did not bark: evidence for the 1918 influenza pandemic in Senegal', in H. Phillips and D. Killingray (eds) *The Spanish Flu Pandemic of 1918–19: New Perspectives*, London: Routledge.

Echeverri, Beatriz (1993) *La Gripe Española: La pandemia de 1918–1919*, Madrid: Centro de Investigaciones Sociológicas.

Echeverri, Beatriz (1998) 'Spanish influenza seen from Spain', paper presented at The Spanish 'Flu 1918–1998: Reflections on the Influenza Pandemic of 1918 after 80 Years, Cape Town, 12–15 September.

Echeverri, Beatriz (2003) 'Spanish influenza seen from Spain', in H. Phillips and D. Killingray (eds) *The Spanish Flu Pandemic of 1918–19: New Perspectives*, London: Routledge.

Edwards, Vivien (1986) 'Pestilence from abroad? The 1918 influenza epidemic', *New Zealand Medical Journal*, 22 October: 809–12.

Eichel, Otto R. (1923) *A Special Report on the Mortality from Influenza in New York State During the Epidemic of 1918–19*, New York: New York State Department of Health.

Elliott, M. (2001) 'Zanamivir: from drug design to the clinic', *Philosophical Transactions: Biological Sciences* 356(1416): 1885–93.

Ellison, J.G. (2003) '"A fierce hunger": tracing the impacts of the 1918–1919 influenza pandemic in southwest Tanzania', in H. Phillips and D. Killingray (eds) *The Spanish Flu Pandemic of 1918–19: New Perspectives*, London: Routledge.

Elveback, L.R., Fox, J.P., Ackerman, E., Langworthy, A., Boyd, M. and Greenwood, L. (1976) 'An influenza simulation model for immunization studies', *American Journal of Epidemiology*, 103: 152–65.

English, F. (1986) 'Princeton plagues: the epidemics of 1832, 1880 and 1918–19', *Princeton History,* 5: 18–26.

Ensley, P.C. (1983) 'Indiana and the influenza pandemic of 1918', *Indiana Medical History Quarterly,* 9(4): 3–15.

Ewald, Paul W. (1994) *Evolution of Infectious Disease*, Oxford: Oxford University Press.

Eyler, John M. (1987) *Sir Arthur Newsholme and State Medicine 1885–1935*, Cambridge: Cambridge University Press.

Eyler, John M. (1992) 'The sick poor and the state: Arthur Newsholme on poverty, disease and responsibility', in Charles E. Rosenberg and Janet Golden (eds) *Framing Disease: Studies in Cultural History*, New Brunswick, NJ: Rutgers University Press.

Fanning, Patricia (1995) 'Disease and the politics of community, Norwood and the great flu epidemic of 1918', unpublished PhD thesis, Boston College.

Fanning, T.G., Slemons, R.D., Reid, A.H., Janczewski, T.A., Dean, J. and Taubenberger, J.K. (2002) '1917 avian influenza virus sequences suggest that the 1918 pandemic virus did not acquire its hemagglutinin directly from birds', *Journal of Virology*, 76(15): 7860–2.

Farmer, Paul (1992) *AIDS and Accusation: Haiti and the Geography of Blame*, Berkeley: University of California Press.

Fatovic Ferencic, S. and Sain, S. (1991) 'Spanish influenza as a cause of death in Zagreb in 1918', *Lijecnicki vjesnik*, 113(11–12): 444–6.

Fee, Elizabeth (1988) 'Sin versus science: venereal disease in twentieth-century Baltimore', in E. Fee and D. Fox (eds) *AIDS: the Burdens of History*, Berkeley: University of California Press.

Fee, E., Brown, T.M., Lazarus, J. and Theerman, P. (2001) 'The influenza pandemic of 1918', *American Journal of Public Health*, 91(12): 1953.

Fenn, E.A. (2002) *Pox Americana: the Great Smallpox Epidemic of 1775–82*, New York: Hill and Wang.

Figura, S.Z. (1998) 'The forgotten pandemic. the Spanish Flu of 1918 was gravest crisis American hospitals had ever faced', *The Volunteer Leader*, 39(2): 5.

Fincher, Jack (1989) 'America's deadly rendezvous with the "Spanish Lady"', *Smithsonian*, 130–45.

Fine, Paul E.M. (1982) 'Applications of mathematical models to the epidemiology of influenza: A critique', in P. Selby (ed.) *Influenza Models: Prospects for Development and Use*, Lancaster: MTP Press Limited.

Fleming, Alexander (1919) 'On some simply prepared culture media for B. Influenzae', *The Lancet*, 196(25 January): 138–9.

Fleming, Alexander (1929) 'On the antibacterial action of cultures of a penicillium, with special reference to their use in the isolation of B. Influenzae', *British Journal of Experimental Pathology*, 10(June 1929): 226–39.

Fletcher, Maisie (1957) *The Bright Countenance: a Personal Biography of Walter Morley Fletcher*, London: Hodder and Stoughton.

Fokeer, A.F. (1921) *The Spanish Influenza in Mauritius*, Port Louis, Mauritius: Mauritius Indian Times.

Fortman, A. (1976) 'Abstract model and epidemiological reality of influenza A', in J. Berger and Deutsche Gesellschaft feür Medizinische Dokumentation Informatik und statistik. Group of 'Mathematical Models' (eds) *Mathematical Models in Medicine*, Berlin: Springer.

Foucault, Michel (1976) *The Birth of the Clinic: an Archaeology of Medical Perception*, trans. A.M. Sheridan, London: Routledge/Tavistock Publications.

Frank, A.L., Taber, L.H., Glezen, W.P., Geyer, E.A., McIlwain, S. and Paredes, A. (1983) 'Influenza B virus infections in the community and the family. the epidemics of 1976–1977 and 1979–1980 in Houston, Texas', *American Journal of Epidemiology*, 118(3): 313–25.

Franklin, M.M., Bowers, R.H. and Smith, R.B. (1919) *'Influenza blues'* from the musical *A Lonely Romeo*, Detroit: Jerome H. Remick & Co.

French, Roger and Arrizabalaga, Jon (1998) 'Coping with the French Disease: university practitioners' strategies and tactics in the transition from the fifteenth century to the sixteenth century', in Roger French, Jon Arrizabalaga, Andrew Cunningham and Luis Garcia-Ballestor (eds) *Medicine from the Black Death to the French Disease*, Aldershot: Ashgate.

Fritz, Stephen G. (1992) 'Frankfurt', in F.R. van Hartesveldt (ed.) *1918–1919 Pandemic of Influenza: the Urban Impact in the Western World*, London: Edwin Mellen Press.

Frost, W.H. (1919) 'The epidemiology of influenza', *Journal of the American Medical Association*, 73: 313.

Galishoff, S. (1969) 'Newark and the great influenza pandemic of 1918', *Bulletin of the History of Medicine*, 43: 246–58.

Gallagher, Richard (1969) *Diseases that Plague Modern Man: a History of Ten Communicable Diseases*, Dobbs Ferry, NY: Oceana Publications.

Gallatly, James M. and Barber, Eric (1927) *Love is Like the Influenza*. London: Boosey & Co. (Song).

Galli-Valerio, B. (1918) *L'Étiologie et la Prophylaxie de la Grippe ou Influenza*, Lausanne: Edwin Frankfurter.

Gamboa Ojeda, Leticia (1991) 'La epidemia de influenza de 1918: sanidad y política en la ciudad de Puebla', *Quipu*, 8(1): 91–109.

Garner, Cathcart (1921) 'Annual report for the year 1918 (Colonial Medical Report. No. 126 Egypt)', *Journal of Tropical Medicine and Hygiene*, 24(Supplement): 75–88.

Garrett, Eilidh and Reid, Alice (1995) 'Thinking of England and taking care: family building strategies and infant mortality in England and Wales 1891–1911', *International Journal of Population Geography*, 1(1): 69–102.

Garrett, E., Reid, A., Schurer, K. and Szreter, S. (2001) *Changing Family Size in England and Wales: Place, Class, and Demography, 1891–1911*, Cambridge: Cambridge University Press.

Garrett, Laurie (1996) *The Coming Plague: Newly Emerging Diseases in a World Out of Balance*, Harmondsworth: Penguin.

Gavrilovic, Z. (1995) 'The Spanish influenza pandemic in Sajkaska 1918–1919', *Medicinski pregled*, 48: 277–80.

Gear, J.H. (1983) 'The 1918 influenza epidemic', *Adler Museum Bulletin*, 1983: 13–20.

Gernhart, G. (1999) 'A forgotten enemy: PHS's fight against the 1918 influenza pandemic', *Public Health Reports*, 114(6): 559–61.

Gibbs, M.J., Armstrong, J.S. and Gibbs, A.J. (2001) 'Recombination in the hemagglutinin gene of the 1918 "Spanish flu" ', *Science*, 293(5536): 1842–5.

Gill, Clifford A. (1928) *The Genesis of Epidemics and the Natural History of Disease*, London: Baillière, Tindall and Cox.

Gladwell, Malcolm (1997) 'The Dead Zone', *New Yorker*, 29 September: 52–65.

Glezen, W.P. (1980) 'Considerations of the risk of influenza in children and indications for prophylaxis', *Review of Infectious Diseases*, 2(3): 408–20.

Glezen, W.P., Couch, R.B. and Six, H.R. (1982) 'The influenza herald wave', *American Journal of Epidemiology*, 116: 344–402.

Glezen, W.P., Paredes, A., Taber, L.H. (1980) 'Influenza in children: relationship to other respiratory agents', *Journal of the American Medical Association*, 243(13): 1345–9.

Goodall, Brian (ed.) (1987) *The Penguin Dictionary of Human Geography*, Harmondsworth: Penguin Books.

Goto, H. and Kawaoka, Y. (1998) 'A novel mechanism for the acquisition of virulence by a human influenza A virus', *Proceedings of the National Academy of Sciences of the United States of America*, 95: 10224–8.

Gould, Peter (1969) *Spatial Diffusion*, Resource Paper No. 4, Commission on College Geography, Washington, DC: Association of American Geographers.

Gould, Peter (1993) *The Slow Plague: a Geography of the AIDS Pandemic*, Cambridge, MA: Blackwell Publishers.

Gouzien, Paul (1921–22) 'L'Epidémie d'influenza de 1918–1919 dans les colonies françaises', *Annales de Médecine et de Pharmacie Coloniale*, 19: 264–303, 443–78; and 20: 43–73.

Graham, Gillian Elizabeth (1996) 'Does maternal influenza cause schizophrenia? A Northwestern Ontario study', unpublished MA thesis, Lakehead University, Canada.

Graves, Charles (1969) *Invasion by Virus: Can it Happen Again?* London: Icon Books Limited.

Graves, Robert (1998) *Goodbye to All That*, Harmondsworth: Penguin.

Greenwood, Major (1935) *Epidemics and Crowd-Diseases: an Introduction to the Study of Epidemiology*, London: Williams & Norgate.

Gregg, Charles T. (1983) *A Virus of Love and Other Tales of Medical Detection*, New York: Charles Scribner's Sons.

Gribble, Constance J. (1997) '"We hope to live through it": nursing and the 1918 influenza epidemic. Lessons for this century and the next', unpublished MS thesis, Gonzaga University.

Grigg, J. (2002) *Lloyd George: War Leader 1916–1918*, London: Allen Lane.

Grist, N.R. (1979) 'Pandemic influenza 1918', *British Medical Journal*, December: 1632–3.

Guan, Y., Shortridge, K.F., Krauss, S. and Webster, R.G. (1997) 'Molecular characterization of H9N2 influenza viruses: were they the donors of "internal" genes of H5N1 viruses in Hong Kong?' *Proceedings of the National Academy of Sciences of the United States of America*, 96: 9363–9.

Guillaume, P. (1978) 'La Grippe a Bordeaux en 1918', *Annales de Démographie Historique*, 167–73.

Hägerstrand, T. (1952) 'The propagation of innovation waves', *Lund studies in Geography* B, 4: 3–19.

Hagmeier, J. Edwin (1981) 'The Hagmeier family, his medical career, Preston Springs', Oral history tape 019. Kitchener, Ontario: Kitchener Public Library.

Hall, S. and Sample, I (2005) 'Flu feared more than terror attack', *Guardian*. Online, available at: www.guardian.co.uk/birdflu/story/0,,1397304,00.html.

Hamer, William H. (1918) *Report of the County Medical Officer of Health and School Medical Officer for the Year 1918*, London: London County Council.

Hamer, William H. (1919a) *Report of the County Medical Officer of Health and School Medical Officer for the Year 1919*, London: London County Council.

Hamer, William H. (1919b) *Report on influenza by the County Medical Officer of Health*, London: London County Council.

Hamilton, Diane (1992) 'Unanswered questions of the Spanish flu pandemic', *Bulletin of the American Association for the History of Nursing*, 34: 6–7.

Hammer, Margaret Anne Elisabeth (1995) ' "The building of a nation's health": the life, and work of George Newman to 1921', unpublished PhD thesis, University of Cambridge.

Hammond, J.A.B., Rolland, W. and Shore, T.H.G. (1917) 'Purulent bronchitis: a study of cases occurring amongst the British troops at a base in France', *The Lancet*, 94(14 July): 41–5.

Hartwig, G.W. and Patterson, K.D. (eds) (1978) *Disease in African History – An Introductory Survey and Case Studies*, Durham, N.C.: Duke University Press.

Harris, B. (1993) 'The demographic impact of the First World War: an anthropometric perspective', *Social History of Medicine*, 6: 343–66.

Hayden, F.G. (2001) 'Perspectives on antiviral use during pandemic influenza', *Philosophical Transactions: Biological Sciences*, 356(1416): 1877–84.

Heagerty, John J. (1928) *Four Centuries of Medical History in Canada*, Toronto: The Macmillan Company of Canada.

Heiser, Victor (1936) *An American Doctor's Odyssey*, New York: W.W. Norton & Co.

Henrikson, Viktor (1956) *Läkaren Berättar*, Stockholm: Lars Hökerbegs Bokförlag.

Henrikson, Viktor (1959) *A Doctor's Story*, trans. Maurice Michael, London: Michael Joseph.

Herda, Phyllis (1998) 'Disease and colonialism in the Pacific: the 1918 influenza pandemic in Western Polynesia', paper presented at The Spanish 'Flu 1918–1998: Reflections on the Influenza Pandemic of 1918 after 80 Years, Cape Town, 12–15 September.

Herda, Phyllis (1999) 'Re: Influenza nomenclature' (pers. comm).

Herring, D. Ann (1994) ' "There were young people and old people and babies dying every week": the 1918–1919 influenza pandemic at Norway House', *Ethnohistory*, 41(1): 73–105.

Herring, D. Ann and Sattenspiel, Lisa (2003) 'Death in winter: the Spanish flu in the Canadian Subarctic', in H. Phillips and D. Killingray (eds) *The Spanish Flu Pandemic of 1918–19: New Perspectives*, London: Routledge.

Higgins, Andrew (1997) 'Tracking down a mutant virus', *Guardian*, 10 December: 15.

Hildreth, Martha L. (1991) 'The influenza epidemic of 1918–1919 in France: contemporary concepts of aetiology, therapy and prevention', *Social History of Medicine*, 4(2): 277–94.

Hildreth, Martha L. (1992) 'Lyon and Marseilles', in F.R. van Hartesveldt (ed.) *1918–1919 Pandemic of Influenza: the Urban Impact in the Western World*, London: Edwin Mellen Press.

Hirsch, August (1883) *Handbook of Geographical and Historical Pathology*, 2nd edn, trans. Charles Creighton, London: New Sydenham Society.

Hoare, B. (1919) *The Two Plagues: Influenza and Bolshevism*, Melbourne: Progressive and Economic Association.

Hoehling, A.A. (1961) *The Great Epidemic*, Boston: Little, Brown and Company.

Hofheinz, Clara R. (1948) *What is Influenza? Why Be Afraid of It?* Barnes (London): R.W. Simpson.

Honigsbaum, Frank (1970) *The Struggle for the Ministry of Health, 1914–1919, Occasional Papers on Social Administration, no. 37*, London: Bell.

Hoyle, Ethelbert Petrie (1935) *How to Cure Influenza*, London: Homeopathic Publishing Company.

Huntington, Ellsworth (1923) 'Causes of geographical variations in the influenza epidemic of 1918 in the cities of the United States', *Bulletin of the National Research Council*, 6, No. 34.

Hutchinson, George Evelyn (1965) *The Ecological Theater and the Evolutionary Play*, New Haven, CT: Yale University Press.

Hyam, William (1963) *The Road to Harley Street*, London: Geoffrey Bles.

Hyslop, A. (1984) 'A plague on whose house? Ballarat and the Spanish Influenza of 1919', in Harold Attwood and R.W. Home (eds) *Patients, Practitioners and Techniques. Second National Conference on Medicine and Health in Australia 1984*, Melbourne: University of Melbourne.

Hyslop, A. (1995) 'Old ways, new means: fighting Spanish influenza in Australia, 1918–1919', in L. Bryder and D.A. Dow (eds) *New Countries and Old Medicine: Proceedings of an International Conference on the History of Medicine and Health*, Auckland: Auckland Medical Historical Society.

Hyslop, A. (1996) 'Fever hospital', in D. Dunstan (ed.) *Victorian Icon: The Royal Exhibition Building, Melbourne*, Melbourne: The Exhibition Trustees.

Hyslop, A. (1998a) 'A question of identity: J.H.L. Cumpston and Spanish influenza, 1918–1919', *Australian Cultural History*, 16: 60–76.

Hyslop, A. (1998b) 'Insidious immigrant: Spanish influenza and border quarantine in Australia 1919', in S. Parry (ed.) *From Migration to Mining: Medicine and Health in Australian History*, Darwin, NT: Historical Society of the Northern Territory.

Hyslop, Anthea (1998c) '"Lots of people blamed the soldiers": Australian recollections of the Spanish influenza pandemic, 1918–1919', paper presented at The Spanish 'Flu 1918–1998: Reflections on the Influenza Pandemic of 1918 after 80 Years, Cape Town, 12–15 September.

Iijima, Wataru (1998) 'The Spanish influenza in China, 1918–1920', paper presented at The Spanish 'Flu 1918–1998: Reflections on the Influenza Pandemic of 1918 after 80 Years, Cape Town, 12–15 September.

Inglis, Brian (1981) *The Diseases of Civilisation*, London: Hodder and Stoughton.

Instituto Centrale di Statistica (1958) *Sommario di Statistiche Storiche Italiane 1861–1955*, Roma: Instituto Centrale di Statistica.

Irwin, R.T. (1981) '1918 influenza in Morris County', *New Jersey Historical Commission Newsletter*, Trenton, NJ: New Jersey Historical Commission.

James, A.T.S. (1923) *Twenty-five Years of the L.M.S.*, London: London Missionary Society.

Jenkins, Virginia S. (1998) 'The 1918 Spanish flu pandemic: what the American people knew', paper presented at The Spanish 'Flu 1918–1998: Reflections on the Influenza Pandemic of 1918 after 80 Years, Cape Town, 12–15 September.

Johnson, Ace (1939) *Influenza*, Washington, DC: Library of Congress. Audio recording AFC 1939/001 3552b3.

Johnson, N.P.A.S. (1993) 'Pandemic influenza: an analysis of the spread of influenza in Kitchener, October 1918', unpublished MA thesis, Wilfrid Laurier University, Canada.

Johnson, N.P.A.S. (1998) 'Kitchener's forgotten struggle: the 1918 influenza pandemic experience', *Waterloo Historical Society*, 85: 41–67.

Johnson, N.P.A.S. (2001) 'Aspects of the historical geography of the 1918–19 influenza pandemic in Britain', PhD thesis, University of Cambridge.

Johnson, N.P.A.S. (2003) 'The overshadowed killer: influenza in Britain in 1918–19', in H. Phillips and D. Killingray (eds) *The Spanish Flu Pandemic of 1918–19: New Perspectives*, London: Routledge.

Johnson, N.P.A.S. (2004a) 'Scottish 'Flu – the Scottish mortality experience of the "Spanish flu"', *Scottish Historical Review*, 83: 216–26.

Johnson, N.P.A.S. (2004b) 'Measuring a pandemic: mortality, demography and geography', *Popolazione e Storia*, 2: 21–52.

Johnson, N.P.A.S. and Mueller, J. (2002) 'Updating the accounts: Global mortality of the 1918–1920 Spanish influenza pandemic', *Bulletin of the History of Medicine*, 76: 105–15.

Jones, James (1981) *Bad Blood: the Tuskegee Syphilis Experiment*, New York: Free Press.

Jordan, Edwin Oakes (1927) *Epidemic Influenza: a Survey*, Chicago: American Medical Association.

Jorge, R. (1919) *La Grippe*. Lisbon.

Kallir, J. (1998) *Egon Schiele: the Complete Works*, London: Thames and Hudson.

Kanfer, S. (2000) *Groucho: the Life and Times of Julius Henry Marx*, Harmondsworth: Penguin.

Kaplan, Martin M. and Webster, Robert G. (1977) 'The epidemiology of influenza', *Scientific American*, 237 (6): 88–106.

Kass, A.M. (1993) 'Infectious diseases at the Boston City Hospital: the first 60 years', *Clinical Infectious Diseases*, 17(2): 276–82.

Katz, Robert S. (1974) 'Influenza 1918–1919: a study in mortality', *Bulletin of the History of Medicine*, 48: 416–22.

Katz, Robert S. (1977) 'Influenza 1918–1919: a further study in mortality', *Bulletin of the History of Medicine*, 51: 617–19.

Katzenellenbogen, J.M. (1988) 'The 1918 influenza epidemic in Mamre', *South African Medical Journal*, 74: 362–4.

Kearns, G. (1988) 'The urban penalty and the population history of England', in A. Brändström and L.G. Tedebrand (eds) *Society, Health and Population During the Demographic Transition*, Stockholm: Almqvist and Wiksell International.

Kearns, G. (1995) 'Tuberculosis and the medicalisation of British society, 1880–1920', in John Woodword and Robert Jütte (eds) *Coping with Sickness: Historical Aspects of Health Care in a European Perspective*, Sheffield: European Association for the History of Medicine and Health Publications.

Keegan, John (ed.) (1989) *The Times Atlas of the Second World War*, London: Times Books.

Keen Payne, R. (2000) 'We must have nurses: Spanish influenza in America 1918–1919', *Nursing History Review*, 8: 143–56.

Kelm, Mary-Ellen (1998) '"With all kinds of colours going through the sky": First Nations' perspectives on the influenza pandemic of 1918–19', paper presented at The Spanish 'Flu 1918–1998: Reflections on the Influenza Pandemic of 1918 after 80 Years, Cape Town, 12–15 September.

Kelm, Mary-Ellen (1999) 'Re: First Nations nomenclature' (pers. comm).

Kendal, A.P. (1987) 'Epidemiologic implications of changes in the influenza virus genome', *American Journal of Medicine*, 82(Suppl. 6A): 4–14.

Kendal, A.P. and Glezen, W.P. (1998) 'Pandemic influenza and pregnancy: lessons from the past, and considerations about use of live Attenuated vaccines', paper presented at The Spanish 'Flu 1918–1998: Reflections on the Influenza Pandemic of 1918 after 80 Years, Cape Town, 12–15 September.

Kerr, K. (2002) *Unity (1918)*, Vancouver, BC: Talonbooks.

Kilbourne, Edwin D. (1977) 'Influenza Pandemics in Perspective', *Journal of the American Medical Association*, 237(12): 1225–8.

Kilbourne, Edwin D. (1980) 'Influenza: viral determinants of the pathogenicity and epidemicity of an invariant disease of variable occurrence', *Philosophical Transactions of the Royal Society of London. Series B: Biological Sciences*, 288: 291–7.

Kilbourne, Edwin D. (1987) *Influenza*, New York: Plenum Medical Books.

Kilbourne, Edwin D. (1998) 'A virologist's perspective on the 1918–19 pandemic', paper presented at The Spanish 'Flu 1918–1998: Reflections on the Influenza Pandemic of 1918 after 80 Years, Cape Town, 12–15 September.

Killingray, David (1994) 'The influenza pandemic of 1918–1919 in the British Caribbean', *Social History of Medicine*, 7(1): 60–87.

Killingray, David (1996) 'A new "imperial disease": the influenza pandemic of 1918–19 and its impact on the British Empire', paper presented at the Annual Conference of the Society for Social History of Medicine, Oxford.

King, D. Barty (1922) *Studies in Influenza and its Pulmonary Complications*, London: J. & A. Churchill.

King, Francine (1992) 'Atlanta', in F.R. van Hartesveldt (ed.) *1918–1919 Pandemic of Influenza: the Urban Impact in the Western World*, London: Edwin Mellen Press.

Kiple, Kenneth F. (ed.) (1993) *The Cambridge World History of Human Disease*, Cambridge: Cambridge University Press.

Kiple, Kenneth F. (ed.) (1997) *Plague, Pox and Pestilence: Disease in History*, London: Weidenfeld & Nicolson.

Kipling, Rudyard (1995) *Rudyard Kipling: the Complete Verse*, London: Kyle Cathie.

Kirkpatrick, G.W. (1986) 'Influenza 1918: a Maine perspective', *Maine Historical Society Quarterly*, 25(3): 162–77.

Klark, Happy and Brown, A.C. (1918) *The I-N-F-L-U-E-N-Z-A Blues*, McAlester, OK: Brown Music Co. (Song).

Knibbs, G.H. (1920) 'The influenza epidemic of 1918–19', paper presented at the Australasian Medical Congress, *Transactions*, Eleventh Session, Brisbane.

Kobasa, D., Takada, A., Shinya, K., *et al.* (2004) 'Enhanced virulence of influenza A viruses with the haemagglutinin of the 1918 pandemic virus', *Nature*, 431 (7 October): 703–7.

Koblenz, Lawrence W. (1998) 'A judgement in time: medical responses to the 1918–1919 influenza epidemic in the United States', paper presented at The Spanish 'Flu 1918–1998: Reflections on the Influenza Pandemic of 1918 after 80 Years, Cape Town, 12–15 September.

Kolata, Gina B. (1999) *Flu: the Story of the Great Influenza Pandemic of 1918 and the Search for the Virus That Caused It*, New York: Farrar, Strauss and Giroux.

Kunzru, H. (2002) *The Impressionist*, London: Hamish Hamilton.

Langford, C.M. (2002) 'The age pattern of mortality in the 1918–19 influenza pandemic: an attempted explanation based on data for England and Wales', *Medical History*, 46: 1–20.

Langford, C.M. and Storey, P. (1992) 'Influenza in Sri Lanka, 1918–1919: the impact of a new disease in a pre-modern Third World setting', *Health Transition Review*, 2 (Supplementary Issue): 97–123.

Larson, Erik (1998) 'The flu hunters', *Time (Canadian edition)*, 23 February: 30–40.

Lautaret, R.L. (1971) 'Alaska's greatest disaster: the 1918 Spanish influenza epidemic', *Alaska Journal*, 16: 238–43.

Laver, G. and Webster, R.G. (2001) 'Introduction', *Philosophical Transactions: Biological Sciences* 356(1416): 1813–15.

Law, C.M. (1967) 'The growth of urban population in England and Wales, 1801–1911', *Transactions of the Institute of British Geographers*, 41: 125–43.

Lawrence, Christopher (1999) 'Edward Jenner's jockey boots and the great tradition in English medicine 1918–1939', paper presented at the Society for the Social History of Medicine, University of Glasgow, 17 July.

Lawton, R. and Pooley, C.G. (1992) *Britain 1740–1950: An Historical Geography*, London: Edward Arnold.

Lederberg, Joshua (1991) 'Pandemic as a natural evolutionary phenomenon', in Arien Mack (ed.) *In Time of Plague: the History and Social Consequences of Lethal Epidemic Disease*, New York: New York University Press.

Lederberg, Joshua (1997) 'Infectious disease as an evolutionary paradigm', *Emerging Infectious Diseases*, 3(4): 417–23.

Lees, Lynn Hollen (1998) *The Solidarities of Strangers: the English Poor Laws and the People, 1700–1948*, Cambridge: Cambridge University Press.

Léon, Henri M. (1921) *Influenza: its History, Symptomology and Treatment*, London: London College of Physiology.

Levinthal, W., Kuczynski, and Wolff, E. (1921) *Epidemiologie, Ätiologie, Pathomorphologie und Pathogenese der Grippe*, Munich and Wiesbaden: Verlag Von J.F. Bergmann.

Lewis, R. (2002) *Anthony Burgess*, London: Faber and Faber.

Link, A.S. (1984) *Papers of Woodrow Wilson*. Vol. 45. Nov. 11 1917–Jan. 15, 1918, Princeton: Princeton University Press.

Linnanmäki, E. (1998) 'Spanish flu in Finnish cities, 1918–1920', paper presented at The Spanish 'Flu 1918–1998: Reflections on the Influenza Pandemic of 1918 after 80 Years, Cape Town, 12–15 September.

Linnanmäki, E. (1999) 'Re: Early outbreak?' (pers. comm).

Linnanmäki, E. (2000) 'Last outbreak of the Spanish flu in 1920: Influenza in Lapland, Finland', paper presented at the Congress on the History of Medicine, Galveston, TX.

Lister, Frederick Spencer (1922) 'A filter-passing micro-organism associated with epidemic influenza', *South African Medical Record*, XX: 434–6.

Lister, Frederick Spencer and Taylor, E. (1919) *Observations and Experimental Investigations in Epidemic Influenza, Publications of the South African Institute for Medical Research, No. XII*. Johannesburg: Hortors Limited.

Local Government Board (1918) *Memorandum on Epidemic Catarrhs and Influenza*, London: HMSO (signed by Arthur Newsholme).

Local Government Board (1919a) *Memorandum on Pneumonia*, London: HMSO (signed by Arthur Newsholme).

Local Government Board (1919b) *Memorandum on Prevention of Influenza*, London: HMSO.

Löwy, Ilana (1998) 'Yellow fever – the known and the lesser known aspects of experimentation on humans', paper presented at Modern Biomedicine Programme seminar, Department of History and Philosophy of Science, University of Cambridge, 2 February.

Luckingham, B. (1984a) *Epidemic in the Southwest 1918–1919*, El Paso, TX: Texas Western Press, University of Texas at El Paso.

Luckingham, B. (1984b) 'To mask or not to mask: a note on the 1918 Spanish influenza epidemic in Tucson', *The Journal of Arizona History*, 25(2): 191–204.

Luk, J., Gross, P. and Thompson, W.W. (2001) 'Observations on mortality during the 1918 influenza pandemic', *Clinical Infectious Diseases*, 33(8): 1375–8.

McBride, David (1991) *From TB to AIDS: epidemics among urban blacks since 1900*, New York: State University of New York Press.

McConnell, C.P. (2000) 'The treatment of influenza. 1918', *Journal of the American Osteopathic Association*, 100(5): 311–13.

McCracken, Kevin and Curson, Peter (2003) 'Flu downunder: a demographic and geographic analysis of the 1918 pandemic in Sydney, Australia', in H. Phillips and D. Killingray (eds) *The Spanish Flu Pandemic of 1918–19: New Perspectives*, London: Routledge.

McCreery, David (1992) 'Guatemala City', in F.R. van Hartesveldt (ed.) *1918–1919 Pandemic of Influenza: the Urban Impact in the Western World*, London: Edwin Mellen Press.

Macdonald, Peter Horne (1919) *Influenza and Air-Borne Diseases*, Auckland: Whitcombe & Tombs Limited.

McDowell, R.B. (1997) *Crisis and Decline: the Fate of the Southern Unionists*, Dublin: Lilliput Press.

McFadden, S., Prine, B. and Shors, T. (2001) 'Oshkosh in 1918: an interdisciplinary study of the 1918 influenza epidemic'. Available from: www.uwosh.edu/archives/flu/home.html.

McGinnis, Janice P. Dickin (1976) 'A city faces an epidemic', *Alberta History,* 24(4): 1–11.

McGinnis, Janice P. Dickin (1977) 'The impact of epidemic influenza: Canada 1918–1919', *Historical Papers,* 1977: 120–40.

McIntosh, James (1922) 'Studies in the aetiology of epidemic influenza', Special Report Series No. 63, London: Medical Research Council.

McKenzie, Andrea (2000) 'Comparative catastrophe: 1918, influenza and sanctioned memories', paper presented at The Memory of Catastrophe, University of Southampton, 14–17 April.

MacKenzie, J.S. and Houghton, M. (1974) 'Influenza infections during pregnancy: association with congenital malformations and with subsequent neoplasms in children, and potential hazards of live virus vaccines', *Bacteriological Reviews*, 38(4): 356–70.

Mackie, A.H. (1949) *Memories of a Scotch Doctor*, Aberdeen: Aberdeen University Press.

McNeill, William H. (1977) *Plagues and Peoples*, London: Basil Blackwell.

McPherson, Robert S. (1990) 'The influenza pandemic of 1918: a cultural response', *Utah Historical Quarterly,* 58(2): 183–200.

MacPherson, W.G., Herringham, W.P., Elliott, T.R. and Balfour, A. (eds) (1920) *History of the Great War Based on Official Documents. Medical Services. Diseases of the War*, London: HMSO.

McQueen, H. (1976) 'The "Spanish" influenza pandemic in Australia, 1918–19', in J. Roe (ed.) *Social Policy in Australia: Some Perspectives 1901–1975*, Stanmore: Cassell Australia.

McShane, C.K. (1968) 'The 1918 Kansas City influenza epidemic', *Missouri Historical Review,* 63: 55–70.

Mamelund, Svenn-Erik (1998a) 'Estimating the death toll of Spanish influenza 1918–19: the case of Norway', paper presented at The Spanish 'Flu 1918–1998: Reflections on the Influenza Pandemic of 1918 after 80 Years, Cape Town, 12–15 September.

Mamelund, Svenn-Erik (1998b) 'Spanskeskyen i Norge 1918–1920: Diffusjon og demografiske konsekvenser', unpublished Masters thesis, University of Oslo.

Mamelund, Svenn-Erik (2003) 'Spanish influenza mortality of ethnic minorities in Norway 1918–1919', *European Journal of Population*, 19: 83–102.

Mamelund, Svenn-Erik (2004) 'Can the Spanish influenza pandemic of 1918 explain the baby-boom of 1920 in neutral Norway?', *Population*, 59(2): 229–60.

Mamelund, Svenn-Erik (2006) 'A socially neutral disease? Individual social class, household wealth and mortality from Spanish influenza in two socially contrasting parishes in Kristiania 1918–19', *Social Science and Medicine*, 62: 923–46.

Mann, Jonathon M. and Tarantola, Daniel J.M. (eds) (1996) *AIDS in the World II*, Oxford: Oxford University Press.

Marker, Chris (1962) *La Jetée*, Agros Films. (Also published as Marker, C. (1962) *La Jetée: ciné-romain*, New York: Zone Books.)

Marker, Chris (1982) *Sans Soleil* (film).

Marks, Geoffrey and Beatty, William (1976) *Epidemics*, New York: Charles Scribner's Sons.

Martin, G. (1921) 'Cameroun, L'epidémie d'influenza de 1918–1919', *Annales de Médecine et de Pharmacie Coloniale*, 19: 444–8.

Mattock, C., Marmot, M. and Stern, G. (1988), 'Could Parkinson's disease follow intra-uterine influenza? A speculative hypothesis', *Journal of Neurology, Neurosurgery and Psychiatry*, 51: 735–56.

Maurizi, Charles P. (1984) 'Influenza and schizophrenia: a possible connection with the substantia nigra', *Medical Hypotheses*, 15: 163–7.

Maurizi, Charles P. (1985) 'Why was the 1918 influenza pandemic so lethal? The possible role of a neurovirulent neuraminidase', *Medical Hypotheses*, 16: 1–5.

Maximilian, Prince of Baden (1928) *Memoirs*, London: Constable.

Maxwell, W. (1988) *So Long, See You Tomorrow*, London: Secker and Warburg.

Maxwell, W. (1995) *All The Days and Nights*, New York: Alfred A. Knopf.

Meikle, J. (2005) 'UK to buy anti-flu drugs for 14 million', *Guardian*. Online, available from: www.guardian.co.uk/birdflu/story/0,14207,1428292,00. html?=rss.

Melzer, R. (1982) 'A dark and terrible moment: the Spanish flu epidemic of 1918 in New Mexico', *New Mexico Historical Review*, 57(3): 213–36.

Menninger, K.A. (1994) 'Influenza and schizophrenia: an analysis of post-influenzal "dementia precox," as of 1918, and five years later further studies of the psychiatric aspects of influenza. 1926', *American Journal of Psychiatry*, 151(6 Suppl.): 182–7.

Metzger, B.H.M. (2001) 'The League of Nations and human rights: from practice to theory', unpublished PhD thesis, University of Cambridge.

Mihaly, Arpad S. (1998) 'Epidemics resulting from wars – a secret bond between slowness and memory, between speed and forgetting: the "Spanish flu" pandemic of 1919 as experienced by AIF troops quarantined in Port Phillip Bay, Australia', paper presented at The Spanish 'Flu 1918–1998: Reflections on the Influenza Pandemic of 1918 after 80 Years, Cape Town, 12–15 September.

Millard, S. (1936) *I Saw Them Die*, London: George G. Harrap & Co.

Miller, D.L. and Farmer, R.D.T. (1982) *Epidemiology of Diseases*, Oxford: Oxford University Press.

Mills, Ian D. (1986) 'The 1918–1919 influenza pandemic – the Indian experience', *Indian Economic and Social History Review*, 23(1): 1–40.

Ministry of Health (1919a) 'Influenza vaccine: instructions to medical officers of health', London: HMSO, 1919 (signed by George Newman).

Ministry of Health (1919b) 'Memorandum on prevention of influenza', London: HMSO (signed by George Newman).

Ministry of Health (1920a), 'Influenza: hints and precautions', London: HMSO (signed by George Newman).

Ministry of Health (1920b) 'Notification of infectious diseases', circular 85, London: HMSO.

Ministry of Health (1920c) 'Report on the pandemic of influenza 1918–1919', Reports on Public Health and Medical Subjects, No. 4, London: HMSO.

Ministry of Health (1921) 'Incidence of notifiable infectious diseases in each sanitary district in England and Wales during the year 1920', Reports on Public Health and Medical Subjects, No. 5, London: HMSO.

Ministry of Health (1927) Memorandum on influenza (revised edition)', London: HMSO.

Ministry of Health (1928) 'Report of an inquiry into the after-histories of persons attacked by encephalitis lethargica', Reports on Public Health and Medical Subjects, No. 49, London: HMSO.

Ministry of Health (1929) 'Influenza and common colds', circulars 761 and 955, London: HMSO.

Ministry of Health (1935a) 'Memorandum on pneumonia', London: HMSO.

Ministry of Health (1935b) 'Pneumonia', circular 1499, London: HMSO.

Mitchell, B.R. (1992) *International Historical Statistics Europe 1750–1988*, 3rd end, New York: Stockton.

Mitchell, B.R. (1995) *International Historical Statistics Africa, Asia and Oceania 1750–1988*, 2nd edn, New York: Stockton.

Mitchell, B.R. (1998) *International Historical Statistics The Americas 1750–1993*, 4th edn, New York: Stockton.

Mokyr, Joel (1980) 'The deadly fungus: an econometric investigation into the short-term demographic consequences of the Irish famine 1846–1851', *Research in Population Economics*, 2: 233–77.

Mokyr, Joel (1983) *Why Ireland Starved: a Quantitative and Analytical History of the Irish Economy, 1800–1830*, Oxford: Clarendon Press.

Monto, A.S. (2005) 'The threat of an avian influenza pandemic', *New England Journal of Medicine*, 352(4): 323–5.

Mooney, Graham (1987) 'Professionalization in public health and the measurement of sanitary progress in nineteenth-century England and Wales', *Social History of Medicine*, 10(17): 53–78.

Moore, J.S. (1993) '"Jack Fisher's 'Flu": a visitation revisited', *Economic History Review*, XLVI(2): 280–307.

Morton, G. (1973) 'The pandemic influenza of 1918', *Canadian Nurse*, 69: 25–7.

Moss, John P. (1936) 'Influenza' (Letter). British Library.

Mueller, Juergen (1995) 'Patterns of reaction to a demographic crisis. The Spanish influenza pandemic (1918–1919) in sub-Saharan Africa. A research proposal and preliminary regional and comparative findings', Department of History. Staff Seminar Paper No. 6 (1994/95), Nairobi: University of Nairobi.

Mueller, Juergen (1998) 'What's in a name? Spanish influenza in sub-Saharan Africa and what local names say about the perception of this pandemic', paper presented at The Spanish 'Flu 1918–1998: Reflections on the Influenza Pandemic of 1918 after 80 Years, Cape Town, 12–15 September.

Mullen, P.C. and Nelson, M.L. (1987) 'Montanans and "the most peculiar disease": the influenza epidemic and public health, 1918–1919', *Montana: the Magazine of Western History,* 37(2): 50–61.

Müller, Jürgen (1996) 'Die spanische Influenza 1918/19. Der Einfluß des Ersten Weltkrieges auf Auusbreitung, Krankheitsverlauf und Perzeption einer Pandemie (The influence of the First World War on the spread, course of disease and perception of a pandemic)', in Wolfgang U. Eckart and Christoph Gradmann (eds) *Die Medizin und der Erste Weltkrieg*, Pfaffenweiler: Centaurus-Verlagsgesellschaft.

Musambachime, Mwelwa C. (1998) '"A great catastrophe: the blood of the dead soldiers is killing us": African reactions to the influenza pandemic of 1918/1919 in Northern Rhodesia (Zambia) and Nyasaland (Malawi)', paper presented at The Spanish 'Flu 1918–1998: Reflections on the Influenza Pandemic of 1918 after 80 Years, Cape Town, 12–15 September.

Neustadt, Richard E. and Fineberg, Harvey V. (1978) *The Swine Flu Affair: Decision-making on a Slippery Disease*, Washington, DC: Government Printing Office.

New South Wales (1920) 'Report of the Director-General for 1919, including a Report on the Influenza Epidemic, 1919, Sydney: NSW Legislative Council and Legislative Assembly.

New Zealand (1919) 'Report of the influenza epidemic commission', Wellington.

Nicholson, K.G., Wood, J.M. and Zamba, M. (2003) 'Influenza', *The Lancet*, 362: 1733–45.

Niven, J. (1923) *Observations on the History of Public Health Effort in Manchester*, Manchester: J. Heywood.

Noble, Ernest (1918) 'A-TICH-OO!! Good evening. I'm the new influenza', London. Pen and ink drawing with wash. Wellcome Library for the History and Understanding of Medicine Iconographic Collection 16001.

Noll, Kenneth (1989) 'When the plague hit Spokane', *Pacific Northwesterner,* 31(1): 1–7.

North, Sterling and Schoenherr, John (1963) *Rascal, a Memoir of a Better Era*, New York: Dutton.

Norway (annual) *Statistical Yearbooks of Norway*, Oslo.

Noyes, William Raymond (1968) 'Influenza epidemic 1918–1919: a misplaced chapter in United States social and institutional history', unpublished PhD thesis, UCLA.

Noymer, Andrew and Garenne, Michel (1998) 'Long-term effects of the 1918 "Spanish" influenza on sex differentials of mortality in the USA: exploratory findings from historical data', paper presented at The Spanish 'Flu 1918–1998: Reflections on the Influenza Pandemic of 1918 after 80 Years, Cape Town, 12–15 September.

Ó Gráda, Cormac (1994) *Ireland: a New Economic History 1780–1939*, Oxford: Clarendon Press.

Ohadike, D.C. (1981) 'The influenza pandemic of 1918–19 and the spread of cassava cultivation on the Lower Niger: a study of historical linkages', *Journal of African History,* 22: 379–91.

Ohadike, D.C. (1991) 'Diffusion and physiological responses to the influenza pandemic of 1918–19 in Nigeria', *Social Science and Medicine,* 32(12): 1393–9.

Olinto, B. Anselmo (1993) '"Uma Epidemia sem Importância" A Influenza Espanhola e o Colapso do Sistema de Saúde no Sul do Brasil, 1918', *Quipu,* 10(3): 285–303.

Oliver, W. (1919) *Spanish Influenza: All About It*, Melbourne: Speciality Press.

Olm, Kristin (1998) 'The Spanish flu in Saxony', paper presented at The Spanish 'Flu 1918–1998: Reflections on the Influenza Pandemic of 1918 after 80 Years, Cape Town, 12–15 September.

Opie, Eugene L., Blake, Francis G., Small, James C. and Rivers, Thomas M. (1921) *Epidemic Respiratory Disease: the Pneumonias and Other Infections of the Respiratory Tract Accompanying Influenza and Measles*, London: Henry Kimpton.

Osborn, June E. (ed.) (1977) *Influenza in America 1918–1976*, New York: Prodist.

Ott, Katherine (1996) *Fevered Lives: Tuberculosis in American Culture since 1870*, Cambridge, MA: Harvard University Press.

Overy, Richard James (1998) *Russia's War*, London: Allen Lane.

Oxford, J.S. (2001) 'The so-called Great Spanish Influenza Pandemic of 1918 may have originated in France in 1916', *Philosophical Transactions of the Royal Society of London. Series B: Biological Sciences*, 356(1416): 1857–9.

Oxford, J.S. and Al-Jabri, A. (1996) 'Specific antiviral therapy of respiratory viruses', in S. Myint and D. Taylor-Robinson (eds) *Viral and Other Infections of the Human Respiratory Tract*, London: Chapman and Hall.

Oxford, J.S., Sefton, A., Jackson, R., Johnson, N.P.A.S. and Daniels, R.S. (1999) 'Who's that lady?', *Nature Medicine,* 5(12): 1351–2.

Oxford, J.S., Sefton, A., Jackson, R., Innes, W., Daniels, R.S. and Johnson, N.P.A.S. (2001) 'Early herald wave outbreaks of influenza in 1916 prior to the pandemic of 1918', in A.D.M.E. Osterhaus, N. Cox and A.W. Hampson (eds) *Options for the Control of Influenza IV*, Amsterdam: Elsevier.

Oxford, J.S., Sefton, A., Jackson, R., Innes, W., Daniels, R.S. and Johnson, N.P. (2002) 'World War I may have allowed the emergence of "Spanish" influenza', *The Lancet infectious diseases,* 2(2): 111–14.

Page, Melvin E. (1998) 'The 'fluenza on the road to Vua: a Nyasaland case study of a medical crisis and colonial politics', paper presented at The Spanish 'Flu 1918–1998: Reflections on the Influenza Pandemic of 1918 after 80 Years, Cape Town, 12–15 September.

Palmer, E. and Rice, Geoffrey W. (1992) 'A Japanese physician's response to pandemic influenza: Ijiro Gomibuchi and the "Spanish flu", in Yaita-Cho, 1918–1919', *Bulletin of the History of Medicine*, 66: 560–77.

Pankhurst, Richard (1989) 'The great Ethiopian influenza epidemic of 1918', *Ethiopian Medical Journal,* 27(4): 235–42.

Parini, J. (1994) *John Steinbeck: a Biography*, London: Heinemann.

Park, Katherine (1993) 'Black Death', in Kenneth F. Kiple (ed.) *The Cambridge World History of Human Disease*, Cambridge: Cambridge University Press.

Patterson, Karl David (1983) 'The influenza epidemic of 1918–19 in the Gold Coast', *Journal of African History,* 24: 485–502.

Patterson, Karl David (1986) *Pandemic Influenza 1700–1900*, Totowa: Rowman and Littlefield.

Patterson, Karl David and Pyle, Gerald F. (1983) 'The diffusion of influenza in sub-Saharan African during the 1918–19 pandemic', *Social Science and Medicine,* 17(17): 1299–1307.

Patterson, Karl David and Pyle, Gerald F. (1991) 'The geography and mortality of the 1918 influenza pandemic', *Bulletin of the History of Medicine,* 65(1): 4–21.

Pearson, A.B. (1919) 'The influenza epidemic', *New Zealand Journal of Science and Technology*, July: 253–6.

Peiris, M., Yuen, K., Leung, C., Chan, K., Ip, P., Lai, R., Orr, W. and Shortridge, K. (1999) 'Human infection with influenza H9N2', *The Lancet*, 354: 916–17.

Pemberton, John (1970) *Will Pickles of Wensleydale*, London: Geoffrey Bles.

Peterson, Richard (1992) 'San Diego', in F.R. van Hartesveldt (ed.) *1918–1919 Pandemic of Influenza: the Urban Impact in the Western World*, London: Edwin Mellen Press.

Pettigrew, Eileen (1983) *The Silent Enemy: Canada and the Deadly Flu of 1918*, Saskatoon: Western Producer Prairie Books.

Pettit, Dorothy Ann (1976) 'A cruel wind: America experiences pandemic influenza, 1918–1920: a social history', unpublished PhD thesis, University of New Hampshire.

Pfeiffer, Richard (1931) 'Die Aetiologie der Influenza', in R. Dujarric de Rivière *et al.* (eds) *Premier Congress International de Microbiologie*, Paris: Masson.

Phillips, Howard (1987) 'The local state and public health reform in South Africa: Bloemfontein and the consequences of the Spanish 'Flu epidemic of 1918', *Journal of Southern African Studies*, 13(2): 210–33.

Phillips, Howard (1988) 'South Africa's worst demographic disaster: the Spanish influenza epidemic of 1918', *South African Historical Journal*, 20: 57–73.

Phillips, Howard (1990a) *'Black October': the Impact of the Spanish Influenza Epidemic of 1918 on South Africa*, Archives Year Book for South African History, Pretoria: Government Printer.

Phillips, Howard (1990b) 'The origin of the Public Health Act of 1919', *South African Medical Journal*, 77(10): 531–2.

Phillips, Howard (2004) 'The re-appearing shadow of 1918: trends in the historiography of the 1918–19 influenza pandemic', *Canadian Bulletin of Medical History*, 21(1): 121–34.

Phimister, Ian R. (1973) 'The "Spanish" influenza pandemic of 1918 and its impact on the Southern Rhodesian mining industry', *Central African Journal of Medicine*, XIX(7): 143–8.

Pickles, William N. (1939) *Epidemiology in Country Practice*, Bristol: John Wright & Sons.

Pickrell, J. (2001) 'The 1918 pandemic: killer flu with a human–pig pedigree?', *Science*, 292(5519): 1041.

Pitt, B. (1962) *1918 The Last Act*, London: Cassell and Company.

Pool, D.I. (1973) 'The effects of the 1918 pandemic of influenza on the Maori population of New Zealand', *Bulletin of the History of Medicine*, 47(3): 273–81.

Porras Gallo, M.I. (1993a) 'La profilaxis de las enfermedades infecciosas tras la pandemia gripal de 1918–19: los seguros sociales', *Dynamis*, 13: 279–93.

Porras Gallo, M.I. (1993b) 'The Real Academia Nacional de Medicina and the problems surrounding the etiology of influenza in the 1918–19 epidemic', *Cuadernos Complutenses de historia de la medicina y de la ciencia*, 1: 103–28.

Porras Gallo, M.I. (1994a) 'The fight against "avoidable" diseases and the 1918–1919 influenza epidemic in Spain', *Dynamis*, 14: 159–83.

Porras Gallo, M.I. (1994b) 'La prensa madrileña de información general ante la epidemia de gripe de 1918–19', *Medicina e historia*, 3(574): I–XVI.

Porras Gallo, M.I. (1996) 'Repercussions of the influenza pandemic in 1918–1919 on mortality in Madrid', *Boletín de la Asociacíon de Demografía Histórica*, 14(1): 75–116.

Porras Gallo, M.I. (1997) *Un reto para la sociedad madrileña: la epidemia de gripe de 1918–19*, Madrid: Editorial Complutense.

Porter, Katherine Anne (1964) *Pale Horse, Pale Rider: Three Short Novels*, New York: Harcourt Brace & World.

Potter, J. (1997) '"A great purifier": the Great War in women's romances and memoirs 1914–1918', in S. Raitt and T. Tate (eds) *Women's Fiction and the Great War*, Oxford: Clarendon Press.

Potter, J. (2000) '"I alone am left to tell the tale...": memoirs by women on active service, 1914–1919', paper presented at The Memory of Catastrophe, University of Southampton, 14–17 April.

Puklin, Diane A.V. (1992) 'Paris', in F.R. van Hartesveldt (ed.) *1918–1919 Pandemic of Influenza: the Urban Impact in the Western World*, London: Edwin Mellen Press.

Pyle, Gerald F. (1986) *The Diffusion of Influenza: Patterns and Paradigms*, Totowa: Rowman and Littlefield.

Quiney, L.J. (2002) '"Filling the gaps": Canadian voluntary nurses, the 1917 Halifax explosion, and the influenza epidemic of 1918', *Canadian Bulletin of Medical History*, 19(2): 351–73.

Radford, Tim (1995) 'Vaccination warning as winter influenza arrives', *Guardian*, 4 October: 8.

Radford, Tim (1996) 'Flu Lazarus', *Guardian*, 10 October, 'Online' section: 8.

Radford, Tim (1998) 'Scientists find flu killer trigger', *Guardian*, 18 August: 9.

Radford, Tim and Ezard, John (1997) 'Hunt for the Satan bug crosses the world', *Guardian*, 9 October: 2.

Ramanna, Mridula (1998) 'Coping with the influenza pandemic, 1918–1919: the Bombay experience', paper presented at The Spanish 'Flu 1918–1998: Reflections on the Influenza Pandemic of 1918 after 80 Years, Cape Town, 12–15 September.

Ranger, Terence (1988) 'The influenza pandemic in Southern Rhodesia: a crisis of comprehension', in D. Arnold (ed.) *Imperial Medicine and Indigenous Societies*, Manchester: Manchester University Press.

Ranger, Terence (1992) 'Prophetic responses to epidemic in Africa', in Terence Ranger and Paul Slack (eds) *Epidemics and Ideas*, Oxford: Oxford University Press.

Ravenholt, R.T. (1993) 'Encephalitis lethargica', in Kenneth F. Kiple (ed.) *The Cambridge World History of Human Disease*, Cambridge: Cambridge University Press.

Ravenholt, R.T. and Foege, William H. (1982) '1918 Influenza, Encephalitis Lethargica, Parkinsonism', *The Lancet*, 16 October: 860–4.

Reddi, Sadasivam (1998) 'War, influenza and public health: a case study of the influenza of 1919 in Mauritius', paper presented at The Spanish 'Flu 1918–1998: Reflections on the Influenza Pandemic of 1918 after 80 Years, Cape Town, 12–15 September.

Registrar-General (1920) *Supplement to the Eighty-First Annual Report of the Registrar-General, Report on the Mortality from Influenza in England and Wales During the Epidemic of 1918–19*, London: HMSO.

Registrar-General (1921) *Registrar-General Decennial Supplement England and Wales 1921*, London: HMSO.

Registrar-General for Scotland (1919) *Report on the Mortality from Influenza in Scotland during the Epidemic of 1918–19: a Supplement to the Annual Reports of the Registrar-General for Scotland*, Edinburgh.

Reid, Alice (2005) 'The effects of the 1918–1919 influenza pandemic on infant and child health in Derbyshire', *Medical History*, 49: 29–54.

Reid, A.H. and Taubenberger, J.K. (1999) 'The 1918 flu and other influenza pandemics: "over there" and back again', *Laboratory Investigation*, 79(2): 95–101.

Reid, A.H. and Taubenberger, J.K. (2003) 'The origin of the 1918 pandemic influenza virus: a continuing enigma', *Journal of General Virology*, 84(9): 2285–92.

Reid, A.H., Fanning, T.G., Hultin, J.V. and Taubenberger, J.K. (1999) 'Origin and evolution of the 1918 "Spanish" influenza virus hemagglutinin gene', *Proceedings of the National Academy of Sciences of the United States of America*, 96(4): 1651–6.

Reid, A.H., Fanning, T.G., Janczewski, T.A. and Taubenberger, J.K. (2000), 'Characterization of the 1918 "Spanish" influenza virus neuraminidase gene', *Proceedings of the National Academy of Sciences of the United States of America*, 97(12): 6785–90.

Reid, A.H., Fanning, T.G., Janczewski, T.A., McCall, S. and Taubenberger, J.K. (2002) 'Characterization of the 1918 "Spanish" influenza virus matrix gene segment', *Journal of Virology*, 10717–23.

Reid, A.H., Taubenberger, J.K. and Fanning, T.G. (2001) 'The 1918 Spanish influenza: integrating history and biology', *Microbes and Infection*, 3(1): 81–7.

République Française (1921) *Annuaire Statistique*, Paris: Mininstère de Travail, Statistique Générale de la France.

Rice, Geoffrey W. (1979) 'Christchurch in the 1918 influenza epidemic: a preliminary study', *New Zealand Journal of History*, 13: 109–37.

Rice, Geoffrey W. (1983) 'Maori mortality in the 1918 influenza epidemic', *New Zealand Population Review*, 9(1): 44–61.

Rice, Geoffrey W. (1985) 'Crisis in a country town: the 1918 epidemic in Temuka', *Historical News*, 51: 7–13.

Rice, Geoffrey W. (with assistance from Linda Bryder) (1988) *Black November: the 1918 influenza pandemic in New Zealand*, Wellington: Allen & Unwin.

Rice, Geoffrey W. (1989) 'Australia and New Zealand in the 1918–19 influenza pandemic', in H. Attwood, R. Gillespie and M.J. Lewis (eds) *New Perspectives on the History of Medicine. First National Conference of the Australian Society of the History of Medicine*, Melbourne: University of Melbourne.

Rice, Geoffrey W. (1998) 'Japan and New Zealand in the 1918 influenza pandemic: comparative perspectives on responses and crisis management', paper presented at The Spanish 'Flu 1918–1998: Reflections on the Influenza Pandemic of 1918 after 80 Years, Cape Town, 12–15 September.

Riley, James C. (1989) *Sickness, Recovery and Death: a History and Forecast of Ill Health*, Iowa City: University of Iowa Press.

Riordan, Patricia (1986) 'Spatial modelling of epidemiological events: geographical aspects of world influenza epidemics 1945–1977', unpublished PhD thesis, University of Bristol.

Rioux, Denise (1983) 'La grippe espagnole à Sherbrooke et dans les Cantons de l'Est, Collection Histoire des Cantons de l'Est 9', thesis, Université de Sherbrooke, Quebec.

Risse, Guenter B. (1991) 'Epidemics before AIDS: a new research program', paper presented at the AIDS and the Historian: Proceedings of a Conference at the National Institutes of Health, 20–21 March 1989.

Roberts, N.A. (2001) 'Treatment of influenza with neuraminidase inhibitors: virological implications', *Philosophical Transactions: Biological Sciences*, 356(1416): 1895–7.

Rockafeller, N. (1986) '"In gauze we trust": public health and Spanish influenza on the home front, Seattle, 1918–1919', *Pacific Northwest Quarterly*, 77(3): 104–13.

Rodies, K.E. (1998) 'That great call: the pandemic of 1918', *Nursing and Health Care Perspectives* 19(5): 204–5.

Rodriguez, Francisco Herrera (1996) 'Incidencia Social de la Gripe de 1918–1919 en la Ciudad de Cadiz', *Llull* 19(37): 455–70.

Rosenberg, Charles E. (1992) *Explaining Epidemics and Other Studies in the History of Medicine*, Cambridge: Cambridge University Press.

Rosenberg, Charles E. and Golden, Janet (eds) (1992) *Framing Disease: Studies in Cultural History*, New Brunswick, NJ: Rutgers University Press.

Royal Society of Medicine (1918) *Influenza: a Discussion*, London: Royal Society of Medicine.

Sabatier, Renee (1988) *Blaming Others: Prejudice, Race, and Worldwide AIDS*, Philadelphia: New Society Publishers.

Sage, M.W. (1995) 'Pittsburgh plague – 1918: an oral history', *Home Healthcare Nurse*, 13(1): 49–54.

Sage, M.W. (1998) 'Pandemic influenza, Pittsburgh – 1918', paper presented at The Spanish 'Flu 1918–1998: Reflections on the Influenza Pandemic of 1918 after 80 Years, Cape Town, 12–15 September.

Sanford, W.L. (1983) 'The influenza epidemic of 1918 and its effects on the military', *Indiana Medical History Quarterly*, 9(4): 16–22.

Sattenspiel, Lisa and Herring, D. Ann (1998) 'Structured epidemic models and the spread of influenza in the central Canadian subarctic', *Human Biology*, 70(1): 91–115.

Sattenspiel, Lisa and Herring, D. Ann (2000) 'Modelling the influence of settlement structure on the spread of influenza among communities', *American Journal of Human Biology*, 2(6): 736–48.

Sattenspiel, Lisa and Herring, D. Ann (2003) 'Simulating the effect of quarantine on the spread of the 1918–19 flu in central Canada', *Bulletin of Mathematical Biology*, 65: 1–26.

Schickel, R. (1984) *D.W. Griffith*, London: Pavilion.

Schild, Geoffrey C. (1977) 'Influenza', in G. Melvyn Howe (ed.) *A World Geography of Human Diseases*, London: Academic Press.

Schoch Spana, M. (2001) '"Hospital's full-up": the 1918 influenza pandemic', *Public Health Reports*, 2: 32–3.

Schoenbaum, Stephen C. (2003) 'Transmission of, and protection against, influenza: epidemiologic observations beginning with the 1918 pandemic and their implications', in H. Phillips and D. Killingray (eds) *The Spanish Flu Pandemic of 1918–19: New Perspectives*, London: Routledge.

Schofield, Alfred T. (1928) *Behind the Brass Plate*, London: Sampson, Low, Marston & Co.

Scholtissk, C., Koennecke, I., and Rott, R. (1978) 'Host range recombinants of Fowl Plague (influenza A) virus', *Virology*, 91: 79–85.

Scott, K.A. (1988) 'Plague on the homefront: Arkansas and the great influenza epidemic of 1918', *Arkansas Historical Quarterly*, 47(4): 311–44.

Scott, S. (1938) *The Influenza Mystery*, London: Stanley Paul & Co.

'Scrutator' (1890) *The Coming Epidemic. Influenza: Its History, Symptoms, Treatment, &c.* London.

Sebald, W.G. (2003) *On the Natural History of Destruction: with Essays on Alfred Andersch, Jean Améry and Peter Weiss*, London: Hamish Hamilton.

Selby, Philip (ed.) (1982) *Influenza Models: Prospects for Development and Use*, Lancaster: MTP Press.

Sena, Rãjendra-Kumãra (1923) *A Treatise on Influenza with Special Reference to the Pandemic of 1918*, Assam: self-published, Hurmutty Tea Estate.

Shope, R.E. (1931) 'Swine influenza. III: Filtration experiments and etiology', *Journal of Experimental Medicine*, 54: 373–85.

Shortridge, K.F. (1999) 'The 1918 "Spanish" flu: pearls from swine?', *Nature Medicine*, 5(4): 384–5.

Slack, Paul (1985) *The Impact of Plague in Tudor and Stuart England*, Oxford: Clarendon Press.

Smallman-Raynor, M., Johnson, N.P.A.S. and Cliff, A.D. (2002) 'The spatial anatomy of an epidemic: influenza in London and the county boroughs of England and Wales, 1918–19', *Transactions of the Institute of British Geographers*, 27(4): 452–70.

Smith, F.B. (1995) 'The Russian influenza in the United Kingdom, 1889–1894', *Social History of Medicine*, 8(1): 55–73.

Smith, W., Andrewes, C.H. and Laidlaw, P.P. (1933) 'A virus obtained from influenza patients', *The Lancet*, ii: 66.

Snacken, R., Kendal, A.P., Haaheim, L.R. and Wood, J.M. (1999) 'The next influenza pandemic: lessons from Hong Kong, 1997', *Emerging Infectious Diseases*, 5(2): 195–203.

Snacken, R., Lavanchy, D., Wood, J., Kendal, A.P., Haaheim, L.R. and Lighart, G.J. (1998) 'What can be learned from 1918 to help plan for the next influenza pandemic?', paper presented at The Spanish 'Flu 1918–1998: Reflections on the Influenza Pandemic of 1918 after 80 Years, Cape Town, 12–15 September.

Sontag, Susan (1988) *AIDS and its Metaphors*, New York: Farrar, Strauss, and Giroux.

Spears, John V. (1979) 'An epidemic among the Bakgatla: the influenza of 1918', *Botswana Notes and Records*, 11: 69–76.

Spicer, C.C. and Lawrence, C.J. (1984) 'Epidemic influenza in Greater London', *Journal of Hygiene*, 93: 105–12.

Spink, W.W. (1979) *Infectious Disease: Prevention and Treatment in the Nineteenth and Twentieth Century*, Folkestone: Dawson.

Starr, Isaac (1976) 'Influenza in 1918: recollections of the epidemic in Philadelphia', *Annals of Internal Medicine*, 85: 516–18.

Statistics Norway (annual) *Statistical Yearbooks of Norway*, Oslo: Statistics Norway.

Steiner, Z. (2005) *The Lights That Failed: European International History 1919–1933*, Oxford: Oxford University Press, Clarendon Press.

Stöhr, K. (2002) 'Influenza – WHO cares', *The Lancet Infectious Diseases*, 2: 517.

Stöhr, K. (2005) 'Avian influenza and pandemics – research needs and opportunities', *New England Journal of Medicine* 352(4): 405–7.

Stuart-Harris, C.H. (1960) '"Twenty years of influenza epidemics", International Conference on Asian Influenza, Feb. 17–19, 1960', *American Review of Respiratory Disease*, 83, 2(Part 2): 54.

Stuart-Harris, C.H. (1965) *Influenza and Other Virus Infections of the Respiratory Tract*, 2nd edn, London: Edward Arnold.

Stuart-Harris, C.H., Schild, G.C. and Oxford, J.S. (1985) *Influenza: the Viruses and the Disease*, 2nd edn, London: Edward Arnold.

Sweden (annual) *Statistisk Årsbok för Sverige*, Kristiania and Stockholm: Statistika Centralbyrån.

Taksa, L. (1994) 'The masked disease: oral history, memory and the influenza pandemic, 1918–19', in K.D. Smith and P. Hamilton (eds) *Memory and History in Twentieth Century Australia*, Melbourne: Oxford University Press.

Tanner, A. (2002) 'The Spanish Lady comes to London: the influenza pandemic 1918–1919', *The London Journal*, 27(2): 51–76.

Taubenberger, J.K. (1998) 'Genetic characterization of the 1918 influenza virus', paper presented at The Spanish 'Flu 1918–1998: Reflections on the Influenza Pandemic of 1918 after 80 Years, Cape Town, 12–15 September.

Taubenberger, J.K. (2002) 'The 1918 influenza pandemic and lessons for the future', *Inside Influenza*, 2(2): 7.

Taubenberger, J.K., Reid, A.H. and Fanning, T.G. (2000) 'The 1918 influenza virus: a killer comes into view', *Virology*, 274(2): 241–5.

Taubenberger, J.K., Reid, A.H., Krafft, A.E., Bijwaad, K.E. and Fanning, T.G. (1997) 'Initial genetic characterization of the 1918 "Spanish" influenza virus', *Science*, 275(5307): 1793–6.

Taubenberger, J.K., Reid, A.H., Janczewski, T.A. and Fanning, T.G. (2001) 'Integrating historical, clinical and molecular genetic data in order to explain the origin and virulence of the 1918 Spanish influenza virus', *Philosophical Transactions of the Royal Society of London. Series B: Biological Sciences*, 356(1416): 1829–39.

Thalman, Hans (1968) *Die Grippeepidemie 1918/19 in Zürich*. Vol. Neue Reihe Nr. 50, *Zürcher Medizingeschichtliche Abhandlungen*. Zürich: Juris Druck and Verlag Zürich.

Thomas, Christine (1998) '"All at sea": Spanish influenza, maritime quarantine and Australian troopships 1918–1919', paper presented at The Spanish 'Flu 1918–1998: Reflections on the Influenza Pandemic of 1918 after 80 Years, Cape Town, 12–15 September.

Thomson, James C. (1927) *Influenza: the New Treatment Fully Explained*, Edinburgh School of Natural Therapeutics, Monograph No. 1. London: C.W. Daniel Company.

Tomkins, Sandra M. (1989) 'Britain and the influenza pandemic of 1918–19', unpublished PhD thesis, University of Cambridge.

Tomkins, Sandra M. (1992a) 'The failure of expertise: public health policy in Britain during the 1918–19 influenza epidemic', *Social History of Medicine*, 5: 435–54.

Tomkins, Sandra M. (1992b) 'The influenza epidemic of 1918–19 in Western Samoa', *Journal of Pacific History*, 27(2): 181–97.

Tomkins, Sandra M. (1994) 'Colonial administration in British Africa during the influenza epidemic of 1918–19', *Canadian Journal of African Studies*, 28(1): 60–83.

Townsend, John F. (1933) 'History of influenza epidemics', *Annals of Medical History*, V: 533–47.

Tumpey, T.M., Garcia Sastre, A., Mikulasova, A., Taubenberger, J.K., Swayne, D.E., Palese, P. and Basler, C.F. (2002) 'Existing antivirals are effective against influenza viruses with genes from the 1918 pandemic virus', *Proceedings of the National Academy of Sciences of the United States of America*, 99(21): 13849–54.

Underwood, J.H. (1984) 'Effects of the 1918 influenza pandemic mortality experience on subsequent fertility of the native population in Guam', *Micronesica*, 19: 1–10.

Union of South Africa (1919) *Report of the Influenza Epidemic Commission*, Pretoria.

United States of America (n.d.) 'Historical estimates of world population', Bureau of the Census. Available from: www.census.gov/ipc/www/worldhis.html.

United States of America (1920) *Special Tables of Mortality from Influenza and Pneumonia: Indiana, Kansas and Philadelphia, PA, September 1 to December 31, 1918*, Washington, DC: Department of Commerce, Bureau of the Census.

United States of America (1960) *The Study of Influenza: a Translation of Ucheniye O Grippe by Zhdanov et al.* Translated by U.S. Department of Health, Education and Welfare, Public Health Service, National Institutes of Health, Division of General Medical Sciences, Russian Scientific Translation Program. Bethesda, Maryland: U.S. Department of Health, Education and Welfare, Public Health Service, National Institutes of Health, Division of General Medical Sciences, Russian Scientific Translation Program.

van Hartesveldt, F.R. (ed.) (1992) *1918–1919 Pandemic of Influenza: the Urban Impact in the Western World*, London: Edwin Mellen Press.

van Helvoort, Ton (1993) 'A bacteriological paradigm in influenza research in the first half of the twentieth century', *History and Philosophy of the Life Sciences,* 15: 3–21.

Vasold, Manfred (1996) 'The influenza epidemic of 1918: nursing personnel was doubly involved', *Pflege Zeitschrift*, 49(2): 112–15.

Vasold, Manfred (1998) 'The influenza pandemic of 1918/19 in Nuremburg/Germany', paper presented at The Spanish 'Flu 1918–1998: Reflections on the Influenza Pandemic of 1918 after 80 Years, Cape Town, 12–15 September.

Victoria: Board of Public Health (1918) *'Spanish' influenza*, Melbourne: H.J. Green, Acting Government Printer.

Vincent, C.P. (1985) *The Politics of Hunger: the Allied Blockade of Germany, 1915–1919*, Athens, OH: Ohio University Press.

Voigt, Ellen Bryant (1995) *Kyrie: Poems*, New York: W.W. Norton.

Wakimura, Kohei (1998) 'The Indian experience of influenza pandemic 1918–19: why the mortality was so huge?', paper presented at The Spanish 'Flu 1918–1998: Reflections on the Influenza Pandemic of 1918 after 80 Years, Cape Town, 12–15 September.

Wardlaw, H.S.H. (1919) 'The venous oxygen content and the alkaline reserve of the blood in pneumonic influenza', *Proceedings of the Linnean Society of New South Wales*, Part III: 514–24.

Watts, Sheldon (1997) *Epidemics and History: Disease, Power and Imperialism*, New Haven: Yale University Press.

Wauchope, Gladys Mary (1963) *The Story of a Woman Physician*, Bristol: John Wright & Sons.

Webby, R.J. and Webster, R.G. (2003) 'Are we ready for pandemic influenza?', *Science*, 302: 1519–22.

Webster, Robert G. and Laver, W.G. (1972) 'The origin of pandemic influenza', *Bulletin of the World Health Organisation,* 47(4): 449–52.

Webster, Robert G., Bean, William J., Gorman, O.T., Chambers, T.M. and Kawaoka, Y. (1992) 'Evolution and ecology of influenza A viruses', *Microbiological Reviews,* 56(1): 152–79.

Weiler, Jo-Anne (1988) 'One more battle: Kitchener fights influenza, October, 1918', BA Honours thesis, Wilfrid Laurier University.

Weindling, P. (ed.) (1995) *International Health Organisations and Movements, 1918–1939*, Cambridge: Cambridge University Press.

Werner, Barry (1987) 'Fertility statistics from birth registrations in England and Wales, 1837–1987', *Population Trends,* 48: 4–10.

Weymouth, A. (1936) *Who'd Be a Doctor?* London: Rich & Cowan.

White, K.A. (1985) 'Pittsburgh in the great epidemic of 1918', *The Western Pennsylvania Historical Magazine*, 68(3): 221–42.

WHO (1980) 'A revision of the system of nomenclature for influenza viruses', *Bulletin of the WHO*, 58: 585–91.

WHO (1998a) *Fact Sheet No. 188 – Influenza A(H5N1)*. Available from: www.who.ch/inf/fs/fact188.html.

WHO (1998b) *Press release WHO/1: Investigation of Origins of H5N1 Influenza Virus Stepped up in Hong Kong*. Available from: www.who.int/inf-pr-1999/en/pr98-01.html.

WHO (1999a) *Fact Sheet No. 211 – Influenza*. Available from: www.who.int/inf-fs/en/fact211.html.

WHO (1999b) *Fact sheet No. 212 – the WHO Influenza Programme*. Available from: www.who.int/inf-fs/en/fact212.html.

WHO (1999c) *FluNet* (Website). Available from: oms.b3e.jussieu.fr/flunet.

WHO (1999d) *Influenza Pandemic Plan: the Role of WHO and Guidelines for National and Regional Planning*, Geneva: World Health Organisation.

WHO (1999e) *Press release WHO/11: 50 Years of Influenza Surveillance: Much Still to do to Stop a Common Killer*. Available from: www.who.int/inf-pr-1999/en/pr99-11.html.

WHO (1999f) *Press release WHO/17: Increased surveillance for Influenza Should be Continued*. Available from: www.who.int/inf-pr-1999/en/pr98-17.html.

WHO (1999g) *Press release WHO/66: Experts Decide Content of 1999 'Southern Hemisphere' Influenza Vaccine*. Available from: www.who.int/inf-pr-1999/en/pr98-66.html.

WHO (2002) 'Global priorities in influenza surveillance and control', speech by Dr Gro Harlem Brundtland, Director-General. Geneva: World Health Organisation.

WHO (2003) *Fact Sheet No. 211 – Influenza*. Available from: www.who.int/mediacentre/factsheets/fs211/en/.

WHO (2004a) *Avian Influenza Fact Sheet*, Geneva: World Health Organisation. Available from: www.who.int/csr/don/2004_01_15/en.

WHO (2004b) *Estimating the Impact of the Next Influenza Pandemic: Enhancing Preparedness*, Geneva: World Health Organisation. Available from: www.who.int/csr/disease/influenza/preparedness2004_12_08/en/.

WHO (2005a) *Cumulative Number of Confirmed Human Cases of Avian Influenza A/(H5N1) Reported to WHO*, Geneva: World Health Organisation. Available from: www.who.int/csr/disease/avian_influenza/country/cases_table_2005_08_05/en/index.html.

WHO (2005b) *Influenza Pandemic Preparedness and Response*. Executive Board. Geneva. 2005: Executive Board, 115th session, Agenda item 4.17. Available from: www.who.int/gb/ebwha/pdf-files/EB115/EB115_44-en.pdf.

WHO (2005c) *WHO Global Influenza Preparedness Plan. The Role of WHO and Recommendations for National Measures Before and During Pandemics*, Report WHO/CDS/CSR/GIP/2005.5, Geneva: World Health Organisation.

Wilshere, Jonathon (1986) *Leicester's Great Influenza Epidemic 1918–1919*, Leicester: Chamberlain Music and Books.

Wilson, Alistair (1981) 'Oddity remembered: 1918 influenza pandemic', *British Medical Journal*, 282: 1766.

Wilson, S. (1980) *Egon Schiele*, Oxford: Phaidon.

Winter, J.M. (1980) 'Military fitness and civilian health in Britain during the First World War', *Journal of Contemporary History*, 15(2): 211–44.

Winter, J.M. (1982) 'Aspects of the impact of the First World War on infant mortality in Britain', *Journal of Economic History*, 11(3): 713–38.

Winter, J.M. and Baggett, B. (1996) *1914–18: the Great War and the Shaping of the 20th Century*, London: BBC Books.

Witte, W. (1998) 'The influenza epidemic of 1918–19 in Baden – the plague that was not allowed to happen', paper presented at The Spanish 'Flu 1918–1998: Reflections on the Influenza Pandemic of 1918 after 80 Years, Cape Town, 12–15 September.

Wolfe, Thomas (1929) *Look Homeward, Angel: a Story of the Buried Life*, New York: Scribner's.

Wood, J.M. (2001) 'Developing vaccines against pandemic influenza', *Philosophical Transactions: Biological Sciences*, 356(1416): 1953–60.

Woolf, Virginia (1979–85) *The Diary of Virginia Woolf*, Harmondsworth: Penguin.

Woolf, V. (2000) *Mrs Dalloway*, London: Penguin.

Worobey, M., Rambaut, A., Pybus, O.G. and Robertson, D. (2002) 'Questioning the evidence for genetic recombination in the 1918 "Spanish flu" virus', *Science*, 296(5566): 211.

Yuen, K.Y. *et al.* (1998) 'Clinical features and rapid viral diagnosis of human disease associated with avian influenza A H5N1 strain', *The Lancet*, 351: 467–71.

Zhdanov, Viktor Mikhailovich, Solov'ev, V.D. and Epshtein, F.G. (1958) *Ucheniye o Grippe*, Moscow: Medgiz. Read in translation *The Study of Influenza: a Translation of Ucheniye O Grippe by Zhdanov et al.* Translated by U.S. Department of Health, Education and Welfare, Public Health Service, National Institutes of Health, Division of General Medical Sciences, Russian Scientific Translation Program. Bethesda, Maryland: U.S. Department of Health, Education and Welfare, Public Health Service, National Institutes of Health, Division of General Medical Sciences, Russian Scientific Translation Program.

Zinsser, Hans (1919) *A Textbook of Bacteriology*, New York: Appleton and Co.

Zylberman, P. (2003) 'A holocaust in a holocaust: the Great War and the 1918 Spanish influenza in France', in H. Phillips and D. Killingray (eds) *The Spanish Flu Pandemic of 1918–19: New Perspectives*, London: Routledge.

Index